Oral Health and Systemic Disease

of related interest

Case Studies in Personalized Nutrition
Edited by Angela Walker
ISBN 978 1 84819 394 9
eISBN 978 0 85701 351 4

**Personalized Nutrition and Lifestyle Medicine
for Healthcare Practitioners series
Mitochondria in Health and Disease**
Ray Griffiths
Foreword by Lorraine Nicolle
ISBN 978 1 84819 332 1
eISBN 978 0 85701 288 3

**Personalized Nutrition and Lifestyle Medicine
for Healthcare Practitioners series
Biochemical Imbalances in Disease
A Practitioner's Guide**
Edited by Lorraine Nicolle and Ann Woodriff Beirne
ISBN 978 1 84819 033 7
eISBN 978 0 85701 028 5

ORAL HEALTH AND SYSTEMIC DISEASE

A Clinical Guide for Nutritional Therapists and Functional Medicine Practitioners

Rose Holmes

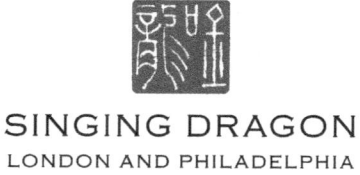

SINGING DRAGON
LONDON AND PHILADELPHIA

First published in Great Britain in 2022 by Singing Dragon,
an imprint of Jessica Kingsley Publishers
An Hachette Company

1

Copyright © Rose Holmes 2022

All rights reserved. No part of this publication may be reproduced, stored in a retrieval system, or transmitted, in any form or by any means without the prior written permission of the publisher, nor be otherwise circulated in any form of binding or cover other than that in which it is published and without a similar condition being imposed on the subsequent purchaser.

Disclaimer: The information contained in this book is not intended to replace the services of trained medical professionals or to be a substitute for medical advice. The complementary therapy described in this book may not be suitable for everyone to follow. You are advised to consult a doctor before embarking on any complementary therapy programme and on any matters relating to your health, and in particular on any matters that may require diagnosis or medical attention.

A CIP catalogue record for this title is available from the
British Library and the Library of Congress

ISBN 978 1 84819 411 3
eISBN 978 0 85701 366 8

Printed and bound in Great Britain by CPI Group

Jessica Kingsley Publishers' policy is to use papers that are natural, renewable and recyclable products and made from wood grown in sustainable forests. The logging and manufacturing processes are expected to conform to the environmental regulations of the country of origin.

Jessica Kingsley Publishers
Carmelite House
50 Victoria Embankment
London EC4Y 0DZ

www.singingdragon.com

I would like to thank my family, particularly my mother Marie Santoro, and my daughter Teresa and son Thomas, for their patience and encouragement during the three years' process of researching and writing this text.

This book is dedicated to my late Dad who supported and encouraged me during my nutrition qualifications and I know would have been so proud of his eldest daughter – the one whose first degree was in Humanities instead of something 'practical and useful'.

Finally, I would like to recognize the support given by my dearest friend José Antonino Sousa Da Graça.

Acknowledgements

The research and writing of this book have been enabled by guidance originally given during my formal study of nutrition at CNELM (and previously at ION). In particular by professor Dr James Neil, lecturer who patiently and expertly supervised my BSc dissertation on circadian rhythm disruption and taught me to go back to basics when considering a daunting project.

Writing a book is certainly a daunting project and the subject chosen for this book on oral health is one that has, perhaps, not been discussed much until recently by nutritionists; I first became intensely interested in the connections between oral health and systemic disease almost half a decade before publication of this book.

I am fortunate that my work for Rio Health Products as their education and training manager provides opportunity to regularly write articles and create and present webinars on various topics. The practitioner webinar I presented for Rio Health mid-2017 on mouth and dental health was the 'spark' for this particular research journey and, ultimately, the writing of this book. I thank Rio Health for providing these opportunities.

Thank you also to Claire and everyone at Singing Dragon for your encouragement and guidance in this project – as I have already said, writing a book is certainly a daunting project. A special mention also to Lorraine Nicolle for her early involvement in this book. Lorraine, you have my heartfelt gratitude for *all* the learning opportunities you have provided me with over the years. Your expertise is deservingly highly respected and acknowledged by so many nutrition professionals.

Thank you, also, to the many people who were generous with their time and expertise including Dr Marilyn Glenville, Leo Cashman, Dr Jerry E Bouquot, Dr Johann Lechner and Dr Shabir Pandor.

Contents

Preface 9
1. What Is a Healthy Mouth? 13
2. Protecting Oral (and Systemic) Health 21
3. Anatomy and Gleeking 29
4. Taste Matters 31
5. Sugars in Health and Disease 43
6. Dysbiosis and Inflammation 53
7. Glycation and 'Silent' Inflammation 63
8. Oral Health Issues 71
9. Perio-Systemic Links 93
10. Ageing, Hormones, Satiety and Loss of Taste 107
11. Functional Dentistry and Personalized Well-Being 121
12. Oral Hygiene Alternatives 125
13. Oral Healthcare Ingredients 131
14. Dental and Oral Optimal Health: Diet 143
15. Supplement Considerations 155
16. Oral Hygiene Considerations 167
17. Lifestyle Options 183

18. Research Directions. 189

19. Oral Health: A Missing Link in Functional Medicine 199

    Appendix 1: Reducing Fluoride Exposure. 203

    Appendix 2: Periodontitis 207

    Appendix 3: Oral Healthcare Products 209

    Appendix 4: Information and Resources 213

    Glossary and Abbreviations 219

    Endnotes 241

    Subject Index 295

    Author Index 312

Preface

Readers may think this book is about dental health. To some extent it is – but only in part. The subject goes far beyond the health of teeth. The only part of the human skeletal system that can be seen, teeth are relied on to chew food, are used to form certain sounds for communication and are understood to be an outward indication of health (and beauty, evidenced by the value placed on a smile).

The word 'dental' means relating to teeth – not just the teeth themselves. The supporting structures include the gingiva, periodontal ligament, cementum and alveolar bone. This book *is*, in part, about dental health but, in fact, in some ways it is more about other features inside the human mouth and how they impact whole-body health (e.g. saliva and salivary immunoglobulin, with important implications for immune health, and taste buds which are now known to be found throughout the human body).

'Taste ability' is a life-and-death function of the oral cavity. The body requires sufficient caloric content to avoid malnutrition and permit survival and reproduction, as well as the ability to detect toxic substances that might result in death. The oral cavity has this important role in 'taste ability'. Taste perception, however, is now known to be body-wide, with potential systemic impact, including an association with respiratory and reproductive health.

Most human sampling of the outside world is through the gut, with food being the biggest daily immune challenge faced by humans. The oral cavity is the gateway to the gut, and, like the gut, the oral cavity has a microbiome with unique features. The environment of the oral cavity changes frequently and is subjected to extremes – both hot and cold foods/drinks, dry and saliva soaked. In addition, there are bacteria, altered pH and the pressure of biting forces with which to contend.

Humans generally eat several times a day, consciously deciding (most of the time) what will be placed into the mouth, often with perceived taste an important determinant. Overeating is not uncommon. Issues of satiety relate to taste perception as well as having implications for disease states such as diabetes and obesity. These and other chronic health conditions show strong associations with periodontal conditions, exhibiting a bi-directional relationship with oral health.

Common considerations for this bi-directionality include high levels of inflammation, poor detoxification and compromised immune health. When looking at why an individual has a health condition – whether that is gingivitis, periodontal disease, type 2 diabetes, cardiovascular disease, cancer or Alzheimer's disease – consideration of these factors is essential.

From a personalized health viewpoint, we need to consider the multi-systemic bacterial dysbiosis (gut, oral cavity, lungs, skin, etc.) commonly found in individuals with less-than-optimal health. Many chronic health conditions relate to a breakdown in basic border control, with resulting inflammatory and immunological reactions at gateways to the body. The widespread occurrence of dental caries, gingivitis and periodontal disease is an indication of this, and oral health must be considered as a potential contributory factor in poor systemic health. Oral inflammation is one of many risk factors – an important one, since inflammation can be unlimited, whilst the immune system has limited ability to fight inflammation and infection.

According to a 2017 review of the worldwide prevalence of periodontal disease (20–50% of the global population), its risk factors and associations with systemic diseases, robust evidence demonstrates association of periodontal diseases with systemic diseases such as cardiovascular disease (CVD), diabetes and adverse pregnancy outcomes.[1]

In July 2019, the *Lancet* published the first of two papers in a series on oral-health in which the 'global public health challenge' of 'largely preventable' oral diseases was discussed. Key messages included recognition of oral health as 'an integral element in overall health and well-being' and of oral diseases having 'substantial effect'. Reforms suggested by the authors included lessening the division between dental and general healthcare, and they presented 'a unifying framework that places oral diseases in a broader context and directly links them to other non-communicable diseases (NCDs)'.[2]

A truly integrative approach recognizes the interconnectedness of all body parts and systems. In considering the functional medicine approach, oral health must be a consideration, yet is often overlooked.

Personalized nutrition includes communication to clients about how to choose genetic signalling for health, instead of for dysfunction and disease. And it includes considering the individual as a whole – not forgetting oral cavity health and considering the impact of dental hygiene, toothpaste ingredients, mercury amalgam fillings, wisdom teeth extractions, teeth whitening procedures, reduced saliva production and other factors. The impact of sugar, sweeteners, acidic foods and carbohydrates needs consideration as do the effects of oral piercings, tooth clenching/grinding and medications that cause dry mouth. Equally, oral conditions such as bad breath, loss of taste and recurrent mouth ulcers may indicate the need to investigate other dysfunctional processes.

The contribution to an individual's health of diet, lifestyle, genetics and mindset needs consideration, alongside recognition of factors such as pervasive inflammation in multiple body systems. Whilst increasing numbers of people show interest in organic foods and natural therapies like nutrition, naturopathy and acupuncture, mouth health treatments are still primarily addressed (relatively unquestioningly) through conventional dentistry – even by most natural therapists. The reasons are unclear, but may relate to insufficient information about oral health, or insufficient exposure to relevant natural therapists such as biological dentists, or lack of confidence in questioning some aspects of conventional dentistry or in parting from the norm in this less-understood health profession.

There is a real need for health practitioners to have a greater understanding of the role oral cavity health may play in the overall health status of individuals. With this would come greater respect for biological dentistry, whose practitioners train conventionally and practise with an understanding of the impact of periodontal health on whole-body health. It should also lead to an improved, more integrative approach by natural health practitioners, and within functional medicine, from which individual clients should benefit.

Written from a nutritionist's point of view, this book is written for practitioners. One of its aims is improved oral health literacy. Health literacy is an important predictor of individual health. The impact of oral health literacy (and improved maternal health literacy which impacts childhood and whole family oral health) should not be underestimated, especially in light of the worldwide prevalence of dental caries, gingivitis and periodontal disease.

Very importantly I must declare that I am not a dentist, nor do I have any dental medicine background. I have, however, like many others, had experience of dental pain, dental treatments and concerns about the implications of these treatments. My nutrition science qualifications and interest in whole-body health have prompted this research journey, which has been an interesting one, including revisiting anatomy textbooks, exploring media coverage of the subject, investigating historical aspects of mouth hygiene, inspecting commercial websites, questioning general perceptions, attending international conferences, and discovering information and viewpoints of professional associations, government and international agencies, and activist groups. Primarily, the research has involved reading hundreds of scientific studies on the subject. I hope readers will find an informative, interesting and useful text which explores and presents varying viewpoints alongside robust scientific evidence where it exists – remembering, of course, that funding impacts the availability of research.

I aim to present a balanced view and have found a number of organizations and individuals helpful in providing information. These include (but are not limited to): the Oral Health Foundation (an independent charity dedicated to improving oral health and well-being around the world, 'providing expert, independent and impartial advice' on all aspects of oral health), the Holistic Dental Association (HDA, established in 1978 to provide support and guidance to practitioners of holistic/alternative dentistry), DAMS (Dental Amalgam Mercury Solutions, whose Executive Director Leo Cashman kindly sent me several documents), the BDA (British Dental Association, professional association and trade union for UK dentists) and the IAOMT (International Academy of Oral Medicine and Toxicology, whose UK co-founder, Dr Shabir Pandor, MFGDP, LDSRCS, MFHom, DipHomotox(Hons), inspired the title of Chapter 19). Materials were also kindly provided by Dr Jerry E Bouquot and Dr Johann Lechner.

— Chapter 1 —

WHAT IS A HEALTHY MOUTH?

Before looking at disease processes affecting the mouth, it is important to understand what constitutes a healthy mouth and its significance for whole-body health.

A healthy mouth is important for efficient chewing, for speaking and for smiling. It is also important for immunity and disease prevention. The mouth is an important gateway to the body, and the lips, whilst also a tactile sensory organ and important erogenous zone in kissing and intimacy, are the point at which the gateway to the digestive tract is accessed. Mouth health may have an impact beyond digestive and immune health, on psychological, social and expressive aspects of individuals.

Role of the oral cavity

The primary role of the oral cavity is as the entry point to the digestive tract. All food and drink begin the journey through the alimentary canal via the oral cavity; here food is tasted, moistened and prepared for passage so that it can ultimately be digested and absorbed as nutrient for the whole body.

Each part of the oral cavity has a role. Taste buds sample incoming food for toxins. The salivary glands provide saliva to lubricate the oral cavity, and to moisten and initiate the breakdown of food. The tongue and muscles participate in manoeuvring food, and the teeth break it into smaller pieces. The jawbone, muscles, tongue and teeth all contribute to effective mastication.

The healthy function of all parts is necessary for optimal chewing capability. Whilst an ability to deal with solid foods is desirable, it is not essential; efficient chewing capability facilitates a more diverse diet which may facilitate (but doesn't always guarantee) healthier, potentially optimal, intake of nutrients.

Oral cavity health has implications for systemic health and for disease progression. Optimal nutrition, psychological function and immune function are best facilitated by aspects of mouth and dental health: the ability to access (chew) a varied, healthy diet, to communicate readily (speak) with others, to smile (confidence and self-esteem) and to defend and protect against immune assaults.

Perhaps more importantly, the oral cavity has a role in providing first line defence – protecting the body against microbes and toxins in food, drink and air. The mouth is where items we ingest as food first meet and interact with our body cells, along with the nasal cavity, where we first encounter inhaled air; oral and nasal cavities provide quick, almost immediate, access to our internal environment. Sampling by immune cells of ingested food and inhaled air informs and alerts the immune system to make an appropriate response.

Our border control

Immune response is also informed by microorganism sampling in the oral cavity. The oral microbiome, in common with other human microbiomes in the gastrointestinal tract, vaginal canal, mammary glands, conjunctiva and skin, may include bacteria, fungi and viruses. These microorganisms can be commensal (co-existing without harming human hosts), pathogenic, or have a mutualistic relationship with their human hosts. Immune system response is informed by both the qualitative and quantitative presence of microorganisms. Oral microbiome dysbiosis, like gastrointestinal microbiome dysbiosis, may negatively impact health both locally and systemically.

Our microbiome is our border control – essentially important for providing protection against all invaders. If the border (epithelial lining whether in the mouth or gut) is 'leaky', microbes and food particles may cross barriers that were meant to prohibit such passing; membrane permeability can allow bacterial translocation causing immune response, and translocation of food molecules causing inflammation and 'allergic' response. It is not uncommon for more than one 'border' (gut, oral, blood–brain, blood–cerebrospinal fluid) to be compromised. Oral microbiome health is an important component of a healthy mouth and healthy body; its importance should not be underestimated.

Commensal bacteria adhere to the dental pellicle, a protein-rich biofilm that forms seconds after teeth are cleaned, and is involved in regulating reactions between tooth surfaces, saliva and erosive acids[1] – helping protect teeth. Glycoproteins in the pellicle allow bacterial adherence and formation of dental plaque. Bacterial co-aggregation, the process by which genetically distinct bacteria become attached to one another, contributes to formation of multi-species biofilms[2] and, thus, of dental plaque; increased species diversity within biofilm associates with gingival inflammation and development of periodontal disease.[3]

In dental biofilm, bacterial proliferation and growth can occur; acids corrosive to dental enamel are produced as acidogenic bacteria consume fermentable carbohydrates, and disease processes initiate.[4] Maintaining a healthy oral environment requires qualitative and quantitative limitation of microbial species to prevent inflammatory processes and demineralization.

Healthy saliva, which contains numerous defence proteins, can provide tooth-remineralization ingredients[5] as well as antimicrobial components such as sIgA and lysozyme.[6] Sufficient production of saliva is essential for oral and systemic health and the common side effect of dry mouth caused by many prescription medications may have a negative impact on dental health, immune health and all-body health.

Tongues talk

Associations between oral cavity health and systemic health have a long-standing tradition. Less than a hundred years ago it was common for physicians to use a tongue depressor along with the request to 'open and say ahhhh' to gain a glimpse into a patient's oral cavity, ascertain their general health and discover possible 'clues' to factors affecting patient health.

Examination of the tongue, a principal diagnostic method in traditional Chinese medicine (TCM), used for centuries, is a powerful means by which information about pathology might be obtained without causing injury to the body. Chinese medicine considers the tongue to reflect physiological functions and pathological changes of the body.

TCM AND TONGUE DIAGNOSIS

In Chinese medicine, major aspects of the tongue (body colour, shape and coating) are considered to be important visual indicators of a person's overall harmony or disharmony, and thus of physiological function. Tongue inspection (as per Western medicine) and tongue diagnosis (as per Chinese medicine) have value in self-diagnosis too, which makes these important and exceedingly valuable tools in ascertaining the health/disease (and harmony/disharmony) state and a useful gauge for monitoring improvement/decline in both acute and chronic conditions.

The characteristics of a normal 'healthy' tongue (of a body 'in harmony') can be described using five primary aspects: colour, shape, moisture, coating and spirit.

1. Body colour should be pale red (or pinkish) and 'fresh-looking'.

2. The shape should be supple, not stiff, not cracked, not quivering, nor swollen or thin.

3. It should be slightly moist.

4. The coating should be thin and white.

5. The normal tongue should have 'spirit'; its colour should be vibrant and vital, particularly at the root.

In tongue diagnosis of Chinese medicine, each of these aspects has clinical significance to the whole body.[7] Certain parts of the tongue are considered to reflect the health of other body parts. In Chinese medicine, correspondences amongst various body parts are related to the channels (meridians).

Although TCM practices will not be specifically covered in these chapters, TCM evaluation and therapies may benefit in many oral cavity health issues. Efficacy of TCM for xerostomia[8] and oral lichen planus,[9] for example, have been assessed and its use can decrease severity of these oral health conditions.

The Ayurvedic holistic system of medicine also considers that each section of the tongue connects with different body organs, making the tongue a window to the inner system and useful for understanding health status.

Tongue diagnosis in TCM and Ayurvedic holistic systems looks at correspondences between the tongue and other parts of the body or of certain internal body systems. Whilst this book will not cover the interesting and specialized subject of tongue diagnosis, it is recognized by this author and other health professionals to have relevance to personalized nutrition for oral cavity and systemic health, and some basic aspects of tongue diagnosis that are common to both Western medicine and Ayurveda/TCM are discussed, as this book investigates and describes scientific research of correspondences with, and connections between, the oral cavity and systemic (body system) health.

What teeth reveal

Teeth can also reveal much about health – and, as with tongue diagnosis, have been used in holistic treatments like tooth reflexology.

TOOTH REFLEXOLOGY

Holistic treatments like reflexology (aka zone therapy outside the UK) consider the connections between parts of the body and look to restore homeostasis by stimulating movement of energy. Reflexology charts can be found for a number of body parts (e.g. feet, hands, ears) showing correspondence between sections of them and internal organs/body systems. According to these principles, acupressure points can be used – to relieve dental pain for example.

Tooth reflexology, applying pressure to specific areas of teeth, can be used to have a beneficial effect on health elsewhere in the body. The first molar, for example, may have a reflexive relationship with the pancreas and stomach, and pain/inflammation in this area may indicate the need for altered diet/lifestyle with respect to pancreatic health (perhaps avoidance of excessive sugar).

Although meridians are part of the TCM system used for centuries, tooth meridian charts have been criticized by some as not scientifically based, with charts greatly differing.[10] Dental health most certainly reveals health/disease aspects, and associates with whole-body health; meridian tooth charts may offer suggestions but cannot be considered scientific diagnostic tools.

Dental health is an important component in oral cavity health and for many people would be the first factor/aspect that might be thought of when hearing the term 'oral health'. There could be a number of reasons for this. A smile is a very visible indication of an individual's state of well-being, if not health, and, whilst smiling involves facial muscles and lips, we primarily consider the human smile as revealing teeth – or sometimes lack of teeth (e.g. toothless grin of babies and some elders). Dental (and gum) health may also be indicative of an individual's diet and lifestyle as well as personal hygiene.

Teeth are also, to some extent, a visible indication of age. Teeth and bones of the human body mature at fairly predictable rates, making these useful indicators of age. Up to age 21 (when permanent teeth have finished erupting), teeth are the most accurate age indicators.[11] There is a 'normal' pattern of tooth eruption and loss of milk teeth which can be indicative of health. When compared with tooth eruption, dental development (in relation to stages of mineralization) is a more reliable indication of age (in children) and is less affected by nutritional and endocrine status.[12,13] Dental (and skeletal) information is used in forensics for this reason.

Over time, teeth will show wear and alter in colour and in other ways; oral health in older individuals may also be impacted by changes in gingiva, dental enamel, saliva and immune health. And for many, multiple medications may impact aspects of oral health. Receding gums and dry mouth can be common complaints in some older individuals, but other, less immediately noticeable alterations occur with age: lower secretion of sIgA,[14,15,16,17] altered mineralization of bone/teeth[18] and connective tissue changes.[19]

Whilst these age-related changes may impact oral health, poor oral health is not a given in old age; neither are age-related diseases, which have been shown to be associated with poor oral health, a given in old age. The New England Centenarian Study (NECS), which collects data on centenarians and centenarian offspring (and offspring referent cohort) to assess the incidence of age-related diseases and mortality, found approximately 45 per cent of centenarians do not experience age-related diseases until after the age of 80 years and another 15 per cent do not have age-related diseases associated with increased mortality risk until after the age of a hundred.[20] Furthermore, centenarians (at earlier ages 65–74) and their offspring were found to exhibit better oral health than their respective birth cohorts.[21]

In older people there is an association between having retained most or all of the teeth and longevity – it can often indicate good health.[22] However, retained teeth can sometimes hide underlying problems. Some types of dental procedures may affect health in other ways: mercury amalgams and cavitations due to root canals, for example, may increase toxic load systemically, with negative health effects.

Although it can affect longevity, becoming edentulous (losing all teeth) is not a predictor of decreased longevity, but it is preferable to remain dentate. Ninety-four percent of centenarians in Japan are edentulous according to Professor Tatsuo Watanabe,[23] who found that eating and talking were important pleasures for these individuals. Research has shown that people can chew with 20 teeth[24] and that might ensure at least the possibility, if not the actuality, of a healthy diet throughout life and into older age. Functional oral health affects ability both to eat and communicate, and this is vital in overall well-being and confidence in older age.

Age impacts oral cavity health in other, non-dental ways. The cell epithelial layer on the tongue surface, for example, shows 30 per cent reduction in thickness between the ages of 16 and 98.[25] The oral health of older individuals may be impacted by these general body changes relating to connective tissue health. Their greater age would mean longer exposure to potentially damaging toxins and microorganisms. And, as mentioned above, older individuals have greater likelihood of being on prescription medication or polypharmacy which carries its own risk of oral side effects, including increased potential for dry mouth and taste changes – common complaints in older individuals.

Taste matters
Our ability to taste is, in part, determined by receptors on taste buds within the oral cavity. Ion channels and GPCR (G-protein coupled receptors) interact with the nervous system; so, ability to experience the five primary tastes – sweetness, bitterness, saltiness, sourness and savouriness – requires healthy 'working parts';

our ability to experience 'flavour' is more complex, involving also our sense of smell – another sense that can be affected by age.

Taste (and flavour) perception is an important part of our enjoyment of food (thus quality of life) as well as having an important protective function related to the role of the oral cavity as gateway to the digestive tract and the rest of the body.

Features of an optimally healthy mouth

So, to summarize – the features of an optimally healthy mouth include:

- the facility to consume (and readily digest) a wide variety of healthy foods
- a healthy balanced oral microbiome
- sufficient healthy saliva
- well-functioning barrier defences
- healthy oral mucosa and tongue
- healthy dental gums and teeth
- absence of effect from toxic components, alongside well-functioning detoxification systems to deal with toxins
- capacity to taste
- capacity for unguarded smiling.

Healthcare providers of all types can potentially increase the chances of their clients/patients in getting as close as possible to these ideals by understanding and communicating the implications of poor (or less-than-optimal) oral health on systemic health. Client compliance to recommended diet and lifestyle change is often higher when the reasons for change are better understood. And health practitioners may find specific dietary and lifestyle recommendations, alongside guidance on supplements and oral healthcare ingredients, useful for clients with oral health issues as well as for numerous other (particularly inflammatory) health conditions.

— Chapter 2 —

PROTECTING ORAL (AND SYSTEMIC) HEALTH

It is unsurprising that a healthy oral microbiome would confer the greatest potential for oral health; what is becoming increasingly evident is that a healthy oral microbiome also gives the greatest potential for systemic health. This is why good oral health is a must for healthcare practitioners to discuss with their clients.

Good oral health is associated with a variety of factors – some of them better understood by the general public than others – including avoidance of sugar (in its various forms), dental hygiene habits (frequency, timing, technique) and decisions about extractions (including wisdom teeth). Two very important, possibly less publicly understood, factors relevant to oral (and systemic) health relate to the status of saliva and the oral microbiome. Both confer protection. Safeguarding them is an important protocol aim.

Microbial ecology is an important aspect of oral health. Homeostasis and species composition are important factors for maintaining healthy oral ecosystems;[1,2] loss of homeostasis and balance may result from a caries-causing, high-sugar diet.

Saliva also has a role in maintaining oral homeostasis,[3] and its many local and systemic effects may be taken for granted unless or until something goes wrong. As a seromucous coating, saliva lubricates, protects and provides an oral tissue barrier against invading microbes (bacteria, fungi, parasites and viruses) and irritants (e.g. potential carcinogens from smoking, exogenous chemicals and desiccation from mouth breathing[4]).[5]

Saliva is a complex, unique biologic fluid; its many constituents commonly have multiple functions, each interacting and contributing to its protective functions: buffering capability, bacterial clearance and mineralization/demineralization balance. Salivary health is essential for these roles.

As with other immune defences, invasive bacteria can overwhelm the protective functions of saliva; safeguarding salivary health and the oral microbiome is important for oral cavity health and likely impacts whole-body health. Indeed, oral pathogenic bacteria have been found in non-oral tissue. Healthcare practitioners need to know this and remember that inflammation is inflammation, in whichever body tissue it occurs.

Oral microbial ecology

The moist, warm oral environment is ideally suited for the growth of microorganisms. Altered salivary pH associates with chronic generalized gingivitis/periodontitis[6] as well as caries. Critical pH range for caries development is 5–5.5, when acids may diffuse through tooth plaque/pellicle, contributing to demineralization.[7,8] The pH of gingival crevices in health is just below neutral and rises to above pH 8 in disease. Production of collagenase and hyaluronidase, impacting connective tissues, is optimal at or below neutral pH. At more alkaline pH, tissue damage may result[9] since alkalinity in gingival crevices and periodontal pockets may encourage colonization by periodontopathogens.[10]

The mouth has a wide range of ecological niches and oxidation-reduction potentials, with the gingival crevices and approximal surfaces of teeth generally having low redox potential and highest concentration of obligately anaerobic bacteria. Redox potential also varies during plaque formation, which results in lower redox potential and thus an increased number of obligately anaerobic bacteria found during plaque formation.[11]

Salivary components include non-specific defence factors (e.g. mucins, lysozyme, lactoferrin) as well as secretory immunoglobulin A (sIgA), the principal specific defence factor in saliva. Each has potential impact on oral ecology with salivary flow rate also impacting.

Host defence mechanisms, hormonal changes and genetic factors also impact oral ecology.[12] Oral microbiota composition is affected by tooth eruption, altered dietary habits, and stress.

Stress also affects oral ecology and alters immune function.[13] Salivary secretion rate of sIgA decreases significantly in high-stress conditions.[14]

External factors such as diet (e.g. sucrose fermentation), oral hygiene and antimicrobial agents may impact oral microbial ecology. Drugs (especially xerogenic pharmaceuticals), disease and disease treatments (e.g. radiotherapy treatments for head/neck cancer) and antibiotics may unbalance oral microbiota.[15] Other factors which might impact oral microbiota include dentures,[16] smoking[17] and oral contraceptives.[18] Awareness of these oral health risks should inform treatment protocols.

Biofilm communities

Dental pellicle is a naturally occurring biofilm with a protective role, defending against invading microbes. Healthy microbial composition is diverse yet stable, with predominant microorganisms preferring neutral pH.[19] Disrupted microbial homeostasis may result in initiation of disease processes.

Teeth, which are non-shedding surfaces,[20] have a greater propensity for undisturbed, established and therefore more diverse biofilm communities within ecological niches.[21] If that biofilm community has been exposed regularly to a fermentable carbohydrate-rich diet then its community may include higher numbers and types of problematic cariogenic microorganisms.

Biofilm formation has a protective function, providing 'colonization resistance', but biofilms are also responsible for caries, gingivitis and periodontitis – some of the most prevalent human infections.[22]

Biofilm in the gingival crevice, if not continually removed by brushing/flossing, eventually stimulates an inflammatory response which increases gingival crevicular fluid (GCF) secretion. This proteinaceous fluid provides nutrients for periodontopathogenic organisms, allowing proliferation, altering the biofilm community to one dominated by Gram-negative anaerobes, as well as inducing over-production of inflammatory mediators which ultimately may result in breakdown of tooth-supporting tissues.[23]

Bacterial species

Only 29 of the hundreds of bacterial species found in gingival crevices were also detected in intestinal/faecal samples. The most common intestinal species are not found in periodontal flora.[24]

More than 700 bacterial species have been detected in the healthy oral cavity; 149 predominant species were detected in nine oral cavity sites. Most sites had 20–30 different predominant species and there is a distinctive, highly diverse, site- and subject-specific predominant bacterial flora of healthy oral cavities.[25]

However, many species found in healthy oral microbiomes from clinically healthy teeth are also found in disease states. The change of status from commensal to invasive may occur in overgrowth conditions – in a manner similar to what may occur with infection by *Candida albicans* whereby this commensal fungus can become problematic and invasive with overgrowth due to, and additionally contributing to, dysbiosis.

Mouthwatering defence: saliva

A very dilute fluid,[26] clear, slightly acidic with pH 6–7, containing both inorganic and organic compounds,[27] saliva has no microbiota of its own and is composed of microbes shed from biofilms on oral tissues, disproportionally from tongue biofilm,[28] alongside proteins and glycoproteins which can both support and antagonize biofilm formation.[29]

Salivary functions are numerous, and saliva must both facilitate detection of nutritious foods and defend the mucosa from infection by the myriad of microorganisms in the mouth,[30] which could potentially include any organism in nature since the mouth is the gateway to the human body.[31] Functions of saliva can be broadly categorized as: limiting microbial adherence,[32] facilitating taste/digestion, buffering/clearance, maintaining tooth integrity, lubricating/protecting and providing antimicrobial activity,[33,34] with many constituents performing more than one function.[35]

Regarding functions associated with food/taste, molecules in food must be solubilized to be tasted[36,37] and saliva has diverse enzymatic composition and activity[38] including amylolytic,[39] proteolytic[40] and lipolytic[41,42] activities. Saliva enhances taste and initiates the digestive process via salivary amylase and lingual lipase.

Saliva is important for clearance of both food debris and undesirable microorganisms, which can be carried out via desquamated epithelial cells, each carrying approximately 100 microorganisms.[43]

As an important component of the human immune system, saliva is rich in antimicrobial peptides and a number of defence factors which limit bacterial growth or kill them directly.

Most of these salivary defence proteins/peptides are present in low concentration in whole saliva but with multi-functional effect that is likely cumulative and/or synergistic.[44]

Some salivary proteins such as statherins, agglutinins, glycoproteins, histadine-rich proteins and proline-rich proteins (PRPs) aid aggregation or 'clumping' of bacteria;[45] 'clumping' processes reduce bacterial ability to adhere to oral cavity hard/soft tissue surfaces, so facilitate control of microbial colonization.[46]

Secretory IgA is the main antibody to microorganisms in saliva[47] and the largest (and crucial) immunologic salivary component.[48] One of its most important defence mechanisms relates to its ability to inhibit bacterial adherence.[49] SIgA plays a major role in protecting mucosal surfaces against colonization and possible invasion by pathogenic microorganisms.[50]

Salivary components also ensure repair. Elevated collagenase activity is found in periodontitis, and salivary TIMP (tissue inhibitors of metalloproteinases/MMPs) levels have been found to be decreased in periodontitis.[51]

WOUND HEALING

Mouth wounds (e.g. from cheek-biting and tooth extraction) may heal quicker, and with less scarring, than those to external skin,[52] possibly due to salivary mucus which protects oral mucosa from desiccation.[53] Salivary VEGF (vascular endothelial growth factor) may also have a role in mucosal wound healing and may be an essential stimulus for oral mucosal tissue repair.[54]

Hyaluronic acid (HA), and sometimes hyaluronidase and hyaluronidase inhibitors, are present in saliva; HA is thought to function as lubricant as well as for wound healing re microtraumas from mastication.[55]

Melatonin, also present in saliva, may also have a role in tissue repair. Both HA and melatonin levels may decrease with ageing; supplementation may be warranted.

Salivary glands

Saliva is produced primarily (approximately 90%) by three pairs of major salivary glands: parotid, submandibular and sublingual. The rest is produced mainly from minor salivary glands with whole saliva also containing GCF, expectorated bronchial/nasal secretions, serum/blood derivatives from oral wounds, mucosal transudations, food debris, viruses and fungi, desquamated epithelial cells and other cellular components.[56]

There are between 600 and 1000 minor salivary glands which line the oral cavity and oropharynx, including in the lips, tongue, buccal mucosa and palate, each having a single duct.[57] These numerous glands mainly secrete mucus, providing oral cavity salivary coating. Minor salivary glands provide many protective components, and their value and contribution should not be underestimated.

One quarter of labial minor salivary gland secretion proteins were not detected in major salivary secretions. These novel salivary components in minor salivary gland secretions may be critically involved in processes influencing infectious diseases, as well as dental caries and periodontal disease.[58]

The minor salivary glands can also produce 30–35 per cent of the IgA that enters the oral cavity. So, whilst they are considered 'minor' glands, their protective function to oral cavity (and whole-body) health appears to be greater than their categorization as 'minor' and their low volume contribution suggest. Indeed, the highest levels of sIgA are found in the minor salivary glands.[59]

Gingival crevicular fluid (GCF)

Whereas saliva bathes the supragingival oral environment, GCF bathes the subgingival environment.

GCF is an inflammatory exudate,[60] with amounts often found to be directly proportional to the severity of inflammation.[61] There is increased GCF flow in gingivitis[62] as well as increased proportions of putative periodontal pathogens.

Sex hormones in pregnancy, ovulation and contraceptives may increase GCF flow, as can smoking.

Saliva-associated communicable diseases

There are several infectious conditions transmitted via saliva and some are referred to as 'kissing diseases', for example mononucleosis, considered to be caused by Epstein-Barr Virus (EBV). Other viruses (e.g. human cytomegalovirus (hCMV)) can spread via infected saliva.[63]

Periodontopathogenic bacteria can spread through saliva; practitioners should remember that periodontal disease is communicable.

SARS-COV-2/COVID-19

Full understanding of the COVID-19 pandemic, caused by infection with SARS-CoV-2 (severe acute respiratory syndrome coronavirus-2), occurring at the time of writing, has yet to be ascertained. SARS-CoV-2 spreads easily, with high virulence, through saliva aerosols which can remain viable in air for three or more hours.[64]

Evidence indicates oral mucosa as an initial entry site for SARS-CoV-2, and that oral symptoms, including loss of taste/smell and dry mouth, may be early symptoms of infection.[65] Emerging evidence indicates salivary glands as potential reservoirs for SARS-CoV-2, explaining the presence of asymptomatic infections.[66] Oral cavity ulcers/blisters also may associate.[67]

Sialogogues

Although highly variable and very individualized, the average daily flow of whole saliva in healthy individuals varies between 1 and 1.5 litres.[68] Constituents differ according to the originating gland and may vary according to flow rate; whole protein content (important in microbial defence) increases proportionately with increased flow rate.[69]

Head and neck radiotherapy can have a serious and detrimental effect on the oral cavity including altered or dysfunctional salivary glands and, as with some prescription medication, xerostomia.

Supporting salivary flow via use of botanical sialogogues may prove beneficial for clients on xerostomic pharmaceuticals, undergoing radiotherapy or experiencing reduced salivary flow for any other reason.

Nutritional support for oral border control

Therapeutic support for factors discussed in this chapter include minimizing xerostomic medications, considering oral probiotics use, including sialogogues where necessary, and using glycan-rich foods to provide the major component sugars of salivary glycoproteins (like agglutinin)[70] and mucins[71] that impact salivary defence actions.

For their ability to impact redox status and counter reactive species, include antioxidant-rich foods,[72,73,74] and consider glutathione supplementation, which has been shown to benefit periodontitis management.[75] Glutathione is an important redox regulator in inflammatory processes.

Where necessary in cases of dysbiotic oral microbiome, consider using botanical anti-microbials and detoxification support as well as oral probiotics.

EFFECT OF EXERCISE ON SALIVA

Although measurement of salivary response to exercise is influenced by other factors, including hydration and measurement/testing methods, exercise as stress was found to significantly decrease salivary flow rate whilst increasing α-amylase activity and sIgA concentration (but not sIgA secretion rate); a three-hour rest was found to be adequate for recovery in terms of saliva secretion and α-amylase and sIgA responses.[76] Decreased salivary secretion rate (and its impact on sIgA in particular) has been implicated as a potential risk factor for repeated respiratory infection in athletes.[77,78]

— Chapter 3 —

ANATOMY AND GLEEKING

Understanding the component elements of the oral cavity is an important part of understanding both the processes of 'normal' development and function of this important body region, and its impact on status within the continuum of whole-body health and disease. Interrelatedness of body systems is an important consideration when exploring potential personalized protocols for optimal oral cavity (and systemic) health.

Many nutritionists will not have learned much about oral anatomy in their formal training. The subject is considered perhaps as a specialism of dentists, dental hygienists and associated professional groups. Teeth and dental health are highly relevant to oral cavity and systemic health yet nutritional therapists may not be aware why the taste system is particularly vulnerable to damage at several locations,[1] which neurotransmitters may be involved in taste,[2] or how general anxiety is associated with altered taste perception (which may explain altered appetite).[3] Furthermore, many people still believe the validity of a now-disproven (yet still much-used) tongue map showing taste zones.

An extended version of this chapter (available online) provides background information on oral anatomy for those who want to read about the misleading tongue map, or want to know why periodontal health should be investigated in clients who complain of thirst. It also explains what gleeking is and the rationale for protocols to support salivary and connective tissue health for a wide group of clients, including those impacted by stress.

The oral cavity

The term cavity is defined as 'an empty space within a solid object'. It can also be defined as 'a decayed part of a tooth',[4] alternatively referred to as dental caries. To avoid confusion, only the alternative term 'caries' will be used in this book when referring to the decayed part of a tooth. The term 'oral cavity' will refer to the 'mouth space' – the area between the lips and pharynx/oesophagus through which food passes en route to the stomach and intestines.

— Chapter 4 —

TASTE MATTERS

Whilst the sense of taste is often considered less important than other sensory perception (e.g. vision, hearing), failure to eat will result in starvation and death, so nature protects eating behaviour.[1]

If experiencing food related only to the five primary Western tradition tastes, eating would probably not be such an interesting (and for some, obsessive) pastime. Scientists have found five tastes for which receptors can be found to explain physiological responses to food. In addition to these five primary tastes, chemesthetic qualities of food (i.e. sensations arising from chemical compounds activating receptors associated with other senses such as food temperature and spiciness) affect the experience of consuming food.

In addition to the obvious impact that taste perception has on dietary choices, information presented in this chapter is important for several reasons, including that aspects of taste may be genetically determined, and taste receptors can be affected by pharmaceutical drugs as well as food temperature. Taste research has already revealed much that informs food manufacturers and dietary protocols, and in time may reveal more associations between food response and overall body health.

Gustation and taste buds

Humans are traditionally said to have five senses: sight, smell, sound, touch and taste. Taste is experienced in the mouth/oral cavity via chemical reactions with taste receptor cells on taste buds; flavour (a distinctive taste or essential character) of food and drink is experienced in combination with olfaction and stimulation of the trigeminal nerve (which registers temperature, texture and pain), and is a unified sense.

The gustatory cortex (GC), located in the cerebral cortex, is responsible for taste perception and integration of taste experiences. Taste perception/sensation is the result of a complex network of nerves and nerve impulses that transport information between the oral cavity and brain. Multisensory factors (including visual factors) contribute to flavour sensations; mechanoreceptors, thermoreceptors and chemesthesis (e.g. perceived pungency) are involved.[2] Specialized peripheral receptors and pathways relay taste information via various nerves to the GC, which is activated by food consumption and taste experience.

Chemoresponsive nerve fibres are present in skin and on mucosal surfaces of the mouth, nose and eyes; mucosal surfaces exhibit greater chemesthetic sensitivity compared with external skin. Examples include the stinging/tingling of carbonated beverages, tear-induction of cut onions, coolness of menthol and burn-like irritation of capsaicin in chilli peppers.

Five primary tastes

There are five established basic tastes: sweet, bitter, sour, salty and umami. Although researchers are considering other possible primary 'tastes', currently all other 'flavours' are said to be combinations of these five primary tastes plus other sensations from olfactory and tactile senses.

Flavour perception is considered a distinct concept, integrating taste, smell, chemesthesis (aka trigeminality) and touch (mouth-feel).[3] Olfactory system stimulation by food can be thousands of times stronger than gustatory system stimulation, and blocked olfaction may result in reduced gustation when an individual is suffering from a cold or allergies.

Although taste can be considered, according to its primary function, as a nutrient–toxin detection system,[4] the word tends to denote something far wider, encompassing concepts including flavour.

The five primary tastes are distinguished by taste receptors on taste buds, through interaction with different molecules or ions. Basic tastes are considered either appetitive or aversive depending on the potential effects on the body.[5]

Two primary tastes – saltiness and sourness – are mediated via ion channels. The other three – bitterness, sweetness and umami (savouriness) – are mediated by G-protein coupled receptor binding.

Salty and sour

Sodium is essential for maintaining normal water distribution; its amount reflects the balance between sodium intake and output.[6] Taste perception of salt, therefore, may have health implications and survival benefits.

Sour taste evokes an innate rejection response in humans, which is thought to function as caution against ingestion of acidic food sources, discouraging ingestion of foods which are unripe or may be spoiled by microorganisms.

Aversive responses to sour/acid foods are readily understandable since acids are potentially harmful tissue-damaging substances.[7] The degree to which humans perceive sourness is affected by saliva,[8] which acts as a buffering system.

Whilst salty and sour foods may be appetitive in small amounts, larger amounts may be less so, likely reflecting potential danger.

GPCRs and gustducin

Bitter, sweet and umami tastes result from tastant binding to receptors on plasma membranes that link to G-proteins which then activate several second messengers inside the gustatory receptor cell, resulting in neurotransmitter release. The pattern of resulting nerve impulses accounts for different tastes.

There are several classes of G-protein-coupled receptors (GPCRs) involved in taste: taste receptor type 1 member 1 (T1R1) is involved in umami; taste receptor type 1 member 2 (T1R2) is involved in tasting sweetness; taste receptor type 1 member 3 (T1R3) is involved in tasting both sweet and umami; and bitter-taste receptors T2Rs (aka TAS2Rs).

Although these three tastes use different receptors, they use similar signalling pathways, including TRPM5 (a taste ion channel) and PLC (phospholipase C – a signalling effector of GPCRs).[9] G-protein α-gustducin has a role in all three taste responses.[10]

In addition to presence in some taste receptor cells and its important role in sweet and bitter signalling in lingual epithelium taste buds, gustducin is expressed in gastric and pancreatic cells. Taste receptors have been found in the bladder, brain and airway, as well as in the gastrointestinal tract;[11] many taste-signalling molecules are expressed in intestinal mucosa.[12]

Taste-sensing GPCRs, T1Rs, and gustducin express in brain cells, particularly regarding glucosensing.[13] Bitter receptors are present in brain cells where activation of TAS2Rs may result in increased intracellular calcium, causing secretion of regulatory peptides (e.g. CCK) involved in the regulation of food intake.[14] Brain glucosensors may alter the firing rate relative to glucose concentration.[15]

GPCRS, DYSGEUSIA AND PHARMACEUTICALS

G-proteins function as molecular switches inside cells, participating in signal transmission from outside-the-cell stimuli to the cell interior. Activation of just one G-protein can signal production of thousands of second messenger molecules[16] with high amplification.[17]

Because of their extensive range of involvement in extracellular signalling, GPCRs are popularly targeted for pharmaceutical intervention[18] to address disease states. Approximately 36 per cent of drugs target GPCRs, most commonly antihypertensive and anti-allergic drugs. GPCRs continue to be popular targets for pharmaceutical research and represent the largest class of target structures for NTDs (novel target drugs) approved since 1983. Six out of the 20 drugs (30%) with the highest global sales in 2010 target GPCRs. Sixty-three of 200 drugs (approximately 32%) with highest 2009 sales in the USA targeted GPCRs.[19]

Leaving aside the relative effectiveness of these pharmaceuticals, there may be an unintended impact on other GPCR signalling – including GPCR signalling in the oral cavity. Dysgeusia, xerostomia and stomatitis (inflammation of mouth/lips) are the three most frequent oral side effects with prescription medications.[20] These and other oral side effects are also common during cancer treatment (radiotherapy and chemotherapy).[21,22]

In all cases of xerostomia, stomatitis, dysgeusia and perhaps with some other oral cavity issues, pharmaceutical prescription medications should be investigated first as the cause.

Umami

Glutamate, aspartate and some other amino acids account for the savoury taste known as umami. Glutamate-rich foods such as meat, fish and cheese trigger this taste sensation. Monosodium glutamate (MSG), the purest form of umami flavour,[23] aka sodium glutamate, is an abundant, naturally occurring amino acid which stimulates the umami taste sensation, especially in foods that are also nucleotide rich.[24]

Glutamic acid can only be tasted when in unbound form. Free glutamate is notably found in green tea, seaweed, tomato, potato, Chinese cabbage, soy sauce, Parmesan cheese, sardines, prawns and clams, as well as konbu.[25] Fermented foods also contain high glutamate content. Approximately 20g daily of glutamate from free glutamate in foods is absorbed in the small intestine where it is a major oxidative fuel.[26]

Glutamic acid is one of the two most prominent amino acids in human breast milk (the other is taurine),[27] benefits of which include potential roles in protecting intestinal mucosa integrity and potentiating the immune response.[28] So, umami taste, which is innately liked, is likely learned through breast milk.[29]

Multiple taste receptors are involved in umami sensation.[30] Three umami receptors have been identified: T1R1+T1R3, mGluR4 and mGluR1.[31] These GPCRs are expressed in taste buds.

Bitter

Bitter taste is innately aversive and stimulated by huge numbers of compounds with diverse chemical structures.[32] Many of these compounds are toxic. Many 'healthy' foods are bitter tasting (e.g. brassicas, chicory, dandelion, olives). Bitter compounds such as isothiocyanates in cruciferous vegetables, naringin in grapefruit juice and caffeine in coffee may invoke a strong reaction in some individuals. Perceived bitterness in these foods/drinks may account for dislike/rejection of these by some individuals.

Humans have around 25 functional TAS2Rs,[33] yet thousands of compounds are perceived by humans to be bitter. Our ability to perceive so many bitter substances with such small numbers of bitter taste receptors is linked to the molecular receptive ranges of TAS2R bitter taste receptors. Genetic polymorphisms in these 25 TAS2R receptors[34] may affect the perceived bitterness of foods and drugs.

TAS2R bitter receptors are also found in extra-oral tissues: gastrointestinal tissues,[35] respiratory epithelia[36] and the brain.[37] Those in the gut may provide a defence mechanism against harmful xenobiotics.[38]

EXTRA-ORAL TASTE RECEPTORS

In addition to its expression in taste receptor cells, gustducin is expressed in gastric[39,40] and pancreatic cells.[41] Its presence may be a defence mechanism as bitter taste reception pathways aid prevention of harmful substance ingestion.[42]

Activation of bitter taste receptors, under control of α-gustducin in the gut, stimulates ghrelin secretion, causing a short-term increase in food intake followed by a prolonged decrease in food intake and inhibition of gastric emptying.[43]

The otherwise counter-intuitive suggestion that bitter herbs are beneficial when bitter constituents are generally considered toxic can be explained with reference to this; the long traditional use of bitter herbs in herbal medicine for appetite stimulation and improved digestion can be explained as helping to process food with maximum efficiency and counteract effects of overeating regarding ghrelin stimulation.[44] Furthermore, bitter agents may inhibit stomach contractility, prolonging nutrient presence in the stomach, resulting in early satiety, increasing intervals between meals and reducing overall food intake.[45]

Nutrient sensing in the gut has been actively researched to provide therapeutic methods to address obesity and obesity-related type 2 diabetes (T2D). Research on bitter receptors (regarding ghrelin), umami receptors (regarding protein-induced satiety) and sweet taste receptors (regarding sustained positive energy balance) may further scientists' understanding of metabolic dysfunction associated with obesity; these receptors may be considered as new therapeutic targets.[46]

Taste molecules have a role in the respiratory tract, stomach, intestines, pancreas, liver, kidney, testes and brain as well as gut (stomach, intestines) and oral cavity.[47] Therefore, roles in other health conditions may yet prove interesting. A 2017 review summarizes physiological and pathophysiological roles that extra-oral TAS2Rs play in processes including immunity and reproduction; the authors include a table of affected body systems and diseases.[48]

A 2018 review discusses GPCR bitter and sweet taste receptors in upper airway epithelium, finding that these extra-oral taste receptors in nose and paranasal sinuses detect pathogens and modulate innate immune responses with opposing effects – bitter compounds triggering calcium waves and rapid release of antipathogenic nitric oxide and antimicrobial peptides, and sweet stimulants inhibiting this.[49]

In the gut, bitters help stimulate production of digestive juice and HCl release. Gastric HCl reduces pH and triggers release of intrinsic factor which aids body utilization of essential vitamin B12. Stomach acid is also important for digestion, mineral/protein absorption and immune defence.

So, including a variety of bitter foods is absolutely advocated. Include these for digestive and potential whole-body effect.

For individuals who are not fans of bitter taste, consider these foods a 'bitter pill', with health benefits – a 'work-out' for gut/whole-body health or gentle detox. Bitter foods are considered by herbalists to have an overall alkalizing effect for even greater benefit.

Sweet

One primary sweet taste receptor may be involved in both caloric sweeteners and non-nutritive sweeteners (e.g. stevia), possibly involving different receptor domains.[50]

Whilst bitter tastes are experienced via 20+ receptors, sweet taste is mediated largely by a single receptor.[51] T1R2+T1R3 taste receptors not only initiate oral sugar ingestion but also detect sugar in the intestinal lumen and trigger physiological responses promoting sugar absorption/metabolism. Modulating gut capacity to absorb sugars may be implicated in malabsorption syndromes and diet-associated disorders such as obesity and diabetes,[52] with knock-on effects on periodontal diseases.

Sweetness is usually considered innately appetitive, indicating the presence of carbohydrates (i.e. energy-rich foods), but can be a poor indicator of a plant's food value. Sweet taste is also considered to be highly motivating. Sensing sweetness may have evolved as a way of detecting glucose, the major obligate energetic fuel of brain tissue.[53]

'Supertasters'

'Supertasters' of bitterness (shown to be genetically determined)[54] have a tendency to dislike foods with bitter compounds (e.g. cruciferous vegetables); these taste factors may impact dietary choices and frequency of bitter food consumption.[55] Additionally, 'supertasters' perceive stronger tastes from sweet substances and perceive more burn from oral irritants (alcohol, capsaicin).[56]

'Supertasters' have more fungiform papillae.[57] Women are more frequently 'supertasters' and have more fungiform papillae and taste buds.[58] Evidence suggests there is a hormonal impact on bitter taste variation including from the menstrual cycle, pregnancy and menopause.[59]

AMERICAN PRESIDENTS AND BROCCOLI. IS GENETICS INVOLVED?

Former American president George H.W. Bush declared (1990) that he hadn't liked broccoli since childhood and wasn't going to eat it as president, causing some people to nod in agreement and others (particularly parents trying to persuade children to eat this superfood with a healthful reputation) concern.

Since broccoli, like other cruciferous vegetables, is considered bitter, and the concept of 'supertasters' is closely associated with bitterness, the question is raised: was the former president a 'genetic supertaster'?

Emerging evidence suggests many TAS2Rs contain polymorphisms. Variations in one of these taste genes, TAS2R38, influences sensitivity to bitterness.[60] TAS2R38 variations are associated with intake of both vegetables and alcohol; other genetic polymorphisms may impact sweet and umami tastes and ingestive behaviour relating to food odours, astringency and creaminess.[61]

Recent research (2018) found that trying more bitter foods changed salivary proteins that affect taste perception, thus perhaps permitting 'learned' behaviour to bitter foods.[62]

Returning to the question of the former president's long-term dislike of broccoli, numerous factors may be involved in addition to brassica bitterness; its allylglucosinolate content may convert into pungent compounds, and dimethyl sulphide content can give a rotting-egg smell when cooked. When over-cooked, brassicas are mushy, slimy and foul-smelling. It is not known what experience this former president had of broccoli, nor if he persisted in 'learning' bitter taste.

Another former American president, Barack Obama, has reportedly said that his favourite food is broccoli, which he admits he didn't used to like when it was served boiled and soft.

What is the moral of this story? Whilst both former presidents made headlines for their broccoli comments, it is probably better public relations to be a good (broccoli-eating) role model who doesn't alienate brassica-growers and other groups. Perhaps more importantly, whilst genetics may be involved, other factors (in this case cooking methods) may be the factor determining ingestive behaviour.

Chemesthetic sensations

Several chemesthetic sensations are associated with taste perception. Many are caused by activation of TRP (transient receptor potential) cation channels.

Trigeminal nerve reactions from substances such as black pepper (piperine), ginger (gingerol), horseradish (isothiocyanate) and chilli peppers (capsaicin) are caused by activation of members of the TRP channel family (e.g. TRPV1, TRPM8, TRPA1).

Sensations of 'hot' or 'spicy', also referred to as pungency or piquancy, are considered as taste sensations. TRPV1 (human vanilloid receptor 1, aka capsaicin receptor) is activated by capsaicin (found in chilli peppers), eugenol (in clove oil), zingerone (in ginger),[63] piperine (pungent alkaloid in black pepper),[64] diallyl sulfides in garlic[65] and allyl isothiocynate (organosulfur compound in mustard, horseradish, wasabi).

Trigeminal receptor activation can also occur from exposure to menthol (e.g. spearmint, peppermint) and ethanol, evoking a perceived sensation of 'coolness' via TRPM8 ion channels.

Isothiocyanate compounds in mustard oil, wasabi and horseradish activate TRPA1, another TRP channel family member for which activation results in the sensation of 'pungency'. TRPA1 is an excitatory ion channel involved in pain pathways, activation of which is accompanied by vasodilation. TRPA1 is also activated by allicin and diallyl disulfide (DADS), constituents in garlic and other *Allium* genus members,[66] as well as by clove, ginger and cinnamon (re cinnamaldehyde).[67] THC (Δ^9-tetrahydrocannabinol), the psychoactive component of cannabis, can also activate TRPA1.[68]

'ADDICTION' TO SPICE

'Spiciness' and 'hotness' are taste/flavour sensations caused by the interaction of capsaicinoids with TRPV1, which acts as nerve cell sensor. TRPV1 is normally activated by physical heat (+43°C) which allows calcium ion flow through ion channels in cell lipid membranes. This sends danger signals, triggering other nerve cells via neurotransmitter release. Capsaicinoids, which also interact with TRPV1, trigger the same reaction, tricking the brain into thinking it is being burned although no heat is present.[69,70]

> The neurotransmitter and neuromodulator, substance P, is one pain-transmitting messenger.[71] The brain responds by releasing endorphins, another type of neurotransmitter which blocks nerves from transmitting pain; dopamine, a neurotransmitter responsible for a sense of reward and pleasure, is also released via inhibition of GABA release.[72] Thus, for some people, eating spicy foods may trigger euphoria similar to a 'runner's high'.[73]
>
> This triggering of TRPV1 gives, for many people, an enjoyable sensation; whilst the body can crave spicy foods, this type of 'addiction' is not a dependence such as experienced with nicotine or caffeine.

Trigeminal pain pathways also appear to be involved in the fizzy sensation of carbonated drinks; all chemesthetic sensations involve similar firing of neurons in the subnucleus caudalis (Vc).[74]

Metallic and other tastes

The aversive metallic/bitter aftertaste that characterizes many artificial sweeteners may involve stimulation of TRPV1 receptors in cells and nerve terminals throughout the oral cavity and is activated by a large range of structurally different chemicals; artificial sweeteners sensitize these channels to acid and temperature.[75]

TRPV1 receptors are also activated by copper sulfate, zinc sulfate and iron sulfate – three salts known to produce a metallic taste sensation,[76] so mineral supplements in contact with lingual surfaces may also elicit a metallic sensation.[77]

Some orally ingested medications may elicit a metallic sensation due to activation of oral cavity receptors;[78] perceived aversion to metallic sensations may vary between patients using these medications due to genetic polymorphisms in the TRPV1 gene.[79] It is not yet known whether metallic is a taste perception or whether activation of TRPV1 in sensory nerve endings of the oral cavity mediates this.[80]

Tannins or calcium oxalate can cause an astringent, puckering sensation of the oral mucous membrane. Rhubarb, red wine, tea, nuts and unripe bananas are foods giving this chemesthetic sensation.

There are also many other contenders of a 'sixth taste' including perception of fat, water, 'starchiness', calcium and magnesium, heartiness/*kokumi* and alkalinity.

Food temperature and flavour perception

Food temperature affects taste experience. Most soups are traditionally expected to be served hot, alcoholic beverages and carbonated drinks cold or iced. Such taste expectations may be important considerations in commercial recipe design.

The temperature at which food is served may affect perceived sweetness and bitterness. High temperatures enhance sweetness perception; increasing food temperature markedly enhances gustatory nerve responses to sweet compounds via TRPM5 channel activation.[81] This has implications for food producers. Ice cream producers, for example, will add very large amounts of sugar to accommodate this. Anyone who has tried to 'drink' fully melted ice cream will attest to its much-increased sweetness, artificially high to accommodate the 'fresh-from-the-freezer' serving temperature.

Beer is also served very cold. The bitter taste is thought to be more apparent when consumed at higher temperatures. Whilst most people seem to prefer the bitterness of beer to be dulled by a chilled serving temperature, other bitter liquid substances (e.g. coffee, tea, cocoa) are often consumed hot by individuals who appreciate/enjoy the bitter sensation.

Oral cavity temperature also appears to impact food tastes. 'Melting effects' of food seem enhanced after a hot mouth rinse, which may be due to enhanced enzymatic action of salivary α-amylase with the raised temperature. The perception of flavour/aroma and the fat after-feel increases with the rise in temperature.[82]

Warmed food gives more aromas, which may stimulate the olfactory nerves, affecting perceived flavours. This has important considerations for the 'neuro-gastronomic' impact of food/eating (see Chapter 17). Strong smells may even confuse the taste buds.

Relevance to nutritional therapy

In addition to inclusion of bitter foods (taste for which can be learned), inclusion of umami-rich foods (e.g. dried shiitake, porcini, morel mushrooms) may benefit health, as umami flavour can increase satiety as well as enhance appetite.[83]

Activation of vanilloid receptors may increase enjoyment of foods and satisfy 'cravings', including black pepper, chilli, cloves, cinnamon, bay leaves, allspice, ginger, garlic, mustard, horseradish and wasabi.

Szechuan peppers and other *Zanthoxylum* genus members (e.g. prickly ash, *Zanthoxylum americanum*) have been used traditionally for trigeminal pain (e.g. toothache).[84]

Sugar-sensing mechanisms are associated with diabetes and with over-eating/obesity and may have relevance in eating disorders. These diet-associated disorders have a knock-on effect regarding periodontal disease. Understanding these connections may inform protocols for associated health conditions. For example, since food temperature affects perception of sweetness, some individuals may get their 'sugar-fix' better by opting for hot desserts rather than ice cream. Reducing sugar consumption impacts oral cavity ecology as well as systemic inflammation.

Practitioner awareness of the potential effects of pharmaceuticals on taste perception and thus dietary choices may help when suggesting protocols to clients. Familiarity with GPCRs and taste perception is important for many reasons, not simply in relation to GPCR-targeting regarding pharmaceuticals; much current research focuses on these receptors in relation to eating disorders and obesity, as well as exercise performance.

More often than not food choices are made according to taste/flavour preferences. Food choices impact health. Taste and flavour matter.

CARBOHYDRATE SENSING: FOOLING THE BRAIN

Since taste and flavour perception starts in the mouth, signalling cascades are initiated when food enters the oral cavity. Those signalling cascades are prior to swallowing of the food bolus. Food that enters the oral cavity but is spat out might conceivably already have initiated these signalling cascades. Researchers have been investigating these possibilities with regard to sports drinks.

Sports drinks are typically high in carbohydrates and designed to supply efficient energy alongside hydration for athletes. They were never formulated for casual gym-goers or individuals exercising for weight loss. Such high-carbohydrate drinks give an energy boost and can cause an insulin rise that limits the rate of fat-burning, which is counter-productive to weight loss aims.

Recent studies looking at the effect of swishing high-carbohydrate drinks in the mouth, then spitting rather than swallowing, suggest that the presence of carbohydrates in the mouth can activate regions of the brain involved in reward and motor control, enhancing exercise performance; there may be a class of so-far-unidentified oral receptors that respond to carbohydrates independently of those for sweetness.[85]

A 2017 study investigating the impact of carbohydrate-mouth-rinsing on performance and cognitive function following fatigue-inducing fencing indicated that maltodextrin solution significantly improved the accuracy of skill-specific fencing performance, although no influence on reaction time was observed.[86]

Studies on carbohydrate-mouth-rinsing so far have investigated the effects on athletes; it is possible that similar benefits for cognitive function and skill performance would also be seen in other areas.

— Chapter 5 —

SUGARS IN HEALTH AND DISEASE

Glucose, although a caries-causative agent, is an important sugar and is a metabolite providing energy to the brain. The dual-edged nature of sugars is demonstrated when improper glucose control by normal metabolic mechanisms results in diabetes. It is evident in its dysregulation, which is a well-understood central risk factor for the development of cardiovascular disease and its negative impact on mouth and dental health. High concentrations of glucose can cause serious organ damage, while low concentrations can cause loss of consciousness and even sudden death due to inadequate energy.[1]

Sugar is a highly emotive subject. We *all* like sugar. Our bodies are programmed to like what gives them energy, allowing them to survive and thrive. However, sugar, in the quantities and manner in which it is consumed in the industrialized world, is undisputedly and recognizably detrimental to good health; sugar contributes to excess, anti-nutritive calories, weight gain, dental caries and generalized inflammation which may promote chronic illness. Such generalized inflammation may have systemic impact. Sugars, by contributing to the production of AGEs (advanced glycation end-products), promote accelerated ageing. And sugar consumption can result in addictive behaviours.

Sugars and other fermentable carbohydrates from the diet are hydrolysed by salivary amylase and metabolized to acids by plaque bacteria, lowering plaque and salivary pH and thus initiating tooth demineralization.[2] Some sweeteners do not have this effect. However, all such dietary sugars and sweeteners, by one or more means, have the propensity to disrupt metabolism and impact health detrimentally.

Whilst consuming sugar-rich foods can wreak havoc in the body, impacting its immune system, reacting with proteins, lipids and nucleic acids to impact function of these important body components, behaving much as a toxin, 'sugars' are also essential to life, providing energy. Glucose, alongside several other somewhat less discussed saccharides (including mannose and fucose[3]) which have been termed 'essential saccharides' by Mondoa and Kitei,[4] have other health-promoting roles. As the glycan component of proteoglycans and glycoproteins, some saccharides can beneficially impact health, and glycans have been referred to as a 'crucial part of a cell's identity'.[5]

Glycans, rather than carbohydrates (a term that generally indicates dietary starches and sucrose-laden foods), should be considered one of four major classes of macromolecules, alongside nucleic acids, proteins and lipids. Glycans are essential for cell structure and function and have critical roles in cell signalling, immunity and inflammation.[6] They may be the largest, most structurally diverse class of molecules in nature and are attached to about half the proteins in the human body.[7]

In addition to Mondoa and Kitei's book, this chapter has been extensively informed by a couple of resources to which the reader may refer for more specific or further information. Dr Marilyn Glenville gives background information and recommendations about the use or avoidance of a number of sugars/sweeteners and recipes in her book *Natural Alternatives to Sugar*.[8] An online resource on sugars and sweeteners provides much information including on the glycaemic index (GI) and the US Food and Drug Administration (FDA) guidelines on the intake of sweeteners.[9]

The information in this chapter (and recommended additional resources) is important because disease-promoting sugars are harmful to oral and whole-body health, whilst glycans are important components of salivary constituents.

Sugars (and sweeteners)

All refined sugars are empty calories (four calories per gram); they provide no nutritional value, although, like all carbohydrates, they provide energy to the body, brain and nervous system. Sugars are harmful to teeth.

Sweeteners can be categorized into groups: sugars, sugar alcohols, natural caloric sweeteners, natural zero-calorie sweeteners, modified sugars, artificial sweeteners and sugar fibres. Factors to consider when choosing a sweetener include taste, aftertaste, calories, effect on teeth, nutritive effect, safety, level of processing involved, effect on blood sugar and suitability for diabetics. Although this book relates primarily to mouth/dental effects, other factors are relevant since whole-body health impacts (as well as is impacted by) mouth/dental health.

An extended version of this chapter is available online.

Sugar alcohols

Sugar alcohols (aka polyols) are naturally occurring carbohydrates, though they typically contain fewer available calories per gram than sugar because the body is unable to fully metabolize them. Contrary to what their name implies, these are neither sugars nor alcohol.[10] Sugar alcohols do not cause tooth decay. Excessive (and sometimes moderate) consumption of sugar alcohols may cause cramps in some people. Sugar alcohol's side effects include digestive effects (due to the body's inability to properly digest, the non-metabolized portion ferments and creates an environment hospitable to harmful bacteria and exacerbates yeast problems). Another side effect of sugar alcohols is that metabolic resources are wasted in the body's attempt to clear the digestive system; this may result in unwanted weight gain.

Xylitol is a much-talked-of five-carbon sugar referred to as a sugar alcohol, which is produced from a naturally occurring substance in plants but requires refining for use as a sweetener.[11]

A potentially beneficial effect of xylitol is its inhibition of *S.mutans* growth by disrupting their energy production processes and starving the bacteria;[12] this is because when caries-causing bacteria such as *S.mutans* and lactobacilli are forced to consume xylitol instead of glucose or fructose, they cannot make the enamel-attacking acids or sticky mucopolysaccharides that encourage adhesion to teeth. Xylitol also decreases the incidence of dental caries by increasing salivary flow[13] and pH[14] and reducing both numbers of cariogenic (*S.mutans*) and periodontopathic (*H.pylori*) bacteria, plaque levels, xerostomia, gingival inflammation and erosion of teeth.[15]

Xylitol consumption can reduce caries and its non-/anti-cariogenic properties may relate to its lack of suitability for microbial metabolism and its physico-chemical effects in plaque and saliva.[16]

Xylitol is recommended by some doctors (for its low GI), although it has also been reported that xylitol can raise BSL (blood sugar level), thus suggesting it should not be used by diabetics.[17] Although some dentists recommend xylitol (for its caries-preventive properties), conflicting reports exist on its beneficial oral effects;[18] the evidence for its benefit to oral health is not conclusive.[19] Other studies show beneficial effect on mutans streptococci, on plaque and caries occurrence when xylitol is consumed three to five times per day with a daily dose of 5–10 grams.[20]

Overall, xylitol remains controversial.[21] It should not be used if following the FODMAP diet for IBS (irritable bowel syndrome). Otherwise, its potential benefit on oral health would possibly justify its use, although not in large amounts and possibly only in toothpaste and chewing gum.

Sorbitol (aka glucitol) is another well-known sugar alcohol which requires little or no insulin, so is often used in foods for diabetics. Sorbitol has the same cautions as xylitol on raising blood sugar levels, however, thus suggesting it should not be used by diabetics,[22] although the effect on BSL is said to be less than for sucrose.[23] Usually made from corn syrup, sorbitol is heavily processed, including hydrogenation, and shows similar side effects to xylitol, so is also contraindicated in IBS. Sorbitol provides 2.7 kilocalories per gram (vs 4 kilocalories for sugars/carbohydrates and 2.4 for xylitol).[24]

When compared with xylitol, sorbitol is less expensive, but also less effective in controlling caries.[25]

Mannitol is, like sorbitol, a hydrogenated monosaccharide; mannitol is commonly produced via hydrogenation of fructose. This sugar alcohol has a very low GI, low caloric value of 1.6 kcals, and is, like xylitol and sorbitol, considered non-cariogenic.[26] Mannitol lingers in the intestines for a long time, causing bloating and diarrhoea.[27]

The diarrhoeal effect of sorbitol is greater than that of erythritol which is not metabolized;[28] over 90 per cent is excreted unchanged in the urine.[29] Although erythritol occurs naturally in some foods including mushrooms, watermelons, pears, grapes and fermented foods,[30] it is usually made from glucose, most commonly from genetically modified (GMO) corn starch, fermented with a yeast called *Moniliella pollinis*.[31] This biotechnological process results in a white crystalline powder with a sweetness of 60–70 per cent relative to sucrose[32] and a caloric value of 0.2 kcal.[33]

Information about erythritol is mixed. Whilst one study with rats indicates this polyol acts as an antioxidant *in vivo*, potentially protecting against hyperglycaemia-induced vascular damage,[34] another study reports a case of allergic urticaria with wheals over the entire body after one glass of beverage sweetened with erythritol.[35]

Other research indicating the positive effect of erythritol includes a 2016 study of the effects of both xylitol and erythritol on gut hormones and gastric emptying; both polyols were found to induce significant delay in gastric emptying and the study concluded that acute ingestion of these stimulates gut hormone release, slowing gastric emptying with little or no effect on insulin release.[36] These same two polyols were looked at in terms of dental caries protection in a double-blind randomized controlled prospective clinical trial of 485 primary school children in a three-year intervention; researchers observed a lower number of cavities in the erythritol group than in the xylitol or sorbitol (control) groups. The time to develop caries lesions was also longest in the erythritol group.[37]

Providing a non-GMO source of erythritol is used, and this is not alongside other artificial sweeteners (which it is often combined with), moderate intake of erythritol may be a better alternative than xylitol or other polyols for individuals without IBS or who are particularly sensitive to allergic reactions. Erythritol may be a more potent inhibitor of mutans streptococci.[38]

Maltilol, mannitol and lactilol are also non-cariogenic,[39] as is glycerol/glycerine (discussed in Chapter 13).

Natural caloric sweeteners

Natural caloric sweeteners are some of the oldest known sweeteners and include honey and maple syrup. They contain nutritive qualities as well as sugar and can be harmful to teeth. Some of them can be better choices than sugar because some contain nutrients or fibre, some have medicinal qualities and they are less likely to contain chemical residues from refining processes.

Honey is considered by many to be one of the best sweeteners. The facts may reveal it is not such a healthy alternative as previously thought. Honey varies in quality. No heat is required in its production but commercial honey is often pasteurized. Blended honeys are often heat-treated, which destroys the natural goodness.

Honey has a great taste, is versatile and has some health benefits, particularly Manuka honey (from New Zealand) and Ulmo honey from Chile which have increased antiseptic properties. However, honey is high in fructose (and glucose), has high GI and is detrimental to teeth. Fructose (all forms), like glucose, causes caries. Fructose and glucose have lower caries production than sucrose.[40] And honey has less caries activity than glucose and fructose.[41] As the sugars in honey are quickly absorbed by the bloodstream, it is not beneficial for BSL (blood sugar level) control or weight loss.

Beneficially, honey has antibacterial activity including against *S.mutans* and *Lactobacillus* (two major cariogenic bacteria).[42] Manuka honey also contains methylglyoxal (MG), thought to give it antibacterial properties. The UMF (Unique Manuka Factor) grading system is used for the unique Manuka factors in this honey. UMF over 10 is considered useful for therapeutic use.

All honey contains hydrogen peroxide, which has an antibacterial effect. The antibacterial effect of normal honey is not long-lasting because it breaks down. The additional antibacterial properties of methylglyoxal in Manuka honey give a further boost. Other grading systems are sometimes used for honey. The MGO level indicates the amount of methylglyoxal in the pot, NPA indicates the non-peroxide level and TA the total activity level.

If honey is to be used, choose organic and raw honey from a reliable apiary.

Other useful non-cariogenic natural caloric sweeteners include yacón syrup

(*Polymnia sonchifolia*)[43] and lucuma (*Pouteria lucuma*).[44] Other natural caloric sweeteners that can cause decay and so should be avoided/restricted include maple syrup, molasses, sorghum syrup, and palm and coconut palm sugars.

Artificial sweeteners

Artificial sweeteners such as saccharin, aspartame, acesulfame potassium and sucralose[45] may not be linked to tooth decay but may have a negative health impact in other ways (including an association with inflammatory bowel diseases (IBDs),[46] waist circumference,[47] metabolic disease/glucose intolerance,[48] and weight gain/T2D/metabolic syndrome/cardiovascular disease)[49] and should be avoided or restricted. Aspartame, which is probably the worst artificial sweetener, is sometimes found in toothpastes.

Natural zero-calorie sweeteners

Not all zero-calorie sweeteners are artificial. Natural zero-calorie sweeteners are not carbohydrates and contain few or no calories. Many have an aftertaste. They are considered harmless to teeth.

Stevia, from the leaf of *Stevia rebaudiana*, a plant native to South America where it has been used for centuries, is perhaps the most well-known natural zero-calorie sweetener. Stevia has many benefits: zero calories, zero GI, and it is 200–300 times sweeter than sucrose. Rebaudioside A, a steviol glycoside, is intensely sweet – at least 200 times that of sugar.

Although stevia is considered to have no calories, it still 'primes the body to expect a corresponding number of calories for the sweetness',[50] thereby increasing appetite and potentially causing weight gain.

Some people do not like the bitter aftertaste in some products. For this reason, stevia is often mixed with other sweeteners.

Stevia's poor digestive tract absorption[51] contributes to its inability to raise blood glucose and its zero calories.[52]

Stevia extracts are non-acidogenic, do not support the growth of *S.mutans*, and reduce its biofilm formation.[53] Ethanol and acetone extracts of *Stevia rebaudiana* show the highest activity against *S.mutans*.[54]

Monk fruit (Luo Han Guo, *Siraitia grosvenori*) comes from China where the fruit has been used for hundreds of years. Monk fruit is a non-cariogenic, zero-calorie natural sweetener with a GI of zero, and no effect on blood sugar. The sweetness comes from mogroside, a substance in the flesh of the fruit. An antibacterial effect has been found against *S.mutans*, *P.gingivalis* and *C.albicans*.[55]

Miraculin is a natural sweetener from the 'miracle fruit' from West Africa.

Miraculin alters the taste buds temporarily so that sour foods taste sweet. Miracle berry (*Synsepalum dulcificum*) contains the molecule miraculin which binds to sweet receptors on the tongue; at neutral pH (pH 7), miraculin blocks the sweet receptors and thus the taste sensation, but at low pH, such as in the presence of acidic foods, the presence of additional protons from the acids bind to miraculin, altering its shape and activating the sweet receptors.[56] This effect, sometimes referred to as 'taste tripping',[57] lasts up to one hour, until saliva washes the miraculin away, and provides a useful means for diabetics to sweeten foods. Miraculin has been used to relieve the side effects of chemotherapy medications that cause food to taste metallic.

GYMNEMA SYLVESTRE

Gymnemic acid in *Gymnema sylvestre*, a woody climbing plant native to tropical forests of Africa, Australia and India,[58] also affects the sweet receptor; but this plant has a different effect to the miracle fruit's 'taste tripping' effect, blocking the sweet receptor and thus the taste sensation, instead of activating it (as with miracle fruit). This cuts off the signal to the brain that leads to sweet cravings since, once filled with gymnemic acid molecules (which have a shape similar to that of glucose), the receptors cannot bind with glucose.

Also known in Ayurveda as gumar, and as madhunashini in Sanskrit (which translates to 'sugar destroyer'),[59] *Gymnema sylvestre* has been used for a variety of ailments; several of its benefits relate to the body's response to sugar. *Gymnema sylvestre* has been shown to suppress sweetness by blocking sugar receptors on the tongue when consumed prior to consumption of a sugary food or beverage, thus making them less appealing,[60] and reducing sugar cravings by encouraging limited intake of sweet foods.[61] *Gymnema sylvestre* is also considered to have anti-diabetic properties, with the ability to help lower post-prandial blood sugar levels in T2D.[62] Studies suggest that gymnemic acid inhibits glucose absorption,[63] including intestinal glucose uptake,[64] and may contribute to favourable insulin levels by increasing insulin production.[65]

To have this sugar-blocking/sugar-craving-reducing effect, *Gymnema sylvestre* should be taken five to ten minutes before a high-sugar meal or snack, although it can take effect in just 30 seconds and last up to one hour.[66] Traditionally, the herb was consumed as a tea from the crushed, ground or soaked leaves of the plant.[67]

Glycyrrhizin is a natural sweetener extracted from the liquorice root. Glycyrrhizin has a strong liquorice flavour, a GI of zero, zero calories and medicinal qualities including benefit as an expectorant and for ulcer treatment. Over-consumption should be avoided as it may increase hypertension if taken in excess.

Several other zero-calorie natural sweeteners are being investigated.

Modified sugars

Modified sugars include HFCS (high fructose corn syrup), refiners syrup, caramel, inverted sugar and golden syrup. They are typically produced by converting starch using enzymes and can be harmful to teeth. Some of these modified sugars, despite sounding natural, make poor choices, healthwise.

HFCS (aka glucose-fructose, isoglucose and glucose-fructose syrup) can contain up to 90 per cent fructose. High intakes of fructose may impact gastrointestinal health, blood glucose control, lipid metabolism and, theoretically, increase production of lipid precursors and increase risk of hypertriglyceridemia.[68,69] HFCS in all forms should be avoided.

Agave syrup is also high in fructose, highly processed and best avoided.

Sugar fibres

Sugar fibres include inulin and oligofructose. They have a prebiotic effect when used in moderation. Excessive (and sometimes moderate) consumption of sugar fibres can cause cramps in some people. Several other sweeteners, including erythritol and yacón syrup, may also have a prebiotic effect.

Beneficial sugars

Salivary (secreted) mucins MG1 and MG2, which have important roles in oral health, coating tooth surfaces and acting as bacterial receptors, are composed of fucose, galactose, mannose, N-acetylneuraminic acid, N-acetylgalactosamine and N-acetylglucosamine,[70] six of the eight 'essential saccharides' discussed by Mondoa and Kitei[71] (glucose and xylose are the others).

These saccharides serve as building blocks for larger molecules called glycoforms (e.g. glycoproteins and glycolipids) which cover the lipid bi-layers of cell membranes, and are utilized for virtually every biological process in the body – immunity, defence, communication and reproduction. Composed of interlocking sugar molecules on the cell surface, glycans are a 'crucial part of a cell's identity, helping it to communicate with other cells and the external environment',[72] and aiding repair, restoration, protection and defence, thus having roles in both health and disease.

The sugar groups in human glycoproteins (for which the principal sugars are these eight saccharides) assist in protein folding, improve the stability of the proteins and are involved in cell signalling. Glycans are also important components of other salivary constituents; for example, glycan epitopes provide secretory IgA with additional bacteria-binding sites, thus enabling sIgA to participate in both innate and adaptive immunity.[73]

Most people can generate other saccharides from glucose. This may not be so when the body is stressed or sick. Supplying all eight may aid those who are unable to find the resources for converting one sugar to another. Some are associated specifically with oral health.

Nutritional therapy relating to sugar

Therapeutic support for factors discussed in this chapter include suggestions to replace caries-causing sweeteners with limited use of, for example, xylitol, erythritol and stevia, and to support immune health with sources of beneficial saccharides where necessary.

These beneficial saccharides are found in *Aloe vera*, arabinogalactan-rich foods (corn, leeks, carrots, radishes, coconut meat, curcumin and *Echinacea*), larch trees, brans, brown rice, whole barley, slow-cooked oatmeal, pectin and breast milk. Other sources are mushrooms: reishi (lingzhi), maitake, *Coriolus versicolor*, *Agaricus blazei* (murill), shiitake (dried or very fresh) and cordyceps (which are rich in glucose, mannose and galactose polysaccharides). Mushrooms should be cooked before eating or the glyco-nutrient molecules tend to remain trapped in the fibrous chitin structure.

Note that whilst glucose and galactose are considered beneficial saccharides, fructose is not.

— Chapter 6 —

DYSBIOSIS AND INFLAMMATION

Optimal oral health is associated with oral microbial homeostasis. The flora of healthy oral cavities, as well as flora in oral diseases, have been studied and, whilst each individual has a uniquely diverse bacterial mix, a healthy oral microbiome commonly includes specific species.

In disease states, microbial homeostasis is proportionally altered, and pathogenic species occur. Distinctive microbial species are also differentially associated with dental caries and periodontal disease since the former constitutes an attack primarily on tooth enamel and the latter on the supporting structures of teeth.

The aetiology of periodontal disease is considered to involve three factors: a susceptible host, the presence of pathogenic species, and the absence of 'beneficial bacteria';[1] in addition, oral plaque (biofilm) is considered an important aetiological factor.[2]

Periodontopathogenic microorganisms may cause disease by tissue invasion (direct action) or via the production of bacterial enzymes/toxins (indirect action) – for example, proteases (which degrade immunoglobulin, collagen fibres, hyaluronic acid)[3] resulting in connective tissue lysis. Hence, nutritional protocols for the maintenance of collagen support oral health.

Plaque accumulation may cause gingival tissue inflammation which environmentally alters gingival sulcus, favouring growth of Gram-negative and proteolytic bacterial species. Periodontal pathogens may dominate, resulting in a greater degree of tissue damage. Tissue inflammation may be the driving force of microbial alteration; controlling inflammatory and immune responses, alongside removing adverse subgingival environmental influences, can help contain oral microbial infection.[4]

Most, if not all, bacteria within periodontal pockets have the potential to damage periodontal tissues. Complex host-driven changes in the local environment may allow commensal flora to switch to opportunistic pathogenic behaviour;[5]

how the host responds may be modulated largely by genetics, immunological and inflammatory responses, stress, diet and a variety of lifestyle and social factors.[6]

In addition to excessive plaque accumulation, there are numerous plaque-independent factors which impact host inflammatory and immune response: immune disorders, altered hormonal balance or systemic diseases such as diabetes.[7] The information in this chapter is important to understand because oral disease processes have a bi-directional association with many non-oral health conditions through processes such as inflammation.

Caries

Dental plaque, a natural biofilm with microbial defence functions,[8] can be removed by brushing/flossing. Hardened dental plaque is referred to as calculus (tartar) and, once formed, is too hard and firmly attached to be removed by toothbrushing. Calculus is caused by the precipitation of minerals from GCF and saliva. Its build-up compromises gingival health and is associated with receding gums, bad breath and gingivitis.

Oral microbial ecology is largely mediated within biofilm. Primary colonizers have receptors that adhere to the pellicle. *Streptococci* can also bind to each other. Cell-to-cell signalling and co-aggregation occurs. Anaerobes (often periodontopathogenic) can colonize in the dense mat of plaque formed. Bacterial co-aggregation capacity impacts both cariogenic and periodontopathogenic processes. Biofilm formation permits an entirely different lifestyle for the community than bacterial existence in planktonic state.[9]

Prime cariogenic bacteria include *Streptococcus mutans*, *Lactobacillus* spp, *Bifidobacterium* spp and *Atopobium* spp. Biofilm formation, implicated in caries processes, can create an environment permissive of dysbiosis, favouring acidogenic/aciduric species and causing pH alteration.

LACTOBACILLI – ADVANTAGEOUS OR DISADVANTAGEOUS?

Lactobacilli are Gram-positive bacteria that convert sugars to lactic acid and are significant components of microbiota of digestive and other body systems. Generally, lactobacilli presence is promoted, and these species, considered generally 'safe', are often included in probiotic supplement mixes.

However, some lactobacilli species, although endogenous, are associated with dental caries,[10] specifically regarding the ability to produce weak organic acids as by-products of metabolism of fermentable carbohydrates and thus contributing to an acid environment in the oral cavity which might promote dental enamel demineralization.[11]

Studies show that consuming specific lactobacilli may reduce the numbers of mutans streptococci in saliva.[12,13] However, some lactobacilli species may sometimes be disadvantageous to oral health.[14]

S.mutans is an ideal caries-causative agent for several reasons. *S.mutans* adheres well to tooth surfaces because it produces glucans which thicken tooth surface plaque and aid acid production and sugar diffusion. Secondly, *S.mutans* produces high amounts of lactic acid which diffuses through pellicle, initiating tooth enamel demineralization. Additionally, *S.mutans* produces extracellular polysaccharides from sucrose (which aids biofilm creation);[15] these polysaccharides provide sugars during periods of low exogenous sugar intake. *S.mutans*, too, can survive/thrive at the low-pH environment of plaque, giving it an advantage over other bacteria.

Why pH is critical

The normal resting pH range for saliva is between 6 and 7. The critical pH range for caries development is 5–5.5, at which point acids diffuse through plaque/pellicle into the liquid phase of enamel between enamel crystals, resulting in crystalline dissolution from tooth structures into the surrounding saliva.[16,17] Salivary clearance and flow rate may impact intraoral pH. Saliva is intimately involved in facilitating demineralization/remineralization processes and so, like pH, has an important role in maintaining tooth integrity.[18]

A shift towards increased proportions of acid-producing and acid-tolerating species (e.g. *Streptococci mutans* and *Lactobacilli*) in lowered pH oral environments encourages further altered microbial mix in biofilm communities, promoting demineralization and development of dental caries. Alongside increased proportions of *S.mutans* and *L.rhamnosus*, proportions of *S.gordonii*, *S.oralis* and *Fusobacterium nucleatum* decrease in oral environments with lowered pH, favouring conditions for dental caries development.[19]

Caries is, thus, a result of an altered environment caused by acid production from dietary carbohydrate fermentation which promotes acidogenic and acid-tolerant species[20] instead of acid-sensitive species associated with 'sound enamel'.[21] The dysbiotic environment alters oral ecology as well as the oral environment and allows opportunistic microorganisms to flourish.

Periodontitis

Oral cavity microbial homeostasis is altered in periodontitis, with a shift from predominantly Gram-positive aerobic microbes (consistent with commensal relationship) to mainly asaccharolytic, Gram-negative anaerobes (consistent with pathogenic flora and disease states).[22] Research suggests that some species involved in disease progression may be commensals that overgrow, as several species have been found to be universally present in both diseased and healthy states.[23]

Whereas dental caries is a bacterial disease of dental hard tissues, periodontal disease is an inflammatory pathologic state of supporting tissues of teeth, and includes gingivitis (which doesn't affect tooth attachment) and periodontitis (which involves the destruction of connective tissue attachment and the adjacent alveolar bone).[24]

Gingivitis (gingival inflammation) occurs when an immune response is triggered in periodontal soft tissues by dental plaque. An early symptom is bleeding gums, a sign of 'leaky gums'. When the oral barrier function is compromised, as evidenced by 'leaky gums', other barriers (e.g. intestinal barrier) might also be compromised (i.e. 'leaky gut').

WHY GUMS BLEED

Bleeding gums is a defining sign of gingivitis. Inflamed dental gums are red, swollen and often bleed when teeth are brushed. Bleeding gums may also be due to tissue injury – e.g. excessive/over-enthusiastic toothbrushing.

Numerous pharmaceutical drugs (e.g. anti-coagulants, methotrexate) may directly or indirectly cause bleeding gums;[25] and vitamin C deficiency may result in bleeding gums due to negative effects on connective tissue.[26]

Interestingly, there is potentially a periodontopathogenic purpose for gums to bleed – not only as a warning sign or consequence of inflammation. The blood benefits some oral bacteria – the ones with potential to do further damage – which can utilize iron in the blood's haemoglobin for growth.

The periodontopathogen *Porphyromonas gingivalis* utilizes cysteine proteases known as gingipains as a virulence factor.[27] Gingipain degrades fibrinogen and hosts' heme proteins, inhibiting blood coagulation and increasing bleeding; this benefits *P.gingivalis* by increasing the availability of hemin used for its growth,[28,29] simultaneously providing heme as a source of iron for other black-pigmented periodontopathogens like *Prevotella nigrescens* and *Prevotella intermedia*. Thus, the periodontopathogenic community flourishes, inviting further damage to oral tissue.

Black-pigmented bacteria transport heme into their cells as a source of iron, storing the dark-coloured porphyrin of haemoglobin. Porphyrin is photosensitive, so light directed at bacteria like *Porphyromonas gingivalis* is absorbed by the porphyrin. Particular broadband light therapy has been shown to rapidly and selectively eliminate black-pigmented periodontopathogens by exciting their endogenous porphyrins.[30]

As an inflammatory response to bacterial products in dental plaque/biofilm, and an oral infectious disease affecting supporting structures of teeth,[31] periodontal disease is both multifactorial and complex, involving destruction of periodontal connective tissue – soft tissue and bone. Destruction of gingival connective tissue, largely composed of type 1 collagen, is mediated by proteolytic enzymes, especially collagenase.

In periodontal disease, the host's inflammatory response to bacterial antigens is both protective and destructive. Tissue damage may be caused in various ways: cytokine production that stimulates connective tissue cell release of metalloproteinases (including collagenases), lysosomal enzymes released from phagocytes, and cytokines that activate bone resorption.[32] Interleukin-1β and IL-6[33] have been used as effective diagnostic markers to evaluate periodontal inflammation.[34]

Caries and periodontal disease are polymicrobial,[35,36] plaque-mediated infections, with current literature indicating that, unlike in the GI tract where a dysbiotic environment is generally a less complex microbiota with singular pathogens, disease initiation in the oral cavity is associated with increased diversity and richness of microbiota compared with that in oral health (which is associated with low diversity and richness of microbial community).[37] A dysbiotic oral microbiome is associated with higher proportions of pathobionts and keystone pathogens (e.g. *Porphyromonas gingivalis*) and is of greater complexity than that in health. Where there is periodontal disease there can be up to 10(5) more bacteria than in a healthy oral cavity.[38]

Increased microbiome complexity of both caries and periodontal disease results from disruption among relatively minor constituents in local microbial communities; these act synergistically to stress the host's ability to respond and protect.[39] Host protection via components such as sIgA is called into action. However, factors such as biofilm ability to function as one unit, and immune response impairment, may result in demineralization (in caries) and/or destruction of connective tissue attachments to teeth via MMP release/activity and alveolar bone loss in periodontal disease.

Periodontopathic ecology

Obligately anaerobic Gram-negative proteolytic bacterial species increase in periodontal disease;[40] these infections may be asymptomatic, with destructive tissue changes clinically observed, a result of inflammatory host response.[41] Inflammatory processes, driven by the microbiota of dental plaque biofilm, may initiate, in susceptible individuals, inflammation in gingival tissues, activating neutral enzymes including collagenases,[42] elastases[43] and metalloproteinases[44] that destroy epithelial and connective tissue tooth attachments, initiating periodontitis and periodontal disease. Disease progression typically includes prolonged periods of disease remission interrupted by occasional clinical relapses.[45] Some acute/rapid forms of periodontal disease may occur in association with other conditions, e.g. hormone changes or suboptimal immune systems.[46]

Periodontitis can occur in otherwise healthy individuals and is statistically associated with various environmental and demographic factors.[47] Socioeconomic, lifestyle and cultural differences may have relevance. A number of non-oral factors are associated with periodontal diseases. Numerous possible warning signs of gingivitis/periodontitis and risk factors for disease initiation/progression are listed in Appendix 2.

Amongst hundreds of bacterial species in the oral cavity, very few are considered periodontopathic. It is likely that no single periodontopathic species singly has the capacity to be responsible for all the destructive events involved in the process and progression of periodontal disease, which is believed to require an 'integrated and orchestrated interaction of selected members of this periodontopathic ecology'.[48]

Whilst no one or handful of microorganisms is entirely responsible, several primarily Gram-negative bacteria have been identified as periodontopathogens. Key Gram-negative periodontopathogens include *Porphyromonas gingivalis*, *Aggregatibacter actinomycetemcomitans* (previously known as *Actinobacillus actinomycetemcomitans*, involved in aggressive juvenile periodontitis),[49] *Prevotella intermedia*, *Fusobacterium nucleatum* (commensal, but potent stimulator of inflammatory cytokines,[50] implicated heavily in adverse pregnancy outcomes),[51] *Bacteroides forsythus* and *Capnocytophaga* species. Gram-positive anaerobe *Peptostreptococcus micros*, several viruses and spirochetes also show an association,[52] as does *Eubacterium nodatum* (putative pathogen strongly associated with periodontitis).[53]

Another bacterial species associated with periodontitis is *Helicobacter pylori*, a helical-shaped, microaerophilic Gram-negative bacillus commonly associated with active chronic gastritis. It may infect the mouth and is associated with periodontitis. The positive detection rate in periodontal pockets of those with gastric diseases is usually higher than in those without gastric disease.[54] There is growing interest in the association between *H.pylori* and oral pathologies including canker sores, halitosis and burning tongue as well as periodontal disease. Studies show that *H.pylori* has three stages/forms (spiral, coccoid and degenerative forms) and is present in oral cavities, although it does not appear to participate in biofilm formation.[55]

Prime players: 'The red complex'

Two 'prime players' in periodontal disease, *Porphyromonas gingivalis* (*P.g*) and *Bacteroides forsythus*, are thought to be associated with 'true' periodontal infection as they are infrequently found in periodontally healthy individuals.[56,57] The odds of detecting these microbes in those with periodontitis is 12.3-fold higher for *P.g* and 10.4 higher for *Bacteroides forsythus*. Several others showed significant but lower ratios.[58]

P.g (previously known as *Bacteroides gingivalis*) can trigger periodontitis even at low numbers and can be transmitted between family members. It resides in subgingival crevices and hacks into innate immune cells there, reprogramming them to self-advantage, thus allowing usually benign bacterial residents to opportunistically rise,[59] causing dysbiosis. Community dynamics are altered and infection of periodontium and supportive structures occurs alongside inflammation.

P.g, an invasive and evasive opportunistic pathogen,[60] has been termed a 'keystone pathogen' as well as a 'potential community activist for disease'.[61] Research continues to focus on its possible direct and indirect influence on systemic diseases (e.g. atherosclerosis, rheumatoid arthritis).[62] Its destructive contribution is such that there has been research into developing a vaccine for immunization against *P.g* to prevent chronic periodontal disease.[63] This 'keystone pathogen' causes damage via numerous virulence factors.

P.g, a black-pigmented, strictly anaerobic, Gram-negative rod, gains metabolic energy by fermenting amino acids (sugars are scarce in deep periodontal pockets) and requires heme or hemin and vitamin K as nutrient for growth to be present.[64] The black pigmentation of *P.g* colonies is associated with the aggregation of heme on its cell surface[65] and with its virulence and capacity to behave opportunistically.[66]

P.g disrupts interleukins, downregulating protective IL-12 and upregulating pro-inflammatory (and bone-resorptive) IL-6, IL-1β and TNF-α.[67] *P.g* shows both pro-inflammatory and anti-inflammatory potential; anti-inflammatory capacity allows it to colonize, invade and establish, whereas, when requiring nutrients, *P.g* is pro-inflammatory. Its virulence factors cause deregulation of innate immune and inflammatory responses.[68] By adapting to its local niche, *P.g* facilitates self-survival.

P.g can be highly destructive (termed pathobiont).[69] Another virulence mechanism includes its outer surface carbohydrate (exopolysaccharide) capsule that inhibits phagocytosis and 'mimics' host tissue to aid immune system evasion. In addition to this anti-phagocytic virulence factor, *P.g* possesses several putative virulence factors including proteases which degrade collagen fibres, immunoglobulins and other proteinaceous components.[70] Three major virulence factors expressed by *P.g* are:

- fimbriae (thin, straight appendages which may bind bacterium to host tissues and saliva-coated hydroxyapatite)[71]

- gingipains (proteinase which can rapidly degrade TNF-α, causing dysregulation of the cytokine network and interrupting the host defence response, including dysfunction of polymorphonuclear leukocytes (PMNs), whose primary function is eradication of bacterial infection)[72]

- lipopolysaccharides (which activate the innate immune system).[73]

Lipopolysaccharides (LPS) of *P.g* is a key factor in the development of periodontitis.[74] LPS, aka endotoxin, is a major component of the outer membrane of Gram-negative bacteria, which initiates local and systemic inflammation.[75] Absorbed into gingival tissues and root surfaces of patients with periodontal disease, LPS is considered a major factor in the pathogenesis of periodontal disease.[76]

Other *P.gingivalis* enzymatic virulence factors also contribute to the induction of chronic periodontitis, including collagenase, gelatinase and hyaluronidase,[77] which have the capacity to lyse periodontal connective tissue. This is why connective tissue support is so important.

P.gingivalis, *Tannerella forsythia* and *Treponema denticola* constitute the 'Red Complex' which Holt and Ebersole (2005) describe as 'a prototype poly-bacterial pathogenic consortium in periodontitis'.[78] *Bacteroides forsythus* (later referred to as *Tannerella forsythensis*[79] and more recently as *Tannerella forsythia*)[80] is a saccharolytic (breaks down carbohydrate for energy), anaerobic Gram-negative rod[81] that has several virulence factors including lipopolysaccharide.[82]

Treponema denticola is a spirochaetal Gram-negative bacterium – slender, helically shaped and flexible. *Treponema denticola* are commonly found in subgingival dental plaque and are associated with periodontal disease. The virulence factors of *Treponema denticola* are many and include their periplasmic flagella (which facilitate translocation in highly viscous environments) and dentilisin[83] (surface protease which induces/degrades IL-1β, IL-6 and TNF-α, thus promoting long-lasting infection).[84] Together its motility and chemotaxis (movement in response to chemical stimulus) enable *Treponema denticola* to rapidly colonize new sites, penetrate epithelial layers and deep periodontal pockets, and interact synergistically with other periodontopathogens including via biofilm formation.[85]

T.denticola and *P.gingivalis* display metabolic symbiosis, responding metabolically in each other's presence, which may explain the enhanced virulence of co-infection by these bacteria.[86]

Non-bacterial periodontopathogens

In addition to bacterial pathogenic species, parasites, viruses and fungi play a role in periodontal conditions. *Entamoeba gingivalis* (one-celled protozoan parasite) has been detected in periodontal pockets; its presence correlates with periodontitis.[87] According to the Centers for Disease Control in the US (CDC), *Entamoeba gingivalis* is also considered non-pathogenic.[88] However, according to a 2011 study, *E.gingivalis* was not detected in healthy gingival pocket sites.[89]

Entamoeba gingivalis displays aggressive behaviour and plays a key role in periodontal disease, perhaps explaining immune system dysregulation and subsequent tissue destruction.[90] Humans are normally their only host and they scavenge disintegrated cells including bacteria. *Entamoeba gingivalis* is transmitted by sharing cutlery and cups and by kissing. It can also be transmitted by coughing onto food. The communicability of periodontal disease means practitioners may wish to investigate the oral health status of family members.

Herpes viruses (which are extremely well-adapted pathogens) have also shown an association with periodontal diseases; bacteria and viruses co-present and may synergistically interact in periodontal disease and a variety of medical infections.[91] Active herpesvirus infections evoke strong immune responses – both adaptive and innate, involving both immune activation and immune suppression.[92] Latent herpesvirus infections are thought to be re-activated by periodontopathic bacteria.[93]

Eight herpes viruses infect humans. Associations between two human herpes viruses and periodontal disease have particularly been noted:[94] cytomegalovirus (CMV/HHV-5) and Epstein-Barr virus (EBV/HHV-4), which typically spreads through bodily fluids, particularly saliva, infecting human B-lymphocytes and epithelial cells and is responsible for infectious mononucleosis (glandular fever).[95] These herpesviruses have been associated with severe types of periodontal disease;[96] EBV and CMV may be contributory causes of periodontitis.[97]

Active herpes virus infections correlate with periodontal disease activity and are potent inducers of pro-inflammatory cytokines; osteoclast activation and matrix metalloproteinases may be involved.[98]

As well as parasitic and viral infections, periodontal diseases may be associated with fungal infection – the most common being *Candida albicans*, frequently referred to as thrush or oral candidiasis.

Implications for nutritional therapy

Practitioners may want to suggest therapeutic support for periodontal connective tissue, especially in disease states, and to support optimal oral cavity health. For this and for caries prevention, consider oral-cavity-appropriate probiotics, addressing gum bleeding and connective tissue support generally (see Chapters 7 and 10).

— Chapter 7 —

GLYCATION AND 'SILENT' INFLAMMATION

Dietary sugar intake affects biomarkers of subclinical inflammation;[1] decreased consumption has been shown to improve some biomarkers of chronic disease.[2] Dietary sugar therefore impacts periodontal health both by creating an environment conducive to caries-formation, and by potentially raising levels of systemic inflammation. Another effect of sugar relates to the formation of AGEs (advanced glycation end-products), formation of which may represent a link between periodontitis and diabetes mellitus.[3] Serum levels of AGEs were found to be significantly associated with periodontal deterioration;[4] AGEs also contribute significantly to oxidative stress and inflammation in diabetes.[5]

Glycation and toxicity (including from sugar/sucrose,[6] mercury amalgam and LPS) contribute to whole-body inflammation levels. Both may be 'silent' and contribute to disease conditions and/or prevent health protocol efficacy.

Glycation and AGEs

Non-enzymatic attachment of reducing sugars (e.g. glucose, fructose, galactose) to proteins/amino acids (especially basic lysine or arginine residues), lipids or nucleic acids is known as glycation.[7] Sugars are covalently bonded to protein or lipid molecules through a Maillard reaction, without the controlling action of enzymes. This difference must be stressed: glycation is entirely different to glycosylation which is an enzymatic reaction.

In glycation, reactions may irreversibly result in protein adducts or protein crosslinks,[8] or can undergo further oxidation and oxidative breakdown reactions resulting in AGEs.[9] Reactive oxygen species (ROS) accelerate AGE formation.

Collagen glycation impairs its function, changing its biochemical properties, resulting in stiffness/decreased flexibility.[10] Glycation of collagen significantly contributes to complications of ageing and diabetes.[11]

AGEs are thought to irreversibly accumulate in periodontal tissue over time, with prolonged hypoglycaemia and/or chronic inflammatory states contributing. Osteoclast activation and bone loss may be the result of AGEs formation in extracellular matrix which may increase ROS production, inducing pro-inflammatory cytokines and metalloproteinase.[12]

AGEs also have a negative effect by interacting with RAGEs (receptors for AGEs), activation of which can directly induce oxidative stress.[13] AGEs present in diabetic gingiva may associate with states of enhanced oxidative stress.[14] RAGE receptors may play a central role in oral infection, exaggerated inflammatory host responses and the destruction of alveolar bone in diabetes.[15,16] The 'perioprotective' effect of vitamin D may be related to regulation of inflammatory cytokines produced by gingival fibroblasts following AGE-RAGE interaction.[17]

A glycated matrix was shown to up-regulate inflammatory signalling similar to the presence of lipopolysaccharides of *Porphyromonas gingivalis*, and periodontal inflammation was shown to lead to matrix glycation.[18] A 2015 study of type 2 diabetic patients found glycaemic control (glycated haemoglobin) associated with periapical inflammation.[19] Treatment of periodontal infection and inflammation reduction is associated with reduced levels of glycated haemoglobin.[20]

AGE formation is increased in diabetes and influenced by smoking and diet;[21] AGEs can be ingested via food or endogenously produced.[22] Inflammation caused by endogenously formed AGEs has been well studied; dietary AGEs also contribute and directly stimulate an inflammatory response from human innate immune cells.[23] Dietary AGEs may substantially contribute to the systemic burden of AGEs.[24] Antioxidants, especially polyphenols, may counteract amplification of inflammation by AGEs.[25]

METHYLGLYOXAL

Whilst reducing sugars are important glycating agents, the most reactive physiological relevant glycating agents are dicarbonyls, particularly methylglyoxal. Endogenously formed dicarbonyl compounds can react with proteins to form AGEs.[26]

Methylglyoxal could also be considered a precursor of AGEs.[27] A potent glycating agent of proteins, nucleotides and basic phospholipids, methylglyoxal, an accumulation of which is cytotoxic, is produced by the body during glycolysis; glutathione and glyoxalase enzymes are part of detoxification systems evolved to deal with endogenously produced methylglyoxal.[28]

Glycating effects by methylglyoxal to low-density lipoproteins (LDL)[29] and amino acids indicate the potentially detrimental impact of methylglyoxal-containing foods despite the generally held public opinion that methylglyoxal-containing

Manuka honey is entirely 'healthful'; methylglyoxal content may also contribute to increased AGEs formation.[30] As the benefit is connected with antibacterial actions, methylglyoxal-rich Manuka honey use is probably best confined to small quantities when such actions may specifically benefit and it is not used to replace sugar.

MMPs and hyaluronidase

Matrix metalloproteinases (MMPs) are key proteases involved in inflammatory processes of destructive periodontal diseases; evidence indicates involvement in cleaving signalling molecules (e.g. cytokines, chemokines, growth factors).[31]

Connective tissue damage can be induced by numerous mechanisms. Gingipains, the arginine/lysine-specific cysteine proteinases that function as major virulence factors of *P.gingivalis*, degrade ECM (extracellular matrix) proteins including collagen, fibronectin and laminin. Alone this may be insufficient to cause destruction of gingival connective tissue, to which matrix-degrading metalloproteinases significantly contribute.[32,33]

Action by MMPs (collagenase, gelatinase) and the mucolytic enzyme hyaluronidase may contribute to the breakdown of periodontal connective tissue and ECM, impacting support for periodontal structure. MMPs can function at neutral pH and their activity can be countered by TIMP (tissue inhibitor of metalloproteinase).[34] An imbalance between MMPs and TIMPs can contribute to the destruction of matrix tissue.[35]

Centella asiatica (gotu kola) has shown potent inhibitory action against MMP-1 enzyme, elastase and hyaluronidase.[36] Both *Centella asiatica* and *Punica granatum* (pomegranate) extracts were shown to significantly improve clinical signs of chronic periodontitis.[37] Hyaluronan may also suppress MMP-1 and RANTES production.[38]

Wound and bone healing

Inflammatory processes are involved in wound healing. Oral cavity environments are warm and moist, with the presence of millions of microorganisms – a challenging environment for wound healing; nonetheless, healing usually satisfactorily results, and with preserved oral function.[39] Wounds may occur during mastication and from burns from food and drink that is too hot, as well as from dental procedures.

Salivary constituents may aid periodontal healing – for example, salivary histatins may exert functions relevant for oral wound healing.[40] Hyaluronic acid, and sometimes hyaluronidase and hyaluronidase inhibitors, are present in saliva;

HA is thought to function as a lubricant as well as for wound healing related to microtraumas from mastication.[41]

Melatonin, also present in saliva, may have a role in tissue repair too.

Factors which may influence oral wound healing include vitamin A status (regarding macrophage numbers, which increase with vitamin A intake, since lack of macrophages leads to reduced collagen synthesis, inhibiting wound healing), chronic corticosteroid administration (which has an inhibitory effect on macrophages), bisphosphate use, smoking, ethanol abuse, diabetes and protein/vitamin deficiencies.[42] An omega-3 fatty acids-rich diet may aid wound healing.

Normal wound healing requires numerous processes to occur in specific sequence; angiogenesis, epithelialization, collagen synthesis and other processes are involved. Healing is initiated by blood clot formation followed by vasoconstriction and platelet activation; cytokines initiate inflammatory reactions for removal of debris, damaged tissue and microorganisms.[43]

Normal wound healing processes start at the moment of injury, with subsequent phases of repair proceeding for much longer in some cases – for example, with bone remodelling following tooth extraction continuing for six months post-extraction.[44,45] Healing involves cytokines, growth factors and matrix metalloproteinases, and, in some areas (e.g. gingiva), healing generally occurs quickly and without significant scar formation.[46] Wound healing following periodontal surgery and dental procedures such as wisdom tooth extraction, root canals or dental implants pose greater risk and may take longer.[47]

Regarding periodontal procedures, wound healing complications include issues around 'sterilizing' root canals, tubules and periodontal ligament and risk of 'dry socket' formation whereby the blood clot that should form after tooth extraction to promote healing either dislodges early or retracts too quickly for some other reason (e.g. smoking, bleeding disorders) during healing.[48]

Regarding healing of teeth, the collagen-containing dentine of teeth is covered with enamel which doesn't have the same regenerative capability as the periosteum of bone. Dental pulp stem cells (DPSCs) (e.g. odontoblasts), however, do assist dentine repair and tooth regeneration.[49] Salivary minerals aid enamel repair; however, the presence of toxins (e.g. heavy metals from mercury amalgam or bacterial endotoxins) chronically disrupts calcium/phosphorous balance in the body. Calcium, required for bone healing, may be mobilized from bone into tissues and urine.[50]

Cavitations

Whereas a cavity is a hole in a tooth, a cavitation is a hole in bone;[51] with reference to dental health this often means where a tooth (e.g. a wisdom tooth) has been removed and the jawbone has not filled in properly. Cavitations may not involve pain.

Whilst the term cavitation has also been used more widely to refer to bone lesions which appear as empty holes in jawbones and holes filled with dead bone and bone marrow, these dead, cavitational areas of inflammatory lesions were until recently mostly referred to as NICO (neuralgia inducing cavitational osteonecrosis) lesions[52] (a jawbone version of ischaemic osteonecrosis). Osteonecrosis is degeneration of bone in cavitation areas and is defined as death of tissue due to poor blood supply. Synonyms of osteonecrosis are inflammatory liquefaction and gangrene.[53] Photographs easily accessible online show osteonecrotic dental tissue as blackened and eroded and it has been described as 'oily black mushy bone'.

The term FDOJ (fatty degenerate osteolysis of jawbone) is now preferred (to NICO) as it is more descriptive of the fatty lumps seen in these cavitational areas.

Mostly, jawbone osteonecrosis (cavitation) is not painful, but, as pointed out in a position paper by the IAOMT, that doesn't negate the presence of a disease process, and if pain was used as an indicator of need for treatment, periodontal disease, like cancer and diabetes, would be left untreated.[54] Jawbone cavitations are indicative of bone marrow defect and may be associated with inflammation but not always with infection. Increasing evidence shows that when FDOJ is present, overexpression of pro-inflammatory cytokines may be the driving force of systemic inflammation.

If cavitation is confirmed, natural antimicrobials and detoxification support may be suggested alongside an anti-inflammatory protocol.

'Silent' inflammation and RANTES

RANTES, a pro-inflammatory chemokine found to be associated with and overexpress in cases of jawbone cavitations, routes various immune cells to sites of inflammation/infection;[55] RANTES is found at high levels in cavitational tissues and is implicated in many serious systemic immune diseases (e.g. cancer),[56,57,58] causing inflammation and immune dysregulation as well as targeting mast cells and having an effect on the central nervous system (CNS).[59]

RANTES is a pro-inflammatory chemokine, now more commonly known as CCL-5, 'chemokine ligand 5'. RANTES has no function in healthy bodies but attracts other cytokines to trauma sites to aid healing, having a detrimental effect via recruitment of immune cells that enhance inflammatory processes.[60] RANTES induces collagen degradation by MMP activation,[61] a key factor in the progression of periodontal disease,[62] serving as a diagnostic biomarker.[63]

TNFα and IL-6 (both seen in periodontal disease) ignite acute inflammation and are usually associated with pain. RANTES differs in that it generally results in 'silent' inflammation; this pattern correlates with the general absence of jawbone pain, but the presence of systemic inflammation, in jawbone cavitations. The 'silent' inflammation that may occur with RANTES overexpression in the jawbone may explain systemic immunological effects in cases of ischaemic osteonecrosis or cavitations.[64] An understanding of RANTES and its potential to influence systemic health is important and is the subject of current research. For more information, look at published research by Johann Lechner.[65,66,67]

Implications for nutritional therapy

In addition to therapeutic support for periodontal connective tissue in disease states and to support oral cavity optimal health, clients may need support for wound repair. In addition to suggestions in the previous chapter, consider:

- hyaluronic acid
- melatonin
- *Centella asiatica* and pomegranate
- omega-3 fatty acids
- vitamin A status
- reducing levels of whole-body inflammation
- vitamin D.

Pre-appointment client questionnaires should include questions about past and current mouth and dental health to ascertain whether root canals, tooth extractions and/or any other dental procedure or known periodontal condition may be involved in a client's level of inflammation. This is alongside questions to ascertain if the client has mercury amalgams.

Therapeutic implications may include the need for detoxification support and dietary and lifestyle measures to reduce inflammation. Referral to a biological dentist may be indicated.

If cavitations are confirmed (often at the sites of wisdom teeth extraction or root canal treatment), practitioners should consider protocols to improve cell oxygenation (exercise, alkalize, deep breathing/laughing, massage, hydration, glutathione, coQ10, chlorophyll, check iron/B12/vitamin A, green tea, garlic) and reduce inflammation.

Inhibition of RANTES expression (generally) is warranted; research suggests *Andrographis paniculata*, *Glycyrrhiza uralensis* (Chinese liquorice, which contains quercetin),[68] *Forsythia suspensa*,[69] *Isatis indigotica* and *Strobilanthes cusia*[70] may have immunomodulatory activity relating to RANTES regarding viruses. Future research may find similar benefits from these botanicals against RANTES in periodontal conditions.

— Chapter 8 —

ORAL HEALTH ISSUES

Earlier chapters looked at the main microbial infections related to caries and the periodontal diseases gingivitis and periodontitis. This chapter looks at other conditions affecting oral health including halitosis, *Candida*, xerostomia, oral lesions, burning mouth syndrome, lip/tongue piercings and many others.

Some tongue conditions (e.g. geographic tongue, glossitis, hairy tongue) are briefly discussed. Tongue diagnosis is not specifically discussed in this book. This TCM practice, however, is an excellent tool for assessing oral (and systemic) issues; its use is highly recommended.

All oral conditions impacting the tongue's and oral cavity's connective tissue may benefit from protocols supporting its two component proteins: collagen and elastase. Support for salivary health is also important.

Oral candidiasis
Candida albicans is a common fungus found in the gastrointestinal tract, oral cavity and genital area as a harmless commensal. Virtually the entire oro-gastrointestinal tract, from mouth to anus, with the exception of the stomach, is colonized by *Candida* spp. Its ability to thrive in different host niches without causing disease suggests adaptation for commensalism.[1] *Candida* spp are also opportunistic infection-causing pathogens. Mucous membranes, important barriers to *Candida*, can be destroyed or altered systemically by antibiotics, mechanical forces or nutrient deficiency.

Over 20 species of *Candida* yeasts can cause infection in humans. Most common is *C.albicans*. In the mouth the condition is called thrush or oropharyngeal/oral candidiasis. A symbiotic relationship exists between *Candida albicans* and *Streptococcus mutans* that synergizes virulence of plaque biofilms.[2] For this reason, thrush should always suggest dental/oral health assessment.

Risk factors involved in oral candidiasis include nutritional malabsorption, chronic diseases, endocrine disorders (e.g. diabetes), cancer, HIV/AIDS, weakened immune system, broad spectrum antibiotics, corticosteroids (including inhaled), smoking, drugs with xerostomic effect, being post-operative, denture wearing and poor oral hygiene.

Superficial mucosal lesions commonly occur in oral candidiasis. They are characterized by white growths on mucous membranes, with underlying red areas. Symptoms, in addition to white patches on the inner cheeks, tongue and roof of the mouth/throat, may include redness/soreness, a cottony feeling in the mouth, loss of taste, pain while eating and cracking/redness at corners of the mouth. Sometimes, too, there is pain/difficulty swallowing. Soft, creamy thrush patches can be wiped off mucosa, leaving erythema.[3] White oral lesions can have other causes.

C.albicans has a number of attributes that enable commensal existence in human bodies. However, when immunity is compromised, *Candida albicans* can, via its numerous virulence factors, become a pernicious pathogen.

Candidiasis is common in those with salivary hypofunction and those receiving radiation therapy for head/neck cancer.[4] Candidiasis also readily becomes an issue alongside other immune issues such as bacterial infections.

Glossitis

Glossitis is tongue inflammation with swelling and changed colour/surface appearance, which sometimes causes tongue papillae to disappear. Glossitis can be painful, affecting speech and eating.

Glossitis can be acute or chronic; a third type is atrophic glossitis (aka Hunter glossitis) in which tongue colour/texture alter, typically giving a glossy appearance.

Glossitis may make the tongue appear smooth. Other reasons for a smooth tongue include denture-wearing, nutrient deficiencies (iron, vitamin B12, folate) and low-oestrogen states (aka 'menopausal glossitis').[5]

Causes include allergic reactions, irritants which aggravate tongue papillae and muscle tissue (including toothpastes and medications, often those treating hypertension), diseases (e.g. HSV), nutrient deficiencies (particularly iron as low myoglobin can impact tongue muscle tissue), and mouth trauma (including cuts/burns/irritation due to dental appliances/interventions).

Risk factors include mouth injury, orthodontic appliances, dentures, herpes, low iron, food allergies, immune system disorder and eating spicy foods.

Improved oral hygiene may help relieve symptoms.

TONGUE BITING

Accidental tongue biting most often occurs during eating but can also occur during sleep. During sleep, facial muscle spasms (more common in children) and bruxism (teeth clenching/grinding) can sometimes result in biting of tongue/cheeks.

Other conditions are associated with tongue biting, including epilepsy, rhythmic movement disorder, sleep apnoea, using MDMA (ecstasy) and Lyme disease.

Whilst most people may have bitten their tongue or cheek at some time in their life, those who do so regularly should talk with a health professional. Regular tongue biting may increase the risk of developing infections, ulcers and scalloped tongue.[6]

Lie bumps and other tongue issues

Lie bumps, properly referred to as transient lingual papillitis (TLP), are painful red and white papillae on the base of the tongue. TLP is harmless and is most likely associated with local trauma (biting/rubbing) or reaction to particular foods. Stress and hormone disruption may also be associated.

Eruptive lingual papillitis (most common in children), often accompanied by fever and swollen glands, may be associated with viral infection and may be contagious.

Generally, lingual papillitis clears within a few weeks. Salt water rinses and cold, smooth foods may provide relief.

Most bumps on the tongue are not serious but, since they can also occur in mouth cancer, those that bleed when touched or are persistent should be investigated. Cancerous bumps more commonly occur on the sides (rather than the top) of the tongue. Oral tongue cancer usually appears on the front part of the tongue.

Another tongue issue is 'strawberry tongue' (red, bumpy and swollen) which occurs in scarlet fever, a contagious bacterial infection that may also cause skin rash, fever and other complications and should be investigated.

Mouth and tongue sores may also occur in the secondary stages of syphilis (a sexually transmitted disease with serious complications if left untreated).

Human papillomavirus (HPV)

Human papillomavirus, a common sexually transmitted viral infection, can infect the mouth and throat as well as the genitals. Oral HPV is mostly spread through oral sex and mouth-to-mouth contact. HPV can also pass from mother to baby.

Although the majority of individuals infected are able to clear HPV viral particles without overt clinical disease,[7] HPV and oral HPV are very common. The CDC states that 'HPV is so common that nearly all sexually active men and women get the virus at some point in their lives'.[8]

Symptoms, when they occur, include growths that are small, hard, white/pink/red, painless, usually slow-growing and anywhere in the mouth, although more frequently on the tongue, lips, soft palate and back/roof of mouth. Squamous papilloma (benign neoplasm, usually a lone irregularly shaped bump) associate with HPV.

Some of the many forms of HPV are associated (although rarely) with oral cavity cancers. Those who develop HPV require medical monitoring and should also have regular dental check-ups to assess for change and abnormal growth.

Cold sores

Several human herpes viruses (HSV, CMV, EBV) are associated with aggressive periodontitis and advanced periodontitis; involvement of these herpes viruses is not yet fully determined.[9]

Cold sores are a visible sign of HSV (herpes simplex virus) infection (aka herpetic stomatitis) and caused by HSV1, which can cause both oral and genital herpes. HSV2 usually manifests as genital herpes. Although cold sores may blister and disappear, the virus remains in the body, able to cause cold sores again, most commonly when the immune system or body is under stress.

Cold sores are not the same as canker sores that occur inside the oral cavity but are small fluid-filled bumps that appear on lips or face (usually near the lips). Tingling, itching or burning may be an indication that a cold sore will soon appear; they can be uncomfortable, painful and unattractive, often lasting for seven to ten days.

Cold sores can spread and are highly contagious until they scab over. For this reason, avoid touching them, avoid kissing and sharing utensils or towels, etc. Replace the toothbrush after an outbreak.

Protocols to avoid and address cold sores include immune-boosting (with probiotics, vitamin E, vitamin C and zinc). Arginine is essential for HSV replication,[10] so avoiding arginine-rich foods like nuts and chocolate may be advised. Lysine may help to reduce symptoms and healing time.[11,12] Anti-viral botanicals (e.g. Chinese skullcap or Andrographis) may help.

Topical application of tea tree (*Melaleuca alternifolia*) or peppermint essential oil may help as these have virucidal activity *in vitro*.[13,14] Lemon balm (*Melissa officinalis*), topically applied, may also be effective.[15,16]

SARS-CoV-2/COVID-19

Use of some medications including ACE-inhibitors and angiotensin II receptor blockers, and comorbidities (e.g. hypertension, cardiovascular disease, diabetes, chronic respiratory disease, chronic kidney disease), are associated with increased infection risk.[17] Some oral conditions (e.g. those with autoimmune aetiology/ linked to compromised immune system/long-term pharmacotherapy) may be aggravated by COVID-19.[18] Corticosteroid use is not recommended with COVID-19; those with immune-mediated oral conditions (lichen planus, pemphigus, pemphigoid) may be affected during viral infection.[19]

Whilst numerous antiviral botanicals and nutrients are associated with prevention, COVID-19 is very much still under research. Note that there is good evidence that improved oral hygiene reduces progression/occurrence of respiratory diseases among high-risk elderly adults in nursing homes,[20] conditions under which COVID-19 has spread rapidly.

Antiviral mouthwashes may benefit.

Mouth ulcers

Mouth ulcers (canker sores) are common in otherwise healthy individuals and are often caused by trauma related to ill-fitting dentures or fractured teeth/ fillings. When due to trauma, mouth ulcers should resolve in about a week. Individuals with mouth ulcers lasting over three weeks or with recurrence should seek further advice to exclude systemic disease.

Mouth soreness due to ulceration is referred to as aphthous stomatitis. There are also non-ulcerative causes of oral soreness; these may have similar causation.

Minor aphthous mouth ulcers are the most common (80% of all aphthae).[21] They are small, round/oval in shape, and less than 10mm across. Lasting seven to ten days, there may be between one and five simultaneously. Minor aphthous mouth ulcers do not leave scars.

Major aphthous ulcers tend to be 10mm or larger, may occur singly or there may be two simultaneously, and tend to last between two and four or more weeks. These ulcers can be very painful; eating may be difficult. Major aphthous mouth ulcers leave scars.

Herpetiform ulcers are tiny pinhead-sized ulcers, 1–2mm across. Multiple ulcers occur simultaneously and may join together in irregular shapes. Herpetiform ulcers last between one week and two months. Despite the name, they are not associated with herpes. Some herpes infections (e.g. chickenpox), however, are associated with mouth ulcers.[22]

The cause of recurring mouth ulcers (affecting at least 20% of the population)[23] should be investigated. Possible causes and triggers include injury, badly fitted dentures, vigorous tooth-brushing, stress/anxiety, hormonal changes, nutrient deficiencies (vitamin B12, folic acid, vitamins B1/B2/B6 and/or iron), medicines (e.g. ibuprofen), nicotine replacement therapy and allergy.

Mouth ulcers can be associated with Crohn's disease, coeliac disease, HIV infection and Behçet's disease; these should be ruled out in all cases of recurring aphthae.

Hand, foot and mouth disease (HFMD) is a contagious viral infection caused by coxsackievirus a16 and enterovirus 71, which causes mouth ulcers, a spotty rash (on palms/feet), fever and sore throat/mouth, and is particularly common in children. HFMD usually clears up within seven to ten days.

MOUTH ULCERS AND *H.PYLORI*

The potential association between recurrent mouth ulcers and *H.pylori* (a gastric ulcer-causative agent) has been considered, particularly as one of the major transmission routes for *H.pylori* is oral–oral;[24] eradication of *H.pylori* from gastric mucosa may not prevent gastric recurrence without elimination of this bacteria from the oral cavity by improved oral hygiene.[25,26] *H.pylori* also appears to cause vitamin B12 deficiency.[27] The authors of a 2014 evaluation of 13 relevant articles believe the action of *H.pylori* in mouth ulcers is due to *H.pylori*-positive gastric disease and iron and vitamin B12 deficiency conditions (anaemia).[28]

Mouth ulcers can be drug induced (e.g. cytotoxic agents, anti-thyroid drugs, nicorandil), or may be a manifestation of disorders of connective tissue, blood (including anaemia), gastrointestinal tract or skin. They may include lichen planus, pemphigus (autoimmune disorder causing blisters on skin/mucous membranes),[29] pemphigoid (a rare autoimmune disorder caused by immune system malfunction, resulting in skin rashes/blistering, sometimes mucous membrane blistering),[30] erythema multiforme (a hypersensitivity reaction usually triggered by infection, commonly HSV, presenting with skin eruption, sometimes mucous membrane involvement),[31] epidermolysis bullosa (a rare inherited skin disorder causing the skin to become very fragile, sometimes causing blisters inside the mouth)[32] and angina bullosa haemorrhagica (painful blood-filled mouth blisters[33]).[34]

Mouth ulcers may also be associated with leishmaniasis, a disease caused by parasites, spread by bites from certain types of sandfly. Some presentations of the disease are mucocutaneous, with ulcers of mouth, skin and nose. Considered a neglected tropical disease, leishmaniasis (aka 'Andean Sickness', 'Dum Dum Fever', 'Jericho Buttons') affects large numbers of people in the Americas, Africa, Asia and Middle East; it is highly prevalent in Sicily (especially in Catania City in 2013[35]) where it had presented major problems for Allied troops fighting in Sicily during World War 2.

There is also some evidence that sodium lauryl sulfate (SLS) toothpastes may irritate and/or damage delicate tissue in the mouth; a significantly higher frequency of aphthous ulcers has been observed in individuals using toothpastes containing SLS.[36]

Mouth ulcers that do not heal should be discussed with a healthcare provider; in some cases mouth cancer (oral carcinoma) can start as a mouth ulcer that does not heal.

Non-ulcerative causes of oral soreness

Erythema migrans (aka benign migratory glossitis, commonly as geographic tongue) is a common condition of unknown aetiology, affecting about 10 per cent of children/adults. Appearing at the top and sides of the tongue, and sometimes on the under-surface, it is characterized by map-like irregular, smooth, red areas of atrophy of filiform tongue papillae in patterns that change. Often there are wavy white lines next to red patches. The tongue is often fissured, and lesions can cause soreness or be asymptomatic.

Occurrence of geographic tongue is thought to relate to the way tongue surfaces self-renew, with top layers coming away unevenly/prematurely. The red areas are thin and may therefore become infected with *Candida* and so feel sore. Geographic tongue is not an infection in itself and cannot be passed to other people but it may run in families. It tends to come and go (often lasting a few days or weeks), often recurring.

Red areas may be painful. Foods (particularly acidic/spicy) may be triggers for pain, though they don't make the condition itself worse.

Erythema migrans is a benign condition. Although there are no reliably effective treatments, zinc supplements may help. And if oral candidiasis is suspected or confirmed, antifungal protocols should be followed.

The lesions seen in geographic tongue are similar to those in Reiter's syndrome (also known as reactive arthritis, a triad of conjunctivitis, urethritis and arthritis occurring after an infection)[37] and psoriasis.[38]

Another non-ulcerative cause of oral soreness is desquamative gingivitis where there is widespread erythema, usually with soreness. This is fairly common and almost exclusively seen in women over middle age. Most usually a manifestation of lichen planus or mucous membrane pemphigoid, desquamative gingivitis symptoms usually include persistent gingival soreness worsened on eating, and red gingivae.[39] Desquamative gingivitis can often be improved with better oral hygiene; conventional medicine sometimes manages with topical corticosteroids.

BURNING MOUTH SYNDROME

Burning mouth syndrome is another non-ulcerative cause of oral soreness. Medically known as oral dysaesthesia, glossopyrosis or glossodynia, it is common in people past middle age and characterized by persistent burning sensation in the tongue. The cause is unclear, but response to topical anaesthesia suggests it is a form of neuropathy.[40] Unlike what happens in ulcerative lesions (where eating typically causes irritation or pain), in cases of burning mouth syndrome relief is sometimes obtained by eating or drinking.

Organic disease should be excluded. Burning mouth is occasionally caused by erythema migrans, lichen planus, a deficiency glossitis (often vitamin B12, folate, iron), xerostomia, diabetes and candidiasis; these should all be excluded. Underlying depression, monosymptomatic hypochondriasis, anxiety about cancer or sexually transmitted disease is more often involved; burning mouth syndrome is more common in Parkinson's disease.[41] Antidepressant agents may be indicated.

Mouth pain, not unlike a burning sensation, might also be caused by sensitivity to tartrazine, ascorbic acid, benzoic acid and propylene glycol as well as from cinnamon aldehyde and menthol.[42]

Since GABA agonists are sometimes used conventionally to address burning mouth syndrome,[43] *Valeriana officinalis*, *Scutellaria baicalensis*, green tea and L-theanine may help.[44]

White oral lesions including lichen planus

White oral lesions were previously known as leucoplakia, a term now restricted to white lesions of unknown cause. Although other causes, including infection, should be investigated, most white lesions are innocuous keratosis caused by cheek-biting, tobacco use or friction.

Infections that cause white lesions include candidiasis, syphilis and hairy leucoplakia. Lichen planus and oral carcinomas can also be the cause.

Keratosis (leucoplakia) is a persistent adherent white patch. It should be investigated and is best removed. Conventional management depends on many factors. If determined to be innocuous, this may include cessation of smoking and/or vitamin A therapy.[45]

Hairy leucoplakia (hairy tongue) is an asymptomatic white lesion typically on the lateral margins of the tongue not removable by wiping. Black hairy tongue in association with chronic use of penicillin may be fungal overgrowth, particularly *Aspergillus*.[46] Hairy leucoplakia is most commonly seen in immunocompromised individuals (e.g. HIV/AIDS) and is associated with EBV. Although there is no known malignant potential, hairy leucoplakia is a predictor of poor prognosis.

Conventional medicine might treat with acyclovir; anti-retroviral agents may be used.[47] Natural anti-retrovirals include cananolides (coumarins), betulinic acid (triterpene), baicalin (*Scutellaria baicalensis*/Chinese skullcap flavonoid), alkaloids (e.g. in *Papaver somniferum*/poppy seeds), lithospermic acid (polyphenolic, e.g. in *Salvia miltiorrhiza*) and phenolics (e.g. in *Terminalia chebula*, *Phyllanthus niruri*, *Curcuma longa*).[48]

Oral lichen planus typically presents as bilateral white lesions in buccal and lingual mucosae and is common, especially after middle age. Although oral lichen planus may be symptomless, less common erosive lichen planus is painful, typically affecting tongue or buccal mucosae on both sides. Lupus erythematosus and other disorders should be ruled out.

There is no single cause; individuals with oral lichen planus should be regularly reviewed in view of the slight risk (about 1%) of oral carcinoma.[49] Some lichenoid lesions may be related to materials used in dental work, hepatitis C infection or be drug induced (e.g. NSAIDs). Conventional medicine often treats the condition with topical corticosteroids to control symptoms. TCM has shown efficacy for oral lichen planus.[50]

Red or pigmented oral lesions and mucous membranes

Red oral lesions are mostly inflammatory in nature; some may be potentially malignant, especially erythroplasia (rare, isolated, red, velvety lesions mainly affecting those aged 60–79). Since these lesions can be dysplastic or malignant, they are best removed.[51]

Widespread redness with thrush may also be erythematous candidiasis, related to corticosteroid or antimicrobial treatments. Cessation of smoking and antifungal agents may aid management.

In denture-induced stomatitis (mild chronic erythematous candidiasis often seen after middle age), the affected area is usually limited to beneath an upper denture, usually occurring when *Candida* spp proliferate beneath dentures. Denture-wearing should be minimized and the infection eradicated. Management may require soaking dentures, adjusting dentures, better oral hygiene and regular oral antifungal agents. Carbohydrate-rich diets and xerostomia may predispose an individual to this problem.

Other red lesions in the oral cavity may be petechiae caused by trauma or suction, or be an indication of scurvy (severe vitamin C deficiency). Localized red patches may also be caused by burns. Avitaminosis may be the cause of either localized red patches or widespread redness which can also be caused by iron deficiency.

Brown or black pigmented oral lesions may be caused by a number of factors. Furred, brown or black hairy tongue is an extreme example of coating due to epithelial, food and microbial debris. More common in edentulous individuals or those with a soft, non-abrasive diet, poor hygiene, smoking, fasting or illness, this may also be seen in those using antimicrobials. In such cases, management may be via improved dental hygiene, tongue brushing, tongue scraper use and increasing dietary fruit and roughage (e.g. pineapple).[52]

A brown tongue is usually caused by poor diet or poor oral hygiene.[53] Tongue diagnosis, widely used in TCM, is not discussed in this book but is a useful diagnostic tool.

Hyperpigmentation of oral mucous membranes/gingiva may be localized or generalized. Hyperpigmentation occurs in all human races. There is no difference in the number of melanocytes between fair-skinned and dark-skinned people; differences relate to the activity of melanocytes.[54]

Pigmentation may be caused by melanin (production may increase due to trauma, hormones, radiation and medications),[55] melanoid (unrelated to melanin, imparts clear yellow shade to skin) and carotene (which gives deep yellow colour to skin) as well as iron (re hemochromatosis, a chronic disease characterized by deposition of excess iron in body tissues).[56]

Melanin pigmentation of oral tissues is not usually considered a medical problem, although individuals may complain of black gums. Underlying conditions should be investigated. Localized pigmentations are often amalgam tattoo but may be malignant melanoma, Kaposi's sarcoma (cancer with skin lesions, usually purple) or otherwise; generalized pigmentations may be genetics (e.g. racial, Peutz-Jegher's syndrome), endocrine (e.g. Addison's disease, pregnancy), post-inflammatory (e.g. periodontal disease), drug-related (e.g. nicotine, antimalarials, antimicrobials, minocycline contraceptive pills, heavy metals exposure to gold, silver, bismuth, arsenic, lead, copper or mercury) or other cause (e.g. haemochromatosis, nutritional deficiencies).[57] Smoker's melanosis refers to discoloured gums (often brown/black) caused by nicotine which can cause melanocytes to produce more melanin than usual. Quitting smoking may help reduce gum discolouration in some cases.[58]

Foods and beverages may also alter oral cavity pigmentation. Chewing of betel nut (psychoactive substance commonly used in parts of Asia and elsewhere) produces copious red saliva (staining teeth/gingiva/oral mucosa) and may induce lichenoid lesions on buccal mucosa; its use with tobacco can cause leucoplakia.[59] Its use may also be associated with fractured teeth.

Halitosis

Whilst halitosis (the medical term for bad breath) can occur normally for a number of reasons, it is an embarrassing problem for some people, sometimes indicating another disease process.

Normal occurrence of halitosis can be caused by smoking and some strong foods/drinks (e.g. garlic, onions, cabbages, spices, coffee, alcohol). Some diets, for example ketogenic diets, low-carbohydrate diets and fasting, may result in halitosis. It is also normal to have halitosis overnight, due to stagnation of saliva in the mouth. Dehydration may also cause halitosis.

Persistent halitosis may come from a build-up of bacteria in the mouth, food debris (especially between teeth), plaque, gum disease, tongue coatings, oral thrush, dental abscess, unclean dentures, tumours in the mouth and xerostomia (dry mouth).

Commonly, the reason for halitosis relates to dental hygiene or a gum/tooth problem, and very often food particles between teeth or germs on the tongue. If improved dental hygiene doesn't address the problem, and the problem isn't likely xerostomia due to prescription medication, other causes of persistent halitosis should be investigated because halitosis may be associated with other health conditions, including several types of cancer. Severe halitosis (with dead tissue smell) may be caused by acute necrotizing ulcerative gingivitis or noma (cancrum oris, a rapidly spreading gangrenous stomatis mainly in malnourishment which destroys tissue structures).

In addition to its association with some medications, persistent halitosis can be associated with acid reflux, *H.pylori* infection, lung infections, diabetes, severe kidney or liver problems, and problems with tonsils, sinuses and nasal passage (e.g. obstruction or polyps, post-nasal drip). A genetic defect in the SELENBP1 gene, which causes absence of the protein that converts sulphur compound methanethiol, causes halitosis.[60] A rare disorder, trimethylaminuria (aka fish odour syndrome) is also associated with persistent halitosis.

Fishy or ammonia/urine-like halitosis is associated with chronic kidney failure. Faeces breath often results from prolonged vomiting, especially with bowel obstruction, and is associated with temporary nasogastric tube placement to drain stomach contents. Fruity breath is associated with exhaled acetones in diabetes mellitus (a sign of ketoacidosis, which is potentially life threatening) or a recent insulin injection.

Oral cysts and dental abscesses

A cyst is a closed sac of tissues; there are a number of commonly occurring types in oral cavities. Dentigerous cysts usually develop close to or on top of the crown of an unerupted (usually wisdom) tooth. Mucocele cysts (mucous cysts) develop on oral cavity soft tissue, often due to trauma or irritation.

Odontogenic cysts are jaw cysts that form from tissues involved in tooth development. These cysts are closed and have a distinct membrane which encloses fluid or gaseous content. Periapical cysts are the most common odontogenic cyst occurring in the oral cavity. These normally form at tooth base due to pulp infection or nerve death. Although asymptomatic, secondary infections of periapical cysts can result in inflammation, pain and damage. Periapical cysts can sometimes develop into an abscess.

An abscess is not a cyst. An abscess is an acute infection manifesting as a swollen area filled with pus. Symptoms may include swelling, fever, fatigue, throbbing pain and an unusual taste/smell inside the oral cavity. Radiating pain (to neck/jaw/ear) may also occur.

Root infections involving tooth decay are often involved in dental cysts. Pulpal necrosis may follow, alongside release of toxins, resulting in periapical inflammation. Failed root canal treatments can result in dental cysts.

Oral swellings

Oral swellings may involve normal cause (e.g. unerupted teeth), inflammatory cause (e.g. abscess, Crohn's disease), trauma (e.g. denture granulomas) or other factors: cystic, fibro-osseous (e.g. Paget's disease, disrupted cycles of bone renewal/repair), hormonal (e.g. pregnancy epulis/gingivitis or oral contraceptive pill gingivitis), drugs (e.g. cyclosporin, calcium channel blockers), developmental (e.g. haemangioma), blood dyscrasias (e.g. leukaemia, lymphoma), neoplasms (benign and malignant) and other (e.g. amyloidosis – a rare, serious condition caused by the build-up of abnormal amyloid protein in body organs/tissue).[61]

Gingival lumps due to erupting teeth are termed pericoronitis; in pregnancy localized swelling of the gingival papillae is referred to as pregnancy epulis. Fibrous lumps and epulis (gingival swelling/growth) can be benign. All gingival lumps should be assessed as some are malignant.

Gingival fibromatosis (gingival overgrowth) can be induced by a number of pharmaceutical medications including anticonvulsants, calcium channel blockers, cyclosporin, erythromycin, oral contraceptives and (chronic/frequent) marijuana use.[62]

Salivary gland swelling may be caused by duct obstruction, sialosis (non-inflammatory, non-neoplastic, recurrent enlargement of major salivary glands, commonly caused by diabetes mellitus and alcoholism), neoplasms, inflammatory conditions (e.g. mumps, tuberculosis, Sjögren's syndrome, sialadenitis), cystic fibrosis, drugs (e.g. protease inhibitors) and deposits (such as amyloid).[63]

Sialadenitis (salivary gland infection, usually viral or bacterial), Sjögren's syndrome and neoplasms are important causes to be excluded. Antimicrobial use may be indicated.

TONSILS

Tonsils and tonsil infections are not specifically discussed in this book. However, tonsil infections and abscesses may affect the oral cavity. Tonsillitis, which affects palantine, not lingual, tonsils, is most often caused by viral infection, and, less commonly, by bacterial infection. Very rarely, a peritonsillar abscess (collection of pus) may form between tonsil and throat wall. Peritonsillar abscess is also known as quinsy. Peritonsillar cellulitis is when the abscess occurs without pus.[64]

Conditions affecting saliva

Conditions that affect salivary flow rates and salivary clearance (e.g. Sjögren's syndrome) and radiation damage to salivary glands (e.g. due to treatment of head and neck cancer) increase susceptibility to dental caries because of prolonged retention of sugar in the mouth. Whilst acid is a strong stimulus of salivary flow, sugar is a relatively weak stimulus.[65]

When radiation treatment fields include major salivary glands, there may be a widespread effect on saliva, including changed quantity, composition and physical properties. Increased doses of radiation are associated with progressive reduction in salivary flow rates, pH and sIgA; reduced salivary secretions often persist after completion of radiation therapy.[66]

Systemic diseases which might affect composition of salivary fluids include cystic fibrosis, multiple sclerosis, graft-versus-host disease (which is characterized by destruction of salivary gland tissues and decreased salivary flow rate), diabetes mellitus (because insulin is able to stimulate salivation, the salivary flow rate is decreased in diabetes mellitus), alcoholic liver cirrhosis, HIV, epilepsy, burning mouth syndrome (most prominent in post-menopausal women) and kidney dysfunction.

Aps and Martens provide a list of pharmaceutical drugs that have an impact on saliva and oral health.[67]

Salivary duct obstruction

The most common cause of salivary gland swelling is sialolithiasis, a benign condition involving the formation of stones (calcific concretions)[68] within major salivary gland ducts,[69] most commonly the submandibular gland,[70] in adults between the ages of 30 and 60 years.[71] The duct may become obstructed causing inflammation from destructive salivary enzymes, bacterial infection (sialadenitis) and sometimes abscess formation.[72] Treatment options may include massage of the duct and sialogogue use, although surgery may sometimes be needed. Natural spasmolytics[73] have also been suggested regarding small calculi.[74] Natural anti-inflammatories may also benefit.[75] 'Milking'/massaging the gland may result in pus discharge.[76] Restoring normal salivary flow is the aim of treatment.[77]

Sialoliths can be single or multiple.[78] Symptoms include pain/swelling, bad breath and foul-tasting mouth[79] and may worsen with stimulation of salivary flow (e.g. with chewing, hunger or smell/taste of food). Although rare, multiple sublingual gland sialoliths may cause dysphagia and speech difficulty.[80]

Predisposing factors for sialolith formation include prolonged stagnation of saliva and infection.[81] The exact pathogenesis of sialolithiasis is not well understood; one theory suggests an accumulation of microscopic stones during secretory inactivity which reduces flow in the duct by obstruction.[82] Another hypothesis suggests bacteria or food debris within the oral cavity may enter salivary ducts over time, acting as a nidus for formation of larger calculi. Stagnation of calcium-rich saliva due to obstruction may result in deposition of tricalcic phosphate salts around the initial nidus.[83] Cases of such 'foreign body' causes of sialolithiasis are considered rare.[84] Gout may predispose to salivary stone formation.[85]

Bacterial infections and resulting endotoxins are important factors in calculi formation. Bacterial toxins may reduce local environment pH which may result in tissue damage; crystallization of salivary ions may occur when tissue-healing processes re-establish the 7.2 pH.[86]

To prevent further salivary stones, hydration and a diet rich in proteins and acidic foods may benefit.[87] Sialogogues are generally recommended therapeutically and prophylactically, although these may worsen symptoms initially.

Xerostomia (salivary hypofunction)

Xerostomia or salivary hypofunction are medical terms for dry mouth. Causes can be dehydration, alcohol (including from mouthwashes), anxiety and mouth-breathing. Radiotherapy can damage salivary glands, and many medications including tricyclic antidepressants, antihistamines, antimuscarinic medications, some anti-epileptic medications, some antipsychotics, antihypertensives, antiretrovirals, bronchodilators, beta-blockers and diuretics may cause xerostomia.

Candidiasis is a common mucosal infection in those with salivary hypofunction.[88]

Sjögren's syndrome (SS), which also commonly affects joints and tear glands, manifests mainly as dry eyes and mouth. In SS, an autoimmune disorder often accompanying other immune system disorders (e.g. rheumatoid arthritis, lupus), mucous membranes and moisture-secreting glands of the eyes and mouth are usually first affected, causing a decrease in tears and saliva. Commonly individuals are aged 40+ at diagnosis, and more commonly they are women. The cause is still unclear; some genes increase the propensity. A triggering mechanism (e.g. viral/bacterial infection) may be necessary.[89]

Due to decreased amounts of saliva in SS, individuals may suffer an increased propensity for dental cavities and oral thrush. Vision problems may also occur due to dry eyes. Other complications are possible in the lungs, kidneys, liver, lymph nodes and nerves.[90]

The dry, irritated mucous membranes in SS may relate to a disturbance in galactose and N-acetylglucosamine.[91] N-acetylneuraminic acid processing is disturbed in SS,[92] and increased serum IgA level is commonly seen.[93] Individuals with SS are thought to retain competence of the salivary immune system even in advanced disease stages;[94] however, xerostomia impacts oral health with associated complications. Galactose, N-acetylglucosamine and N-acetylneuraminic acid may benefit.

Dry mouth can make it difficult to swallow, eat, taste and speak. Mastication stimulates saliva production and can relieve xerostomia, as well as cleansing the mouth. Mucin, a salivary glycoprotein, gives hydrating qualities, allowing optimally moistened membranes.

TCM has shown efficacy for xerostomia.[95] Sialogogues may be useful to increase salivary flow.

SLEEP APNOEA

Characterized by mouth breathing and repeated breathing disruption during sleep, obstructive sleep apnoea (OSA) is associated with periodontal disease.[96] Sufferers usually have oral cavity dryness[97] with consequent impaired salivary cleansing and altered oral microbiome composition. OSA is also associated with systemic inflammation and intermittent hypoxemia which can stimulate increased cytokine production.[98] OSA may thereby, via various mechanisms, increase the propensity for periodontitis.

Other salivary gland disorders

Excessive salivation, sialorrhea, known also as ptyalism or hypersalivation, can be caused by excessive production or decreased clearance of saliva and can contribute to drooling and excessive spitting. Hypersalivation precedes vomiting and is also associated with numerous health conditions: pregnancy, mouth ulcers, gastroesophageal reflux disease, oral infections, serotonin syndrome, liver disease, pancreatitis and problems of the jaw such as fractures, dislocation, myasthenia gravis, rabies, Parkinson's disease and radiation therapy. Hypersalivation can also be caused by excessive starch intake, some medications (e.g. clozapine, pilocarpine, ketamine, potassium chlorate) or toxins (mercury, copper, organophosphates and arsenic).[99]

Many types of infection may impact salivary glands. Paramyxovirus (mumps), inflammation/enlargement of the parotid glands, often results in swelling on one or both sides of the face. Fever and malaise also occur, with extreme throat pain, particularly when swallowing sour foods or acidic juices. Mumps and other infections such as tonsillitis, epiglottitis and retropharyngeal and peritonsillar abscesses may cause hypersalivation due to decreased salivary clearance.[100]

Hypersalivation may occur as an early symptom in Sjögren's syndrome.[101]

Oral mucositis

Oral mucositis, a painful inflammation/ulceration of mucous membranes lining the mouth, is a common side effect of chemotherapy/radiotherapy, especially when radiotherapy involves the head/neck. Those with oral mucositis are more likely to develop other mouth problems including xerostomia and infections.

Oral cancer

The prevalence of oral cancer, which is most commonly oral squamous cell carcinoma and is seen mainly in the developing world, particularly South East Asia and Brazil, mainly in men over middle age, tobacco users and lower socioeconomic groups, is increasing.[102] Uncommon oral malignant neoplasms include lymphomas, malignant melanoma, some odontogenic tumours, Kaposi's sarcoma and others.

Oral cancer may present as a solitary lump, ulcer or white/red lesion. Any oral lesion persisting for more than three weeks should be treated with suspicion. Often sufferers present or are detected late with advanced disease. Earlier diagnosis offers better treatment, a cosmetic and functional outcome, and survival.

Aetiological factors include tobacco use, betel use, alcohol consumption, a diet poor in fresh vegetables/fruit, infective agents (viruses, *Candida*), immune deficiency, and, in cases of lip carcinoma, exposure to sunlight.[103] Those with lung cancer have increased risk for second primary oral cancers.

In cases of radiotherapy to neck/head, both preventive and curative dental treatment should be undertaken beforehand to minimize oral disease and possible adverse consequences of operative intervention. Complications of radiotherapy may include painful mucositis, osteoradionecrosis (potentially serious complication, risk of which increases with high radiation dose, and extraction of teeth after radiotherapy), xerostomia, dental caries, oral candidiasis, bacterial sialadenitis, loss of taste and other complications.[104]

Overall results of an epidemiological study which looked at the protective effects of vegetables and fruit found that fruit intake consistently decreased risk of oral and pharyngeal cancer but did not find this protective effect for vegetables for these cancers (note that the reverse was found for some other cancers).[105]

Orofacial pain (including TMJ) and bruxism

Causes of orofacial pain are varied and can include local diseases, psychogenic pain, referred pain, neurological disorders and vascular disorders. Organic disease must be excluded; if cause of orofacial pain is determined to be psychogenic, a protocol related to mood-boosting may be indicated.

Temporomandibular joint pain dysfunction syndrome (abbreviated TMJ, TMD or TMJD), referred to as myofascial pain dysfunction syndrome or facial arthromyalgia, is a common disorder mainly affecting young women. Referred to by some as a psychogenic disorder,[106] TMJ has also been referred to as a functional pain syndrome[107] and is likely caused by multiple factors. Symptoms vary and are characterized by recurrent clicking in the temporomandibular joint during jaw movement, periods of limitation of jaw movement/locking, and pain in the joint and surrounding muscles.[108]

Bruxism (clenching/grinding of teeth), which is thought to be related to anxiety/stress, often occurs during sleep, with sufferers often waking with pain. TMJ aetiological factors may include muscle overactivity (e.g. clenching/bruxism), disruption of temporomandibular joint and emotional upset.[109] Illicit drug (MDMA, aka ecstasy) use may also associate with bruxism.[110] See Scully and Shotts (2000) for more information about causes of orofacial pain.[111]

Oil-pulling may help strengthen the jaw.[112]

TMJ may play a role in other disorders; for example, sufferers of Lyme disease, a multi-microbial inflammatory infection with systemic multi-symptom and often chronic effect, may have orofacial pain and other oral symptoms. There are specific Lyme borreliosis-associated dental signs and symptoms which are considerations for dental professionals[113,114] and may also guide health practitioners with Lyme patients for management of their condition.

In stage 1 of Lyme disease, the sufferer often has a stiff neck and lymphadenopathy; stage 2 Lyme disease patients often suffer a variety of dental/oral symptoms including TMJ pain, masticatory musculature pain, facial paralysis,

Bell's palsy (one-sided facial nerve paralysis), atypical orofacial pain, difficulty opening the mouth, ear pain when chewing or opening and lymphadenopathy. In stage 3, Lyme sufferers have prolonged arthritis-like symptoms including potentially in the temporomandibular joint.

Lyme sufferers have prolonged arthritis-like symptoms, including potentially in the temporomandibular joint. Lyme disease requires an antimicrobial, detoxification and immune-supporting protocol which is beyond the scope of this book.

Tooth issues

If the jaw is not large enough to accommodate all the teeth, wisdom teeth may be unable to properly erupt, thus remaining below the jawline (i.e. they are impacted). Impacted teeth can be painful, become infected and damage other teeth. Impacted wisdom teeth can be extracted; this can have other health implications.

Malocclusion (tooth misalignment), cleft lip/palate and delayed tooth eruption may impact various aspects of mouth and systemic health but are beyond the scope of this book.

Tooth discolouration

Discolouration of tooth enamel can be caused by a number of intrinsic and/or extrinsic factors. Ageing is one factor; this is caused by the natural thinning of overlying enamel or by darkening of underlying dentine due to formation of secondary dentine which is darker and more opaque than primary dentine.[115]

Other intrinsic factors include medication (e.g. minocycline used to treat acne[116] and tetracycline), excessive fluoride ingestion, severe jaundice in infancy, porphyria, enamel microcracks/defects and thinning of enamel layer.[117] Professional bleaching procedures may help reduce intrinsic stains, although with differing speed and effect; brown fluorescence may only be moderately responsive, and tetracycline stains (usually yellow, grey) are slowest.[118,119] Fluorosis may result in yellow or white staining.

Tetracycline administered during development is associated with staining of dental hard tissues, possibly due to its ability to form complexes with calcium ions on the surface of hydroxyapatite crystals within bone and dental tissues.[120] Dentine stains more heavily than enamel.[121] Tetracycline should be avoided during pregnancy, breastfeeding and in children until after age 12.[122] Staining is yellowish/brown-grey in appearance.[123,124]

In addition to fluorosis and tetracycline staining, several other systemic factors and metabolic diseases that affect developing dentition and cause discolouration include alkaptonuria, congenital conditions, root resorption, ageing and injury.[125]

Staining may also occur due to iron supplementation, eugenol and phenolic compounds used during root canal therapy, and removal of long-standing amalgam restoration[126] (due to migration of tin into tubules).[127]

Foods, beverages and smoking are able to intrinsically and extrinsically stain teeth.[128] Coffee, tea, wine and cola commonly have this effect; other culprits include carrots, oranges, chocolate and liquorice. Extrinsic staining can also be due to poor dental hygiene and even mouthwash ingredients (e.g. chlorhexidine is associated with increased tooth staining,[129,130] often green/brown). Most extrinsic staining can be removed by routine prophylactic procedures as well as being responsive to bleaching.[131] Fluoride gels may stain grey.

Understanding the cause of tooth discolouration is important for determining an appropriate treatment plan.[132] Although many people have heard of tooth bleaching, much of their exposure to the subject is via advertisements on electronic media and newspaper/magazine articles; many will be unaware of safety issues of these products/procedures,[133] having high expectations in line with (sometimes aggressive) marketing claims. There are suggested contraindications,[134] and professional opinion should be sought before use of whitening products.

A number of product types are available alongside whitening rinses and toothpastes. Natural methods of whitening include baking soda (ideal because it has a low, not excessively abrasive, effect as well as acid-buffering components) and activated charcoal.

Oral piercings

Oral piercings are not a new phenomenon; there is history of ritual tongue piercing in Mayan and Aztec cultures, either for honouring gods or to inflict pain.

Contemporary oral piercings (of tongue, lip, cheek or uvula) are considered an expression of style. Piercings can, however, be dangerous. Such 'body art' can make chewing, speaking or swallowing more difficult, may increase drooling, damage tongue, gum or fillings, and lead to allergic reactions. Oral piercings can interfere with dental X-rays and lead to uncontrolled bleeding, gum disease and long-term infections. The jewellery (e.g. barbells, most commonly worn on the tongue) may chip teeth or cause choking or create a need for root canal treatment if it breaks in the mouth or tissue. Tongue piercings generally cause more dental issues than lip piercings, with gingival recession similar for both.[135] Chipping of front teeth is the most common complaint.[136] Other common complaints include pain, damage to tooth enamel, scars and excessive salivation.[137]

Blood-borne infections are a potential complication and tongue swelling could cause airway obstruction. Tongue piercing is a risk factor for *C.albicans* colonization (even in the absence of jewellery).[138]

Some health conditions may impair healing after a piercing, and this should be considered beforehand. Vaccines for tetanus and hepatitis B should be up to date if oral piercing. Healing time for lip piercings can be one to three months.

For four to six weeks after piercing, cleanse the mouth at least 12 times daily (and always after eating/smoking/drinking) with sea salt water for one minute. Avoid use of hydrogen peroxide and mouthwashes with alcohol content. Avoid all oral sex activity and open-mouth kissing during this time. Avoid sharing cups, plates and eating utensils (avoidance of contact with saliva from others). Avoid touching the piercing and wash hands beforehand if touching is necessary. Reduce swelling with ice or drinking ice water.[139] Salty, spicy/acidic foods and hot drinks are also not advised during healing.

Once the tongue is healed, jewellery should be removed nightly and the tongue brushed.[140]

Nerve damage

Numerous nerves, including the vagus nerve, are involved in taste and oral health, and when damaged they may impact both oral and systemic health. Nerve damage may contribute to reduced saliva secretion, chewing/swallowing difficulty and speech issues, and may associate with viral infections, Lyme disease and burning mouth syndrome (which may be a form of neuropathy).[141]

The chorda tympani (CT), a branch of the facial nerve, is directly involved in transferring taste information from tongue fungiform papillae. The CT is particularly susceptible to damage because its path is meandering – through the middle ear, where damage is extremely common (e.g. in middle ear infection,[142] dental anaesthesia and procedures, head trauma, herpes zoster infection and stroke).[143]

Taste-related nerve damage can have long-term consequences for perception of bitterness as the nerve fibres conveying this important taste perception are small and unmyelinated, and susceptible to invasion by pathogens (e.g. viruses).[144]

Taste issues

Taste loss (ageusia), reduction of taste (hypogeusia) and dysgeusia (abnormal taste) are widespread and commonly associated with many health conditions (e.g. Alzheimer's disease, Bell's palsy, epilepsy, Parkinson's disease, diabetes mellitus, hypothyroidism, allergic rhinitis, sinusitis, influenza-like infections and many others)[145] as well as being strongly associated with various therapies such as radiation therapy[146] and some drugs (methotrexate, dexamethasone, antihypertensives, antimicrobials and antiproliferative agents).[147]

Smell disorders and taste disorders can be the result of similar factors and sometimes loss of smell is perceived as loss of taste. Taste disorders can be caused by taste bud injury as well as upper respiratory and middle ear infections, exposure to certain chemicals (e.g. insecticides) and some medications (including some common antibiotics and antihistamines), head injury, some surgeries to ear, nose and throat, radiation therapy for cancers of head/neck, dental surgery, especially of third molar (wisdom tooth), and poor oral hygiene.[148] Taste alterations can also occur in relation to hormonal change (e.g. pregnancy and menopause), xerostomia and in ageing.

Health of the oral cavity, taste cells and nerve fibres have important effects on dietary choices, food nutrient quality, blood sugar level and weight regulation. Taste dysfunction can resolve on its own after several months. If cut or crushed, nerve fibre injury can result in the disappearance of taste buds which, if the nerve fibre is allowed to grow back, may reappear.[149]

Levels of gustin correlate with hypogeusia.[150] Gustin is a zinc-metalloprotein which may have a role in taste bud growth and function,[151] and is described as a taste bud trophic factor.[152] Zinc therapy thus may be a useful taste restorative. A variety of other potential means of naturally addressing taste loss are discussed in later chapters (primarily Chapter 10).

── Chapter 9 ──

PERIO-SYSTEMIC LINKS

Inflammation is a defining characteristic of periodontitis, which means around (*perio*) the tooth (*dontal*) inflammation (*itis*). Periodontitis significantly increases risk for various conditions including diabetes, cardiovascular disease (CVD), respiratory diseases and preterm delivery of low birth-weight infants.[1] These and many other health conditions have shown to be associated with periodontal conditions, and various inflammatory markers have been suggested as links for this bi-directional association.

Evidence of the systemic spread of oral commensals and pathogens (specific strains) to non-oral body sites and the resulting inflammation and extra-oral infection is increasing.[2] Specific oral bacterial species are associated with specific systemic diseases: aspiration pneumonia, bacterial pneumonia,[3] bacterial endocarditis,[4,5] preterm low birth-weight[6] and osteomyelitis in children.[7] Whilst these associations are well documented in literature, this chapter focuses on broader health conditions. They are important because these bi-directional associations may contribute to common health conditions, yet generally be overlooked.

Although with age there is increased susceptibility to inflammatory or degenerative pathologies, including periodontal disease, this may relate less to age *per se* and more to age-dependent alterations in innate immunity and the inflammatory status of the host.[8]

Many of the disease conditions that are associated with periodontitis are lifestyle-related comorbidities. Awareness of these associations by practitioners and clients may give them a greater incentive to address oral inflammatory processes, as well as other oral cavity factors.

This chapter presents evidence of bi-directionality of these perio-systemic associations; they are largely mediated by inflammation which triggers cytokine cascades with widespread systemic effect.

With gum disease affecting nearly half (45%) of UK adults,[9] these bi-directional associations with other health conditions suggest that greater consideration of oral health in protocols is warranted.

Diabetes and glycaemic control

Periodontitis was declared the sixth complication of diabetes in 1993 in a study that concluded that Pima Indians (from Arizona, USA, a community with the world's highest prevalence of T2DM)[10,11] were 15 times more likely to be edentulous if type 2 diabetic; periodontal disease incidence was almost three times higher in those with T2DM than in non-diabetic individuals, and diabetic persons with retinopathy were almost five times more likely to have advanced periodontal disease than those without retinopathy.[12]

Periodontal disease was found to be a strong predictor of mortality from diabetic nephropathy and ischaemic heart disease in Pima Indians with T2DM.[13] Those with T$_1$D also showed increased periodontal breakdown; those suffering T$_1$D for more than ten years showed greater loss than those with less than ten years' history. Both types of diabetes were found to be predictors of periodontal disease.[14]

The bi-directionality of this relationship is succinctly summarized in a 2015 study investigating links between glycaemic control/diabetes and periodontal health: 'Poorly controlled diabetes predisposes to periodontitis. Periodontitis contributes to both the worsening of diabetes control and development of diabetes.'[15] Periodontal disease is more prevalent in diabetics, and symptom progression may be rapid.

Mechanisms proposed as an explanation for bi-directional connections between diabetes and periodontal disease include:

- hyperactive inflammatory response in diabetes and bacterial challenge of periodontal infection resulting in exaggerated inflammation and periodontal tissue destruction

- elevated AGEs receptors with diabetes and increased AGEs levels in periodontal disease which activate these receptors, resulting in increased levels of pro-inflammatory cytokines (e.g. IL-6, TNF-α)

- increased fibroblast apoptosis, which may account for delayed wound healing in diabetes

- altered immune responses in diabetes, with functions regarding phagocytosis and neutrophil chemotaxis impaired, which may predispose diabetics to more severe periodontal disease.[16]

Other proposed explanations for this link between diabetes and periodontal disease include microvascular disease, changes in GCF composition and altered collagen metabolism.[17] Reduced peripheral blood flow in diabetes may reduce blood flow to gum margins. Functionality of, and immune response to, red blood cells damaged by consistently high blood sugar and AGEs are altered, thus potentially impacting autoimmune reactions.

Periodontitis in diabetes mellitus may be more serious and unmanageable due to stimulation of periodontal ligament fibroblasts, up-regulation of RAGEs and accumulation of AGEs that negatively impact periodontium regeneration and wound healing.[18] (Periodontal ligaments connect teeth to the alveolar bone; they are involved in periodontium regeneration.)

Regarding the wider impact of inflammatory and immune response, a variety of inflammatory mediators may simultaneously present with periodontal microbes to challenge both inflammatory and immune response.

Oral cavity inflammation impacts blood sugar regulation by triggering a pro-inflammatory state resulting in the release of inflammatory mediators into the bloodstream; in addition to this indirect effect, inflammation can directly impact pancreatic insulin production by beta cells. The way cells respond to insulin is affected by mediators, and insulin resistance may result. Insulin has a potent acute anti-inflammatory effect, reducing intranuclear NF-kB and decreasing generation of reactive oxygen species[19] so that when pancreatic beta cells no longer produce sufficient insulin – that is, in a state of insulin resistance — anti-inflammatory and ROS-reducing benefits of insulin may be chronically absent.

Inflammation has been investigated as a link since periodontitis is a low-level systemic infection with the potential to affect glycaemic control in diabetics. A 2012 review found that periodontal therapy given to those with T2DM assists in the amelioration of inflammatory biomarker levels (e.g. interleukins, TNF-α, C-reactive protein) and glycaemic status.[20]

Diabetes and periodontal disease commonly occur in the same individual in wider populations, and a 2017 study of cytokine ratios in these groups, individually and together, showed that both the levels of various pro-inflammatory markers (e.g. HbA1c, TNF-α, IL-1β, IL-6) and ratios of these inflammatory markers with IL-4 and IL-10 (which are generally considered protective cytokines) were highest in participants having both T2DM and chronic periodontitis.[21]

The complexity of the chronic inflammatory response (IL-1β, IL-6, TNF-α, MMPs) generated by diverse periodontopathogens and their numerous bacterial products (e.g. endotoxins), coupled with the complex cascade of tissue-destructive pathways involved, result in unusually destructive periodontal breakdown in diseases like diabetes that can exaggerate host response to local microbial factors.[22]

Salivary flow rate, which helps establish a protective environment against dental caries, was found to be significantly lowered alongside levels of salivary calcium, phosphate and fluoride in those with diabetes; decreased salivary flow rate, combined with poor glycaemic control and significantly increased HbA1c (glycated haemoglobin), has been found to be associated with high numbers of dental caries.[23]

The salivary level of chromogranin A (CHGA), an acidic glycoprotein in secretory vesicles of neurons and endocrine cells[24] and a biological marker of sympathetic nerve activity,[25] increases in response to physical and psychological stress;[26] both psychological stress and salivary chromogranin A level are associated with periodontitis.[27] CHGA is also a pro-hormone; pancreastatin is a CHGA-derived peptide that exerts multiple, potentially dysglycaemic actions and may be important in the regulation of insulin secretion and the pathogenesis of diabetes mellitus.[28]

A 2016 study found that T2DM patients were more prone to periodontal tissue damage than to caries risk; results also suggest high concentrations of salivary CHGA are associated with worse periodontal parameters and with T2DM, and could thus be related to the pathogenesis of both diseases.[29]

Obesity

A 2010 systematic review and meta-analysis of association between chronic periodontal disease and obesity found that a higher prevalence of periodontal disease should be expected among obese adults.[30] Periodontitis was found to be more common in those with serum HDL cholesterol concentrations <60mg per decilitre (1.6 mmol/litre) and associated with obesity; periodontitis may be exacerbated by some obesity-associated conditions, such as metabolic syndrome, dyslipidaemia and/or insulin resistance.[31]

High levels of prime inflammatory mediator TNF-α may explain the susceptibility of obese individuals, who are demonstrated to express two and a half times more TNF-α mRNA in fat tissue,[32] to more severe periodontal disease.[33] TNF-α has been shown to suppress insulin action by various mechanisms.[34,35,36,37,38]

Periodontitis may induce the initial stages of white adipose tissue (WAT) inflammation, promoting subsequent development of insulin resistance.[39] TNF-α and IL-6 may be common aetiological factors for destructive periodontal disease associated with obesity and metabolic syndrome; inter-organ inflammation may be involved.[40] Salivary/serum TNF-α levels correlate with clinical parameters in metabolic syndrome patients with periodontitis.[41] Adipokines like TNF-α provide a pro-inflammatory state that may link with oxidative stress in conditions like metabolic syndrome and periodontitis, thus bi-directionally influencing one another.[42]

The obesity hormone leptin, which is secreted by adipocytes and is found in saliva,[43] has been shown to negatively interfere with the regenerative capacity of periodontal cells and may be the link between obesity and compromised periodontal healing.[44] Leptin has, however, also been shown, when topically applied, to promote wound healing in the oral mucosa by accelerating epithelial cell migration and enhancing angiogenesis,[45] which VEGF (vascular endothelial growth factor) has also been shown to do.[46]

Disrupted circadian rhythm abolishes the normal diurnal pattern of leptin, and promotes metabolic conditions and obesity.[47] Melatonin, the hormone that regulates circadian sleep–wake cycles, is synthesized and secreted by the pineal gland and released into saliva, and has powerful antioxidant effects as well as an immunomodulatory role, also stimulating the synthesis of type 1 collagen fibres and promoting bone formation.[48] Melatonin may be beneficial to oral cavity health where it is thought to function as an antioxidant and anti-inflammatory agent.

MELATONIN AND ORAL HEALTH

Melatonin is synthesized in the pineal gland and gastrointestinal tract from which it passes into the circulatory system.[49] Melatonin from the blood into saliva (where it is found at levels between 15 and 33 per cent of those in plasma) also contributes to oral cavity protection regarding tissue damage via the action of different receptors and may help suppress oral diseases including periodontal disease, herpes and oral cancer.[50]

Melatonin is highly lipophyllic and enters all body cells.[51] This important hormone participates in many important body processes; levels decline gradually with ageing, and deficiency may contribute to reduced antioxidant protection.[52]

Melatonin and its receptors are found in the oral cavity. A 2017 review found that melatonin could play a role in the homeostasis of periodontal tissues, concluding that antioxidant, anti-inflammatory, immunomodulatory and osteogenic actions on maxillar bone metabolism indicate melatonin as a potential therapeutic strategy for periodontitis, especially in light of its widespread therapeutic effects in the context of other (perio-)systemic conditions.[53]

An earlier review indicated the potential role of melatonin in protecting the oral cavity from tissue damage from oxidative stress, and its potential to aid alveolar bone regeneration through stimulation of type 1 collagen fibre production and modulation of osteoblastic/osteoclastic activity.[54]

Mechanisms of action for melatonin include the involvement of various membrane receptors and receptor-independent activity (by directly scavenging free radicals); its presence in the oral cavity may contribute to beneficial effects in oral cavity HSV. As a known oncostatic agent, melatonin may have a beneficial effect in oral cancer.[55]

The severity of periodontitis in morbid obesity is associated with the inflammation-sensitive plasma protein orosomucoid,[56] levels of which are associated with tissue destruction.[57]

Obesity, diabetes and periodontitis are thought to link in a 'triangular relationship', and research suggests that periodontitis may adversely affect glycaemic control, whilst also stimulating inflammatory changes in adipose tissue, creating a 'self-generating cycle of morbidity' linking these three health conditions metabolically.[58]

Metabolic syndrome

Insulin resistance and central obesity are component conditions of metabolic syndrome alongside hypertriglyceridemia, low HDL (high-density lipoprotein) and hypertension; it is not surprising that severe periodontitis is also associated with metabolic syndrome,[59] and metabolic syndrome was found to be associated with the incidence of tooth loss among middle-aged adults in a retrospective study of 2107 participants in Japan.[60]

Hyperlipidaemia affects both periodontitis and diabetes via its effects on insulin secretion and the production of pro-inflammatory cytokines TNF-α and IL-1β,[61] and may be the linking factor between periodontitis and cardiovascular disease – two diseases with common risk factors. Periodontal infections result in bacteraemia and endotoxaemia and promote systemic inflammatory and immune responses that may impact systemic health; virulence factors expressed by periodontal pathogens may affect atherosclerotic events.[62]

Atherosclerosis, which is characterized by lipid accumulation, chronic inflammation and endothelial dysfunction, has been shown to be associated with multiple bacterial and viral pathogens, including periodontopathogens via direct and indirect mechanisms; various infectious agents have been found in atherosclerotic plaque and these accelerate atherosclerotic lesion progression.[63]

Studies indicate an association between amounts of periodontopathogenic microorganisms and numerous markers including LDL and hs-CRP (high-sensitivity CRP); periodontal treatment may reduce atherosclerosis risk.[64]

An association between CVD (cardiovascular disease) and oral health has been demonstrated by a large body of evidence. Since periodontal disease often occurs due to poor oral hygiene and excess sugar consumption, both periodontal treatment and dietary alteration may be required.[65]

Periodontal disease is likely to cause 19 per cent increased CVD risk, with higher relative risk of 44 per cent in those aged 65 or over.[66] Any increased risk of CVD or other serious health condition due to periodontal disease potentially has a profound impact since such a large percentage of the world's population has some level of periodontal disease. An association has also been found with coronary heart disease and early atherogenesis.[67]

Statistically significant increases in CRP levels have been found in periodontal disease, and the extent of this increase depends on disease severity. The positive correlation between CRP and periodontal disease has been suggested as a possible underlying pathway regarding the observed higher CVD risk in periodontal patients.[68]

C-REACTIVE PROTEIN

C-reactive protein (CRP) participates in systemic response to inflammation and is regulated by cytokines like IL-6, IL-1β and TNF-α.[69] CRP is both extremely sensitive and non-specific, and is thus produced in response to many forms of injury or infection.[70] As part of the innate immune system response to bacterial infections, CRP is an important marker of systemic bacterial exposure from periodontitis.[71]

Its structure enables CRP to recognize pathogens and damaged host cells and, by activating complement cascades, facilitates their removal.[72] In response to tissue injury or infection, serum concentration of CRP may increase more than 10,000-fold,[73] returning rapidly to baseline levels with homeostasis recovery.[74] As its level appears to tightly correlate with inflammation severity, CRP is considered a non-specific, exquisitely sensitive systemic marker of inflammation and tissue damage.[75]

CRP is associated with smoking, obesity, coffee consumption, triglycerides, diabetes and periodontal disease.[76]

The CRP level can be assessed via a blood test. More recently a test that measures high-sensitivity (hs-CRP) has become available and is often used to assess CVD risk. Since CRP levels are associated with a variety of health conditions, these tests may aid overall inflammatory risk assessment.

Cerebrovascular and pulmonary links

As with cardiovascular health, periodontal disease is an important risk factor for cerebrovascular accidents (CVA); there is a significant associated risk with periodontitis of developing cerebrovascular conditions, especially non-haemorrhagic stroke.[77] The CVA relative risk tends to be higher for periodontitis than for edentulousness, supporting the theory that periodontal pathogens are important factors.

The possibility of confounding factors, such as the association of periodontal status with socioeconomic status and health-risk lifestyle/behaviours, is also considered in relation to the association of cerebrovascular disease with periodontal health (e.g. medical service use may be impacted, so that incident CVAs are more likely to be missed and potentially the effects of periodontal disease may be underestimated).[78]

Higher levels of inflammatory mediators, especially hs-CRP, in GCF (gingival crevicular fluid) and lower numbers of teeth associated with COPD (chronic obstructive pulmonary disease) may reflect the systemic effects of this disease on periodontal tissues.[79] Smoking is a common risk factor for COPD and periodontitis. However, high prevalence of periodontitis in COPD patients appears to be independent of possible risk factors for periodontitis (e.g. pack years smoked, age, BMI, corticosteroids use, bone mineral density).[80]

Asthma, too, has been found to be associated with periodontal disease, with inflammation the hypothesized link.[81]

Connective tissue destructive diseases

In their discussion of the bi-directional connection between periodontitis and diabetes, Manikandan and Ajithkumar discuss a hypothetical 'two-hit' model of induction of chronic destructive periodontitis (to explain how bone and connective tissue destructive diseases in one location may communicate with tissues in the periodontium) whereby hit one is generated by periodontopathic subgingival biofilm and microbial products (e.g. endotoxin), and hit two is generated by a systemic inflammatory response characterized by elevated biomarkers (e.g. CRP, IL-6, MMP). Hit two involves bone and connective tissue destructive diseases (e.g. in joints in rheumatoid arthritis, in the skeletal system in post-menopausal osteoporosis) and increased circulation of biomarkers of systemic inflammation.[82]

Elevated pro-inflammatory mediators (e.g. IL-6) in junior rheumatoid arthritis[83] are cited as an example. IL-6 regulates immune and inflammatory responses and bone metabolism, with potential involvement in the pathogenesis of infection, autoimmunity and malignancy.[84] The association between rheumatoid arthritis (RA) and periodontitis may be related to the periodontal pathogen *Porphyromonas gingivalis* against which RA patients with severe periodontitis have a more robust antibody response than non-RA controls.[85] RA patients with severe periodontitis also have less healthy pocket epithelium and a tendency to a higher inflammatory state than controls.[86]

The relationship among postmenopausal osteoporosis, tooth loss and alveolar bone loss[87] is a second example. Potential pathways involve increased MMP (collagenase, gelatinase) gingival activity in response to oestrogen deficiency. Gingival collagenase activity parallels changes in periodontal bone loss and reflects trabecular bone density changes.[88]

A third example is the relationship of destructive periodontal disease to acute-phase response, in particular with respect to CRP, looked at by Craig *et al.*; those with chronic destructive periodontitis exhibited 100 per cent higher levels of serum CRP than those with mild, less destructive periodontitis.[89]

TNF-α, a cytokine involved with CRP in acute-phase response, has been shown to exacerbate pre-existing periodontal disease by inducing production (in gingival fibroblasts) of MMPs involved in connective tissue destruction (IL-1β and IL-17 are also involved in this),[90] and by stimulating the host response to cause osteoclastogenesis and thus bone resorption.[91]

Periodontal status has been investigated in relation to bone status since both osteoporosis and periodontitis are characterized by bone resorption. These two diseases have shared risk factors: age, hormonal change, smoking, genetics, nutrient deficiencies (calcium, vitamin D).[92]

A 2016 Taiwanese population-based cross-sectional study including 35,127 osteoporosis patients and 50,498 healthy controls showed that periodontitis is associated with increased risk of osteoporosis, and that osteoporosis is associated with a six-fold increased risk of periodontal inflammation; the study concluded that good oral hygiene may be crucial for preventing disease progression in osteoporosis.[93]

An earlier cross-sectional study in Korea (321,103 cases of periodontitis in 1,025,340 samples) found periodontitis significantly and positively correlated with most lifestyle-related comorbidities, particularly osteoporosis.[94]

Prevalence and progression of periodontal disease in older men was investigated with respect to bone metabolism biomarkers in the Osteoporotic Fractures in Men (MrOS) study which recruited 5994 men of 65+ years in six clinical sites in the USA. Bone turnover biomarkers, for example CTX (C-telopeptides which are a measure of fragments derived from type 1 collagen degradation, thus indicative of osteoclastic activity), were found to be associated with periodontal progression; other bone metabolism biomarkers, for example parathyroid hormone (PTH) and 25(OH)D, were associated with severe periodontal disease.[95]

A 2017 cross-sectional study of 492 post-menopausal women found that women treated with oestrogen (some of whom also received progestin, calcium and vitamin D supplements) for at least six months had a lower prevalence of severe periodontitis than women not receiving this treatment.[96]

Investigations to determine the pathology of periodontitis found a potential role of bone morphogenetic protein-1 (BMP1) in maintaining homeostasis of periodontal formation possibly via procollagen-1 and dentine matrix protein-1 (DMP1), and impacting the extracellular matrix environment.[97] BMP1 is a metalloprotease known to induce bone and cartilage development.[98] Procollagen-1 forms when glycine and proline initially combine as a three-dimensional stranded structure, and is later modified to form the triple helix structure of collagen. DMP1 is a major and highly expressed ECM protein with a key role in osteogenesis, regulating bone development, mineralization and phosphate metabolism; glycosylation of DMP1 is a key posttranslational modification process during development.[99] These proteins may have important roles in maintaining periodontium.

These studies demonstrate an association between various connective tissue destructive conditions and periodontal diseases, with inflammation (and lifestyle factors) having input, and suggest benefit from connective tissue support protocols.

Erectile dysfunction, infertility and pregnancy outcomes

Periodontitis significantly and positively correlates with many lifestyle-related comorbidities including CVD, hypertension, diabetes, obesity and rheumatoid arthritis (RA), and particularly strongly associates with osteoporosis and erectile dysfunction.[100]

The relationship between chronic periodontitis and erectile dysfunction may relate to promotion of endothelial dysfunction via increased systemic levels of inflammatory cytokines such as TNF-α.[101] Additionally, unexplained male infertility has shown an association with periodontal and caries status.[102]

Interestingly, taste receptors and components of the transduction cascade are expressed during phases of spermatogenesis as well as in mature spermatozoa, suggesting that sperm 'taste' cues in their natural microenvironment; clearer understanding of the precise role of taste receptors in human male fertility may inform future research and treatment options.[103]

Adverse pregnancy outcomes also associate with periodontal disease; a 2013 systematic review found a modest but significant association with low birth-weight and preterm birth, and a significant association of maternal periodontitis with pre-eclampsia.[104] Studies indicate that maternal periodontal infection can lead to placental-fetal exposure and, when associated with fetal inflammatory response, can lead to preterm delivery, with the added complication (from maternal periodontal infections) of possible long-term effects on infant development.[105]

A meta-analysis of randomized trials looking at the effects of periodontal disease treatment during pregnancy on incidence of preterm births found treatment reduced rates of preterm birth and may reduce the incidence of low birth weight.[106]

Neuroinflammation

Low-grade inflammation (e.g. from chronic periodontitis) can also impact nervous tissue and initiate neurodegenerative processes. Neuroinflammation is thought to be a significant factor in neurodegenerative diseases such as Alzheimer's disease[107] and Parkinson's disease.[108]

An association between tooth loss, caries and periodontal disease is found in Parkinson's disease (PD); a clinical study in Japan found patients with PD had fewer remaining teeth, more caries and a higher incidence of deep periodontal pockets.[109]

An association between cognitive decline and tooth loss was shown in a 13-year longitudinal study of Chinese older adults; those with fewer teeth tended to show a quicker rate of cognitive decline.[110] Several possible mechanisms are discussed alongside the inflammatory effects of periodontitis including poor nutrition due to tooth loss and decreased masticatory function (mastication may be effective in sending sensory information to the brain for maintaining hippocampal learning and memory functions).[111]

Research shows an association between periodontitis and increased cognitive decline in Alzheimer's disease, likely mediated through the effects on systemic inflammation.[112] *Porphyromonas gingivalis* has been thought to play a role[113] but neuroinflammatory mechanisms from a systemic inflammatory response triggered by periodontitis are more widely discussed;[114] in particular CRP has been shown to be associated with periodontitis.[115]

Studies using animal models and post-mortem human brain tissues (AD subjects) show *P.gingivalis* (and/or its product gingipain) can translocate to the brain, suggesting investigation of an association between oral exposure to *P.gingivalis* and neuroinflammation/neurodegeneration and confirming formation of amyloid plaque,[116] which has shown a protective role.[117]

In addition to these neuroinflammatory factors, mercury exposure from dental amalgams may cause some of the same biochemical effects as seen in Alzheimer's.[118] Effects of fluoride–aluminium compounds may also be a factor in Alzheimer's disease development.

Gut inflammation

Chronic inflammation is a common factor in many gut and periodontal conditions. Inflammatory bowel diseases are associated with dysbiosis of salivary microbiota.[119] Salivary *Klebsiella* spp have been shown to colonize in the gut where they strongly induce TH1 cells, eliciting severe gut inflammation.[120]

Liver cirrhosis is also associated with gut dysbiosis, with 54 per cent of problematic bacterial species originating in the mouth.[121]

Helicobacter pylori also commonly infect the gut and mouth, where it is even more difficult to eradicate and from where it easily re-infects the gut.[122]

The connection between translocated periodontopathogen (e.g. *P.gingivalis*) and their potential to contribute to gut dysbiosis via endotoxemia and inflammatory mediators is discussed by Olsen and Yamazaki,[123] and suggests a possible mechanism for periosystemic links elsewhere in the body.

Immune factors

With regard to other immune issues, an association was found between human herpes virus (HSV, cytomegalovirus, EBV) and aggressive periodontitis.[124]

HIV (human immunodeficiency viruses) infection, which causes substantial irreversible damage to mucosal barriers and hyper-immune activation, is associated with the prevalence of oral mucosal infections and dysregulation of oral microbiota; this impaired oral immunity may predispose HIV patients to periodontal diseases associated with systemic inflammation.[125]

Lastly, and very briefly, a mention of the perio-systemic link with cancer. Researchers found 59 per cent greater risk of pancreatic cancer in those with *Porphyromonas gingivalis* in their oral microbiome.[126] A 50 per cent increased relative risk was also found regarding *Aggregatibacter actinomycetemcomitans*. A link has also been found between *P.gingivalis* and oesophageal squamous cell carcinoma.[127] Poor oral health is a risk factor for squamous cell carcinoma of the head/neck with the most pronounced associations for sites closer to the dentition.[128]

Breast cancer risk may be 11 times higher in those with poor oral health or gum disease according to a survey of 3273 individuals aged 30–40.[129] Another study of 73,737 women concluded that periodontal disease was associated with increased risk of postmenopausal breast cancer, particularly among former smokers who quit in the past 20 years (oral microbiome of those with periodontal disease differs with smoking status).[130]

A 2019 pilot study of 160 women (80 with breast cancer and 80 healthy age-matched women) looking at the association between breast cancer chemotherapy, oral health and chronic dental infections found breast cancer patients showed higher risk for missing teeth and more apical lesions (which appear in bone surrounding portals of exit from infected root canal systems), particularly those of endodontic origin without root canal.[131]

General statements by practising biological/holistic dental practitioners suggest that all cancer patients have mouth/dental issues and that none have 32 perfect teeth.[132] It has also been suggested that dental infection shares lymph drainage with breast – described as 'hot lines' from the mouth to the breast.[133]

There is evidence of a robust association between circulating CRP levels and cancer risk.[134] An association between CRP and periodontitis is also evident. No causality is proven, only association. The same appears to be true of other inflammatory markers. YKL-40, an acute-phase protein which may have a role in cancer cell proliferation, survival and invasiveness,[135] is found in periodontal disease (increased levels in both serum and GCF) and in inflammatory diseases such as RA, T2DM and coronary artery diseases.[136]

Tooth loss shows a significant positive association with risk of some cancers including oesophageal, lung and head/neck cancers.[137] An association was also found between the number of decayed, missing or filled teeth (DMFT) and depressed levels of all classes of immunoglobulins, indicating that those with immune dysfunction also have greater susceptibility to dental caries and greater frequency of harbouring *S.mutans*.[138]

There may also be an association between 'dead' teeth and cancer. Dr Issels, a German physician, recommends extraction of root canal teeth for terminal cancer patients. Over a period of 40 years treating 16,000 cancer patients, he has found that 90 per cent of them had between two and ten dead teeth in their mouths.[139] He has had a 24 per cent total remission rate with these 16,000 patients.[140]

Summary implications for nutritional therapy

Evidence for an association between periodontal disease and a wide range of diseases/conditions exists. Inflammation and increased oxidative stress are implicated in disease. The disease that manifests may depend on the degree, duration and location of inflammation/oxidative stress in the body. The nature of the pro-oxidant/toxic substance(s) (periodontopathogenic bacteria, bacterial endotoxins, fluoride, pesticides, heavy metals and mercury) involved in the inflammation/oxidative stress also play an important part in disease determination.

There is increasing evidence that periodontal disease conditions are associated with and contribute to other health conditions (e.g. soft gums in metabolic disorder, kryptopyrroluria, involving compromised haemoglobin formation and loss of vitamin B6, zinc and other nutrients).[141,142] This is particularly pertinent since periodontal disease is a preventable condition. With gum disease affecting nearly half (45%) of UK adults,[143] these bi-directional associations with other health conditions suggest greater consideration of oral health in protocols is warranted.

Oral health protocols may benefit alongside client-relevant, condition-specific protocols, and should be included prophylactically if not already needed therapeutically.

— Chapter 10 —

AGEING, HORMONES, SATIETY AND LOSS OF TASTE

This chapter looks at the impact of ageing, hormones, taste perception and satiety on oral health and gives protocol suggestions throughout for these and general connective tissue support.

Ages of life

The mouth and teeth can cause problems at any time during life – from infants cutting teeth, impacted wisdom teeth at young adulthood, and during ageing, when various natural processes impact both mouth and dental health.

Hormonal changes during pregnancy[1] and puberty are known to affect oral ecology due to increased steroid hormones in plasma and therefore in GCF and saliva. Unbalanced hormone secretion during puberty may promote gingivitis,[2] and the effect of increased oestrogen production in young women at puberty, during ovulation and pregnancy may influence cellular proliferation, differentiation and growth of keratinocytes and fibroblasts as well as stimulating inflammatory mediators with resulting increased gingival inflammation and bleeding impacting microbial ecology.[3]

Fluoride exposure in pregnancy may associate with birth of babies with Down syndrome,[4] and may affect human male fertility.[5] Studies indicate IQ deficits in children exposed to excess fluoride; four human studies indicate fluoride can enter and damage fetal brains.[6] These are important considerations for those seeking to become pregnant.

Infant oral health may be impacted by breastfeeding, for example by beneficially providing high levels of sIgA and controlling early infections by *Streptococcus mutans*.[7] Although prolonged breastfeeding may potentially contribute to a higher caries rate,[8] it may also promote deposition of calcium and phosphate ions on tooth surfaces; overall, bottle feeding has raised more concern.[9]

Childhood caries causal factors include addition of sweeteners to bottles and, generally, inclusion of sugar/sweet foods. Other causal factors relate to the initial age of infection with cariogenic bacteria (greater caries risk with earlier infection); enamel of newly erupted teeth is vulnerably immature and likely affected by prenatal/perinatal insults. A strong social gradient associates with dental caries experience, particularly in young children.

A review of evidence for the aetiology and prevention of early childhood caries[10] lists the following evidence-based preventive advice, which includes: reduction of frequency of sugar intake, use of fluoride toothpaste in absence of water fluoridation, encouragement by parents of infants/toddlers to learn self-maintenance of oral health, and reduction of behaviours which increase risk of early transmission of *Streptococcus mutans* (e.g. tasting the child's food, cleaning the child's 'soother' in parents' mouths, sharing cups/utensils).

Secretory IgA concentration in saliva increases five-fold between birth and age two.[11] During the first two years of life, the infant is adapting to its surroundings and developing an immune response. Although salivary sIgA increases during this period, commensal oral bacteria elicit a limited secretory immune response.[12] Humoral immunity to commensal oral bacteria may aid homeostasis and oral tolerance.

Older ages

In contrast, salivary sIgA concentrations and saliva flow are significantly lower in the elderly than in the young.[13] Altered concentration and/or activity of organic salivary components, particularly concentrations of sIgA and mucins (two important salivary defence factors),[14] may impact immune function, inflammation, oral health and whole-body health.

Other physiological changes during ageing may also impact these health parameters. The epithelial layer of cells on the surface of the tongue, for example, shows a 30 per cent reduction in thickness between the ages of 16 and 98.[15] During ageing, too, the number of taste buds, acini and the protein biosynthesis activity of saliva decreases,[16] thus potentially impacting salivary function and taste.

Risk of both tooth decay and gum disease increases with age; gingiva is affected by thinning of the epithelium and diminished keratinization in ageing.[17] Older individuals may have a greater likelihood of mouth sores, *Candida* or HSV infections. Age-related alterations (e.g. increased staphylococci, lactobacilli, yeasts and opportunistic pathogens) in oral microbiota may occur.[18] Oral microbiome support should be considered for all older clients.

Although teeth are very resilient, with molars, for example, able to deal with large amounts of pressure, they are not indestructible and may show wear, including cracks, with age. The outer layer of enamel wears away and biting edges flatten. Nerves at the core of the tooth may lose sensitivity with age.

Over time, enamel can be dissolved by acidic foods and carbonated drinks, weakening the protection previously provided. Yellowing of dentine inside the tooth may occur and, with thinning of the protective enamel coating, overall tooth colour may be affected. Enamel may also become stained by tobacco, wine, coffee and tea.

With age, there is often a greater likelihood of multiple medications, some of which may detrimentally affect oral health; many affect saliva and are associated with xerostomia, bad breath and swallowing difficulties. Other medications and/or disease conditions may affect gum health, increase inflammation and/or impact immunity.

Denture-wearing (and other dental interventions) may alter oral ecology. In addition, altered dietary habits, hormones, stress and other age-associated changes may impact oral microbiota; immune function may be less optimal.

With age, too, there is the potentially cumulative effect of AGEs and increased likelihood of inflammaging (i.e. chronic inflammation which potentially contributes to age-associated conditions); one source of inflammaging may relate to harmful substances produced by oral (and gut) microbiota in cases of 'leaky' mouth/gut;[19] altered microbiota are associated with increased age.[20]

Menopause

Falling oestrogen levels during the menopause may impact the susceptibility of dental gums to plaque, thus increasing the probability of caries, gingivitis and periodontitis. In addition, the menopause may affect bone health, reducing attachment and the relative anchorage of teeth to the jawbone.[21] Dry mouth, burning mouth and candidiasis may also be associated with the menopause.[22]

Oestrogen, progesterone and testosterone have been linked with periodontal pathogenesis and wound healing.[23] Oestrogen receptors are found in oral mucosa and salivary glands[24] where their presence is thought to suggest a biological role.[25] Oral microcirculation has been evaluated to show significant differences in post-menopausal women, correlating with periodontitis, and suggested to predispose to inflammation.[26]

The most significant oral issues in menopausal women are related to oral dryness; salivary flow rate is decreased in the menopause, although salivary pH and some salivary constituents seem to be unaffected.[27] Reduced salivary flow may increase the propensity to experience numerous oral issues including gingivitis, dental caries, taste alteration and periodontitis.

For post-menopausal women with periodontitis, hormone replacement therapy (HRT) was shown to influence interleukin levels, accelerating healing.[28] The effect of HRT on saliva has also been studied and its use may increase salivary flow when used alongside calcium and aldendronate (a bisphosphonate).[29] A systematic review on the cost of dental care in postmenopausal women with osteoporosis found that those who did not receive HRT had a greater incidence of adverse dental outcomes.[30] However, there are only a small number of studies examining the effect of the menopause on oral symptoms, and the effect of HRT on symptom alleviation and oral health improvement is controversial.[31] Natural hormone-balancing therapies alongside sialogogues may prove beneficial.

Lip changes for both sexes

Lips of both men and women are affected in ageing. Soft tissue changes include loss of collagen and elastin, reduced glycosaminoglycans (including hyaluronan) resulting in water loss/dry skin, epidermal thinning with flattening of the dermal-epidermal junction, alterations to perioral fat compartments which alter fat distribution and droop, and development of perioral wrinkles (due to reduction in soft tissue volume/elasticity and repeated muscle activity).

A number of structural lip changes also occur including loss of curves of the lip, drier lips, more noticeable wrinkles/folds, partial loss of Cupid's bow, thinning of vermillion border, and changed exposure of teeth; the lower lip becomes thinner and rolls inward, and the upper lip loses volume, lengthens and inverts.

In addition to these changes there are changes to jaw angles, tooth wear that results in the flattening of incisal edges affecting the smile arc, and effects from tooth loss and/or denture-wearing.[32]

Not only are lips redder in younger people than older individuals,[33] oestrogen levels and facial femininity also associate with fullness of lips; full lips are sometimes considered to be more sexually attractive than lips that are less full, and a 2012 study found that oestrogen levels and facial femininity are associated with maternal tendencies and thus, it is surmised, men's preference for facial femininity relates to her likely fertility and his reproductive strategy.[34] Changes in oestrogen level, especially at menopause, may hugely impact a woman's sense of self. Such physiological changes, especially alongside (unisexual) changes in dental health and regenerative capacity regarding collagen, can further impact emotional well-being and have significance in relation to the concept of 'beauty' in older age. Self-esteem and confidence (and the smile) may thus also be impacted by the health of lips and teeth. This may impact client mental health.

HYALURONIC ACID

Hyaluronic acid (HA), aka hyaluronan/hyaluronate, is a large, naturally occurring molecule described as being able to retain a thousand times its weight in water and as such is responsible for plumping skin and lips, maintaining healthy synovial fluid in joints, making up a large percentage of vitreous humour gel fluid in the eye and in the ECM of connective tissue including gingivae.[35,36]

Hyaluronic acid is the simplest of GAGs (glycosaminoglycans), composed of repeating alternating units of glucuronic acid and N-acetylglucosamine.[37] Its linear, rope-like structure allows hyaluronan to bind up to a thousand times its weight in water, thus providing cushioning, elasticity and lubrication to various body parts.

Cell receptors for HA are varied and widely distributed, including in mucous membranes,[38] which is why the oral cavity allows easy absorption.

HA is a key element in both hard periodontal tissue (alveolar bone/cementum) and soft periodontal tissue (gingiva/periodontal ligament).[39] With roles in tissue healing and regeneration, its large size and capacity to absorb large amounts of water allow HA to provide buffering action to the bite force on periodontal ligament.[40]

HA exhibits many beneficial effects in the treatment of periodontal disease including anti-inflammatory, anti-oedematous, anti-hyaluronidase and antibacterial effects.[41] HA is also used for gingivitis[42] and for its involvement in dental implant osseointegration.[43] Topical application for oral ulcers may also be effective;[44] its use has been suggested in a formula for dry mouth.[45] Levels of HA decrease with ageing.[46]

HA is synthesized by (three types of) hyaluronan synthases and degraded by hyaluronidases. *Centella asiatica* may stimulate the production of HA.[47]

Telomere length

Telomere length is also associated with ageing. These protective caps on the ends of chromosomes shorten as humans age, with quicker shortening associating with quicker ageing. Sugar intake has been shown to be associated with shorter telomere length and may accelerate cell ageing.[48]

Inflammation and oxidative stress also cause telomere shortening;[49] shorter telomere length and oxidative stress were found to be associated with periodontitis.[50]

Taste and smell perception in ageing

Altered taste/smell functioning is common in the elderly, with impairments due to a variety of factors: ageing, disease, medication use and environmental exposure. Such losses are of concern because they may contribute to malnutrition and weight loss as well as increasing vulnerability to food poisoning and possibly decreasing quality of life.[51] In older age, altered taste/smell is incorrectly attributed to external sources (i.e. 'food doesn't taste or smell the same as it used to') unlike altered vision or hearing, which is correctly attributed to physiological changes. Furthermore, older individuals may be consciously aware of taste/smell impairments.

The most common causes of smell disorders (which may also impact nutrient choice) include viral infections, head injuries, nasal obstructions and normal ageing, whereas drugs are common causes of taste dysfunction.[52]

Many medications induce taste problems, with some causing other oral side effects – for example, xerostomia (dry mouth), which may impact taste sensation as well as potentially impair oral health. Hyposalivation may increase concentration of drugs into saliva; the unpleasant taste of some medications may result in a stress response.[53]

Hyposalivatory drugs include antihistamines, antidepressants and analgesics, according to Handelman et al., who discuss the prevalence of drugs causing hyposalivation in institutionalized geriatrics, finding approximately half of this population received one or more drugs with this potential side effect.[54]

Drugs can also disrupt normal taste stimuli signals, distorting taste perception.[55,56]

Menstrual cycle changes may affect the bitter taste sensation; this may be protective for a woman and her fetus when ingestion of poison (often bitter) might disrupt fetal organ formation. Ability to taste bitterness diminishes in menopause.[57]

Impaired taste and smell perception (e.g. in the elderly) may alter nutrient intake and impair nutrient status and immunity.[58] A variety of medical conditions may induce a loss of taste and/or smell; Alzheimer's disease and cancer are two chronic medical conditions which are highly associated with taste/smell disorders.[59]

Evidence suggests that compensating for loss of taste/smell that occurs with advancing age, via flavour-enhanced food, may improve palatability, intake, salivary flow and immunity in elderly individuals, both healthy and ill.[60]

Dysgeusia

Disrupted taste can occur at any age. In addition to the issues discussed above (e.g. medications, altered hormones) which can be factors at any age, other specific health conditions may be associated, including Sjögren's syndrome, Bell's palsy, multiple sclerosis, renal failure, liver disease and some cancers. Less commonly, epilepsy, migraine headaches, some endocrine disorders (including diabetes and thyroid conditions) and psychiatric disorders (including depression and eating disorders) may be associated.

Infections which may be associated include herpes virus, candidiasis, gingivitis and periodontitis. Evidence of taste/smell loss is thought to be a symptom in largely asymptomatic individuals infected with SARS-CoV-2, the virus that caused the COVID-19 pandemic.[61] Dental procedures and dental appliances may also be associated with dysgeusia, as can exposure to some minerals and other substances (e.g. formaldehyde, benzene, chlorine and paint solvents).

Generally speaking, although commonly occurring, disruption of taste/smell seems to be of less interest to the medical profession than disrupted hearing or sight. Taste/smell issues may not be adequately addressed by the medical profession through lack of knowledge and understanding of these issues.[62] Consequently, patients may turn to nutritional therapists for advice.

SMOKING

Smoking and other oral behaviours show an association with the ability to taste. Smoking appears to impact sensitivity of the salt receptor as smokers require much higher concentrations of NaCl than (non-smoker) controls; this might cause an inadvertent increase in salt intake, contributing to increased risk for CVD, renal and other diseases.[63] Smokers were found to prefer salty and spiced foods, compared with non-smokers' preference for more bland foods; heavy smokers consume significantly more meat and eggs than non-smokers who consumed more fat (in cakes, sweets and chocolate).[64]

Clients who smoke may need to monitor salt intake.

Addressing loss of taste

Possibilities for natural therapies to address alteration of taste include the following substances, many of which may have other beneficial actions and effects on oral health. Many of these substances have strong tastes and smells, which may help to stimulate taste (including to alleviate symptoms of cold/flu that might be altering the sense of taste/smell), some due to anti-inflammatory effects and others because of antimicrobial or immunomodulatory effects:

- *Ginger*: Small pieces of peeled root can be chewed or consumed as ginger tea. Ginger can activate the taste buds and enhance the sense of smell. Anti-inflammatory effects[65] may help in blocked nasal passages.

- *Garlic*: Anti-inflammatory and immunomodulatory effects[66] may help in blocked nasal passages.

- *Cinnamon*: Anti-inflammatory and antimicrobial properties[67] – applying a paste of cinnamon (with a minimum amount of honey or similar) to the tongue for ten minutes may enhance the effect more than simply using it in foods.

- *Peppermint*: Antimicrobial, immunomodulatory and other effects[68] – drink peppermint tea.

- *Curry leaves (Murraya koenigii)*: Anti-inflammatory and antimicrobial effect[69] – add to a glass of water and infuse for 30 minutes before drinking.

- *Cayenne pepper*: An active constituent, capsaicin may help to clear nasal congestion[70] and stimulate saliva secretion.[71] Add cayenne pepper powder to warm water (sweeten with honey or similar as needed) and drink.

- *Apple cider vinegar*: It is sour and acidic so may stimulate the taste buds, and is anti-inflammatory.[72] Add a tablespoon of apple cider vinegar to a glass of warm water and drink.

- *Lemon*: It is strongly acidic so may stimulate the taste buds. Its high vitamin C content may support immune health. Add the juice of half a lemon to a glass of water and drink.

Other therapies that may help in cases of taste loss include the following:

- *Oil-pulling with sesame seed or coconut oil*: An antimicrobial and helps promote oral health.

- *Castor oil*: Ricinoleic acid in castor oil is a powerful anti-inflammatory.[73] Put a drop of warmed castor oil into each nostril.

- *Trachyspermum ammi seeds (aka Ajwain, bishop's weed, carom)*: They have an anti-inflammatory effect.[74] Inhalation of the aroma may help clear nasal passages.

- *Aromatherapy oils (peppermint, eucalyptus, cinnamon)*: Use a bowl of hot water and one or two drops of oil. Bend over the bowl and cover the head with a towel to enable steam inhalation for 10–15 minutes. The oils can also be used in a diffuser.

Nutrients may also help in cases of taste loss. Gustatory dysfunction is associated with deficiencies of zinc or copper, vitamin B12 or B3 (niacin).[75] Olfactory dysfunction is associated with deficiencies of zinc or copper, vitamin B12 (due to nerve damage),[76] B6, B3 (niacin) or vitamin A.[77]

Protocol considerations should include supporting immune function, detoxification, hydration and addressing stress, which may impair the sense of taste.

Satiety and overeating/obesity

The association of obesity with food intake suggests taste perception may be an important consideration in this condition. Obese individuals were found to be more sensitive to salty and sweet tastes and perceived these and sour more intensely than did lean individuals.[78]

Responses to the anticipation and consumption of food may be different in obese individuals, who show weaker activation in the striatum during food intake and so there is possibly an association with an altered release of dopamine.[79] Regulation of dopamine levels may benefit in such cases. Where necessary, levels of dopamine may be boosted by regular exercise, meditation, quality sleep, stress avoidance, listening to music, massage therapy and tyrosine-rich foods. L-theanine in green tea may help to increase dopamine.[80] Adaptogenic herbs such as *Rhodiola rosea* may also influence levels of dopamine and other neurotransmitters.[81]

Taste perception may be altered in depressed/anxious states, which may account for diminished or altered food consumption.[82] Since salivary secretion is controlled by sympathetic and parasympathetic innervations, an autonomic nervous system affected by depressive disorder can alter salivary composition, affecting oral health, increasing vulnerability to oral infection.[83] Ensuring appropriate cephalic response may have implications for satiety as well as weight regulation and oral health.

Texture hardness (during chewing) and sweetness of foods affects the endocrine cephalic response and satiation, according to Lasschuijt *et al.*, who found that sweetness increased overall pancreatic polypeptide response and that hardness increased overall ghrelin response.[84] Cephalic responses, which are both innate and learned, may be affected by inconsistencies between the sensory signal (e.g. the sweetness of artificial sweeteners) and the subsequent post-ingestive effect (here, lack of energy due to nil calories). Chewing stimulates salivation, enhancing orosensory stimulation; the amount and constituents of saliva might be associated with satiation.[85]

The overall flavour pleasantness of satiating (as opposed to sugary/fatty/salty) foods increased with repeated exposure over a period of three to six weeks during a weight loss intervention,[86] indicating that perceived palatability can change. A satiating diet (non-restricted minimum numbers of servings of whole vegetables, whole fruits, whole-grain fibre-rich products and lean protein, alongside one legume meal weekly, moderate fat consumption and flavour consumption of hot pepper or red pepper) resulted in twice the fat loss in obese men classified as having a low- or high-satiety phenotype. Satiety responsiveness improved and compliance was good; overall, the results suggest a non-restrictive, flavour-stimulating, highly satiating diet may be useful to improve body composition.[87]

Current and future satiety/taste research informs nutrition protocols.

LEPTIN AND ENDOCANNABINOIDS

Leptin (an anorexigenic mediator that inhibits hunger and reduces food intake via hypothalamic receptor Ob-Rb) and endocannabinoids have been investigated regarding sugar-addictive behaviours and obesity. Endocannabinoids are orexigenic mediators that act via cannabinoid CB_1 receptors in the hypothalamus, limbic forebrain and brainstem to induce appetite[88] and stimulate food intake. Circulating leptin may modulate sweet taste function at receptor level, with local endocannabinoids becoming more effective modulators under conditions of deficient leptin signalling. Endocannabinoids alter sweet taste response[89] and may play a role in regulating energy balance through their ability to alter taste perception.[90] The effect of phytocannabinoids such as CBD oil on hunger and food intake is the subject of current research; mixed effects have been found.

SWEET SENSING AND OBESITY

Diet-added sugars, initially sensed in the oral cavity, are a driving force behind the obesity epidemic; this is of particular concern during development.[91] Low-calorie sweeteners, also sensed in the oral cavity, have become common replacements for sucrose in an effort to reverse this obesity trend. Dissociating sweetness from energy may disrupt the balance between taste response, appetite and consumption patterns.[92]

Sweet receptors may also be triggered by these non-carbohydrate molecules (e.g. saccharin, aspartame, sucralose). These reactions to artificial sweeteners may involve different mechanisms than for sucrose and natural sugars.[93,94]

Findings that sweet-tasting molecules can interact with different sites within sweet taste receptors offer clarification as to how such a variety of molecules including simple sugars, sweeteners and some proteins can all taste sweet.[95] Studies also show that although sucralose (Splenda, a common artificial sweetener) may activate common taste pathways to those for sucrose, the primary taste cortex and reward circuitry are more activated for sucrose comparatively; only sucrose impacts dopaminergic midbrain areas in relation to the behavioural pleasantness response.[96]

Addictive substances

An innate and universal liking for sweetness is a 'given' and may relate to the role of sweet foods in providing energy and essential nutrients.[97] Tasting sweetness activates pleasure-generating brain circuitry, which has been demonstrated in binge-eating disorders;[98] this same circuitry may overlap with pathways that mediate the addictive nature of opiates and alcohol.[99]

Generally, drug, tobacco and alcohol dependence give rise to increased dental pathology.[100] Opiate use (methadone, heroin) has shown an independent association with dental pathology.[101] Methadone-maintained patients are especially prone to diabetes and weight gain.[102] For sweet cravings, chromium picolinate may be effective in treating binge-eating disorders and depression, based on its potential to improve insulin, dopamine and serotonin function.[103]

Sugar produces the symptoms of addictive substances – binge-behaviour, craving, tolerance, withdrawal, cross-sensitization, cross-tolerance, cross-dependence, reward and opioid effects – and overlaps exist in respect to behaviour as well as brain neurochemistry.[104] Addictive behaviours, including binge-eating and obesity, are not the focus of this book and require specialist protocols.

EATING DISORDERS

Eating disorders, including anorexia and bulimia nervosa, are associated with oral health symptoms as well as altered nutritive status. Oral manifestations may include dental caries, sensitivity, mucosal lesions, gingivitis, periodontitis, xerostomia, dysgeusia and oral pain. Mouth pH may be altered and made worse when vomiting regularly occurs.

Levels of ghrelin, also present in saliva, may be dysregulated in eating disorders, causing aberrations in eating behaviour; a greater understanding of the role of ghrelin in saliva may suggest improved treatment options.[105]

Sugar-craving

Sweet tastes tend to be an indication that food is safe to eat; humans have a natural attraction to sweet tastes. Whilst it is easy to think that sweet cravings are normal, cravings can be the first step to addiction, creating danger little by little. Cravings become more frequent; behaviour alters. Metabolism is also impacted, and the body and brain bear the toll: decreased energy, increased stress, accelerated ageing, worsening health, weight gain and sometimes outright disease.

Self-control mechanisms may be overridden. An association with the release of opioids and dopamine in the brain may result in dependence, or in binge-eating behaviours. Comparisons between sugar and illegal addictive drugs have been made on a variety of levels including sugar's highly processed 'pure' white crystalline form, habit-forming nature, and drug-like psychoactive effects.[106]

Behaviours that indicate when substance use becomes addiction include withdrawal and tolerance as well as consumption of larger amounts than intended, persistent desire/unsuccessful efforts to reduce substance use and continued use despite knowledge of it being a problem. The Yale Food Addiction Scale is a useful resource for determining whether an individual is addicted to sugar. The seven questions in this scale are given in Dr Marilyn Glenville's book *Natural Alternatives to Sugar*[107] in which she also describes a '5-Day Sugar Detox' that may radically change health and well-being, kickstarting body healing. Although this may be challenging for some, it is designed to help control sugar addictions.

Nutritional support

Therapeutic support for factors discussed in this chapter include recognizing that inflammaging and other ageing factors may increase the need for anti-inflammatory, connective-tissue-supportive and other oral-health-supportive protocols in ageing. Post-menopausal women, particularly, should be aware of the need to consider their oral and dental health.

Oral health should be assessed in all clients with hormonal disruption.

CONNECTIVE TISSUE SUPPORT

Hyaluronic acid may be particularly useful regarding connective tissue support for gingivae. *Echinacea* and gotu kola may promote hyaluronic acid.

Other natural support for connective tissue includes vitamin C, flavonoids (particularly anthocyanidins and catechins), vitamin A/beta-carotene, glucosamine, chondroitin, superoxide dismutase (spirulina/barley grass), zinc, copper, manganese, protein (especially amino acids – lysine, glycine, proline, glutamine), glucuronic acid (in globe artichokes) and proteolytic enzymes.

Ensuring optimal dietary protein intake supports connective tissue. Glycosaminoglycan-rich bone broth may be especially beneficial.

Therapies to support telomere length may benefit. A number of nutraceuticals may have benefit including ascorbic acid, selenium, CoQ10, vitamin D, carotenoids, omega-3 fatty acids[108] and homocysteine-lowering B vitamins.[109]

Regarding satiety, support for dopamine regulation via lifestyle and diet is discussed. *Rhodiola rosea* may be beneficial. Umami-rich foods may increase satiety.[110] Including hot pepper alongside the satiety dietary advice above may aid weight regulation.

Regarding the effects of weight loss and/or detoxing from sugar, as the body sheds toxins, side effects may be experienced, including tiredness, interrupted sleep, headaches, light-headedness, upset stomach, unusual bowel movements, spots/rashes/pimples, furry tongue, bad body odour/breath and cravings for sweet-tasting foods.[111] These effects will need to be addressed via lifestyle and other support.

This chapter included a number of suggestions regarding dysgeusia.

— Chapter 11 —

FUNCTIONAL DENTISTRY AND PERSONALIZED WELL-BEING

A dental degree makes all dentists, including holistic and biological dentists, doctors of the mouth and jaw. Dental professionals may choose to practise dentistry that is mercury free or mercury safe (i.e. uses SMART protocols – Safe Mercury Amalgam Removal Technique). Alternatively, they can practise with preventive strategies and understanding of the toxic nature of dentistry (i.e. biological dentistry) or with the aim of making people feel understood, taking into account emotional states (i.e. holistic dentistry).[1] All are conventionally trained professionals who further their knowledge/training.

Acupuncture, homeopathy, kinesiology, use of biocompatible materials, consideration of meridians and use of laser/lights and ozone are common therapies/practices employed by biological dentists.

Biological dentists concentrate on the complete human being, with their viewpoint closely allying the personalized health practices of nutritional therapists and functional medicine practitioners.

The term 'functional dentistry' is just starting to be used. Like functional medicine, functional dentistry is likely to mean 'from an evidence-based mindset'. Many of the practices and mindsets of biological dentistry are in line with those used in functional medicine. 'Functional dentistry' is still an undefined term. It may involve a team approach whereby a range of associated aspects – for example, bruxism, sleep apnoea, spinal health, breathing, dental arch development, awareness of microbiome, and role of diet – would be considered alongside other aspects.

Clearly, what is important – when oral health is so intimately connected with whole-body health, and since whole-body health is so intimately connected to health of the body's individual 'parts' including oral health – is a systematic approach and a (professional) team approach to health.

Crucial to understand regarding functional medicine (and dentistry) is that the client/patient becomes co-therapist, accepting responsibility for his/her own health.

Adjunctive therapies

In addition to its antimicrobial activity (bactericidal, virucidal, fungicidal and parasiticidal), ozone may have the capacity to stimulate blood circulation, immune response[2] and remineralization of recent caries-affected teeth.[3] A 2015 systematic literature review of its application in dentistry discusses the potential of ozone therapy to impact inflammation, pain and wound healing, as well as having antimicrobial action, immune-stimulating action and anti-hypoxic action, and roles in periodontics, prosthodontics, endodontics, implantology and caries prevention/management.[4]

Ozone therapy is minimally invasive, quite economical,[5] painless and atraumatic,[6] eliminates dental phobia,[7] and can be used for sterilizing cavities, disinfecting root canals and periodontal pockets, bleaching discoloured teeth, desensitizing extremely sensitive teeth, enhancing epithelial wound healing, as a denture cleaner and to decontaminate toothbrushes.[8]

Gupta and Deepa (2016)[9] summarize the literature on the applications of ozone in dentistry, providing historical background, generating systems, applications, mechanisms of action, applications, advantages/disadvantages and contraindications – thus providing a good introduction to readers unfamiliar with ozone therapy in oral health.

Homeopathic remedies are sometimes used in dentistry, primarily to improve the psychological or emotional condition of the patient,[10] for example via pain relief. All symptoms are matched to distinct remedies.

Homeopathic mouthwashes with hypericum and/or calendula and homeopathic toothpastes with *Krameria* (aka rhatany/ratanhia) may also be available.[11]

Tissue salts are sometimes suggested, either chewed or allowed to dissolve inside the mouth so that absorption is via mucous membranes. See Appendix 4 for information sources on homeopathy and tissue salts.

Kinesiology is sometimes suggested as potentially useful for TMJ, bruxism and the restoration of worn dentitions.[12]

Most common uses of acupuncture in dentistry relate to their analgesic effect and for the management of TMJ, prominent gag reflex and dental anxiety.[13] Oral acupuncture (in the mouth) is sometimes used by biological dentists.

Effects of emotion and stress

Emotional events, trauma and stressful situations are primary triggers of mouth/dental pain. Negative emotions create stress which results in a cascade effect within physiology and biochemistry, thus causing symptoms. This concept is familiar to nutritional therapists as fight or flight. The body may tense, moving joints out of position and deviating facial alignment. Misalignment, whether from TMJ or from other parts of the body, may result in a cascade effect.

Structural, emotional, neurological, biochemical, mental and nutritional imbalances may all be implicated. The fight–flight reaction may lead to body acidity, an inability to digest foods, muscle tension, and deficiencies of magnesium[14] and zinc[15] as well as B vitamins and vitamin C. In stress, the body is often dehydrated, so is not detoxifying, allowing toxins to build up and essential minerals to deplete. Magnesium deficiency may contribute to muscle tension and various health conditions. Zinc deficiency may contribute to immune issues including allergies and viruses. Shallow breathing may also occur, resulting in body acidity.

The effects of negative emotions and stress on the body should not be underestimated. Several therapies may help address emotional issues and they should be considered as adjunctive therapies in dental/oral issues. Examples include Bach Flower Remedies and ActaLine® therapy. See Appendix 4.

Implications in nutritional therapy

Awareness and understanding of biological dentistry and possible therapies used in this approach generally fit with holistic approaches used by nutritional therapists and similar professionals. Nutritional therapists may wish to link with biological dentists to facilitate referrals; a coordinated approach to inflammatory conditions, for example, may benefit clients and improve outcomes.

— Chapter 12 —

ORAL HYGIENE ALTERNATIVES

Coconut oil pulling and salt water rinses are much discussed online as beneficial means to improve mouth health and clients may already be aware of their use. The use of activated charcoal and clays is potentially confusing due to the number of product types available. Greater familiarity with them may be useful for practitioners.

Practitioners already familiar with the use of CoQ10 for energy and healthy ageing protocols may wish to use oral spray delivery for clients with oral health issues for this added benefit.

Oil-pulling

Oil-pulling is an ancient folk remedy in which oils from plants are held and swished in the mouth for long periods of time for health benefit. It is claimed that toxins and bacteria can be drawn out by this practice and expelled by spitting out the oil. Oil-pulling is thought to strengthen gums and whiten teeth as well as eliminate plaque.[1]

Historically, oil-pulling practices were used to prevent bleeding gums, dry throat, bad breath, decay and cracked lips as well as to strengthen the gums, teeth and jaw. Today, oil-pulling is usually described as a 20-minute process of swishing before spitting out and is recommended in addition to (usually before) tooth brushing. The liquid in the mouth nearly doubles in volume during the swishing as saliva production is stimulated; the consistency of the oil when spat out is described as unpleasant and can be off-putting.

Studies show oil-pulling may reduce plaque index and modify gingival scores.[2] Oil-pulling has also shown positive benefits in treating halitosis.[3,4]

The mechanisms of action of oil-pulling therapy are unclear but several have been suggested.[5] The emulsification process of the oil was found to start five minutes after commencement;[6] due to the agitation of the oil in the mouth, a soapy layer is formed. This and/or the viscosity of the oil may alter bacterial adhesion on tooth surfaces, removing damaged/worn-out cells, preventing bacterial adhesion and plaque coaggregation.[7,8]

In addition to oral health benefits, oil-pulling is thought to support/strengthen the body's immune system – thus conferring health and function to the whole body – possibly via quietening inflammation and shifting toxins.[9]

Oil-pulling is recommended before eating, drinking (including water) or cleaning teeth and can be practised three times daily (always before meals on an empty stomach).[10] The oil should not be swallowed and must be spat out to have the purported benefit. Teeth should be brushed after oil-pulling.

Although there are many advantages of oil-pulling (it is inexpensive, completely harmless and doesn't cause staining or allergic reactions), the American Dental Association does not recommend it as a dental hygiene practice.[11]

Oils popularly used for this practice include coconut, sesame, sunflower, olive and palm oils. Because coconut oil becomes solid at higher temperatures than some other oils, it may have more beneficial effect blended with other oils such as sesame. Sesame oil is recommended primarily in Ayurvedic literature for daily use. Coconut and other oils are suggested for specific issues.[12] Coconut oil has, for example, antibacterial and antifungal activity.[13]

Salt rinses

Salt rinses are an alternative to commercial mouthwashes. They use sea salt or Himalayan salt and are suggested for toothache, healing oral tissues and even, by some, for healing dental caries.[14]

For healthful purposes, unrefined salts must be used. Refined salt has been bleached and put through harsh chemical processes; it may have ferrocyanide and aluminium in it. Some of the chemicals added to refined salt increase shelf life by absorbing moisture; this interferes with the regulatory functions of salt with respect to body hydration. Unrefined sea salts and Himalayan salt do not have these added chemicals, and do boast many natural trace minerals.[15]

Salt has many health benefits and has been used medicinally for thousands of years in a variety of ways. The antiseptic and bactericidal qualities of sea salt benefit plaque removal.[16]

SALT WATER RINSE

To make a salt water rinse dissolve enough unrefined sea salt/Himalayan salt in cold or lukewarm water to make a strong solution (between 0.9% and 27% is

> recommended).[17] Swish the solution vigorously around the mouth allowing the brine to cause salivation. Always spit out a salt water rinse.

Salt is also found in some toothpastes and can be used straight to clean teeth. Salt causes salivation which naturally creates an antibacterial barrier to protect enamel. Salt and baking soda can be used together as a toothpaste to replace/augment use of commercial toothpaste.

Exploring 'the dirt' on clays and charcoal

Activated charcoal, a black powder made from coconut shells or other natural ingredients (e.g. olive pits), is known for its powerful detoxifying power and ability to absorb dirt and impurities. Although its inclusion in toothpastes (and face masks, shampoos, body scrubs and even energy drinks) is currently trending, activated charcoal has been used for hundreds of years for its adsorbent properties.

In rural parts of Africa, charcoal may be used to clean teeth due to the unavailability of other oral hygiene products. But does its undisputed use for treatment of poisoning and overdoses[18] make activated charcoal an ideal toothpaste ingredient for daily oral hygiene?

Also known as activated carbon, activated charcoal is highly porous and thus has a high surface area. It uses adsorption (surface adhesion capacity) which gives it binding capacity. The pores have a magnetic-like capacity to attract unwanted substances and toxins. When activated charcoal binds to acidic elements it can increase the excretion rate from the body,[19] raising oral cavity pH and helping to reduce build-up of acidic plaque.

Some cautions regarding oral cavity use of activated charcoal should be considered. Since it can be gritty, activated charcoal may polish teeth, but may also wear down enamel and should not be used with an aggressive brushing action. Smearing it on teeth with a finger can be an alternative, or gentle circular motions with thorough cleansing afterwards via rinsing. Some suggest use two to three times weekly (or less often) may be sufficient and that daily use may be too much.[20]

Activated charcoal may help to remove stains, favourably impact mouth pH, and may help destroy bacteria that cause bad breath, but results of a 2017 review did not find sufficient clinical and laboratory data to substantiate the safety and efficacy claims for charcoal and charcoal-based dentifrices.[21] Charcoal-containing toothpastes may be most effective as a means to delay recurrence of surface staining after professional cleaning of teeth.[22]

Whilst activated charcoal may help to remove extrinsic tooth staining, it can stain sinks, grout, clothing, etc.; care should be taken, and sinks should be wiped immediately. A suggestion sometimes made is to use two different toothbrushes, one for applying charcoal and one for brushing after rinsing.

Like activated charcoal, bentonite clay has detoxifying capacity. Clays have been used medicinally since prehistoric times, and geophagy (eating substances like clay or chalk) has been mentioned in many famous ancient medicinal texts. Today, clay is being considered in scientific studies for its medicinal potential, for example its antimicrobial benefits, especially in light of 'superbug' MRSA (methicillin-resistant *Staphylococcus aureus*) infections.[23]

Bentonite and montmorillonite clays are the most commonly used clays mentioned for oral health use. White kaolin clay is sometimes used in toothpastes. When compared to other whitening dentifrices (mainly containing hydrated silicas, but also other abrasives – e.g. sodium bicarbonate/calcium carbonate/dicalcium phosphate), the most efficient, assessed for abrasion, polishing and stain removal characteristics, contained refined kaolin clay as the abrasive.[24]

Different types of bentonite are referred to with respect to their dominant element; calcium bentonite, potassium bentonite and sodium bentonite are commonly discussed. All are highly absorbent. Calcium bentonite is the type most commonly seen in oral healthcare products.

Bentonite and montmorillonite clays have absorption capacity as much as eight times greater than other clays.[25] Although these clays are not specifically the same, their properties and abilities are similar and so are considered to be interchangeable.[26] Accordingly, in this book, hereafter, both clays will be referred to as bentonite clay. Bentonite clay is made of the mineral montmorillonite but montmorillonites are not bentonites.[27]

Although it has been suggested that some clays (e.g. kaolin) have a bleaching capability for hair[28] – and alongside bentonite may be referred to as 'bleaching clays'[29] – they are sometimes used in oral care products as a thickener.[30]

Bentonite clay has been studied and reviewed as a natural remedy for numerous benefits to body function; its safety has been demonstrated, including after chronic oral consumption.[31] Bentonite clay has absorptive and adsorptive properties; the negatively charged particles in the clay can bind with positively charged particles (e.g. toxins); some clay minerals act like a sponge in this respect.[32] This benefits teeth/gums by neutralizing oral bacteria and toxins/impurities on tooth surfaces.

Alkalizing minerals such as calcium and potassium are also present in bentonite clay[33] and may raise mouth pH, neutralizing harmful acid as well as potentially aiding remineralization of tooth enamel.

Bentonite clay also contains minerals such as silica[34] (also found in diatomaceous earth) which is mildly abrasive, so may aid dental plaque removal; the superfine particles of bentonite clay may aid teeth polishing. Bentonite clay may aid whitening via its capacity to de-colour.[35]

DIATOMACEOUS EARTH AND ZEOLITE

Like activated charcoal and bentonite clay, diatomaceous earth (DE) is sometimes found in dentifrices. DE is a naturally occurring, soft, easily crumbled, silica-rich rock consisting of fossilized remains of diatoms (silica-rich microalgae). Deposits of DE vary with regard to composition of silica as well as being found in combination with other clays and minerals.

Diatomaceous earth is mildly abrasive and has been used in toothpastes as well as facial scrubs. Diatomaceous earth is more abrasive than bentonite clay, and like the clay can be taken internally (food grade only). The silica content of DE is higher than for bentonite clay. For dentifrices, the preferred diatomaceous silica should contain 94–96 per cent SiO_2, and no solid material harder than the diatomaceous silica which might otherwise damage tooth enamel.[36]

According to Claudia Orgill, author of *Beyond Wheat and Weeds*, in her comparison of DE, bentonite clay and activated charcoal, it is unknown how much of the trace minerals in DE can be absorbed by the body; bentonite clay may be more reliable in this respect.[37]

The potential advantages of DE include possible antiparasitic qualities (although bentonite clay and activated charcoal may also have this quality, DE may be a better option). Both DE and bentonite clay may be useful for *Candida* infections, although the clay may act more slowly.

Zeolites, which form when volcanic lava meets water,[38] are aluminosilicate minerals, but are microporous like these other substances. Zeolite does occur naturally but is also industrially produced; clinoptilolite is a naturally occurring zeolite.

Zeolite, advantageously, releases ortho-silicic acid (a bioavailable form of silicon).[39] Zeolite may also alkalize[40] and easily mixes in water (compared with bentonite clay).

Calcium bentonites are richer in calcium and silica for re-mineralizing the body, and have high montmorillonite content, so may be best all round. When using bentonite clay, always use non-metal utensils due to the high negative charge of the clay which may pull metals from the utensils, lessening the detoxing capacity of the clay.

With respect to daily detoxing, Orgill claims bentonite clay is the better option. Calcium bentonite has been shown to have clinical applications in dentistry.[41]

CoQ10

Co-enzyme Q10 (CoQ10) has several important roles in the body and, in addition to roles related to mitochondrial energy and membrane health, functions as an antioxidant.[42] It has been suggested that CoQ10 counters the negative effects caused by the induction of overproduction of reactive oxygen species by periodontal pathogens, and reduces associated collagen degradation.[43,44]

CoQ10 is known to impact the immune system, improving host defence mechanisms in periodontal disease. A US patent dated 2002 discusses the potential benefits of 100mg CoQ10 over two months in 22 patients with periodontal disease.[45] The beneficial effects from topical application via toothpastes, mouthwashes and lozenges are also discussed by the inventors. Topical CoQ10 in gel form alongside hyaluronic acid[46] or tea tree oil (*Melaleuca alternifolia*)[47] have also shown benefits. CoQ10 oral sprays are available.

Gingival tissue in periodontal disease is often significantly deficient in CoQ10.[48] Topical application of CoQ10 may improve cases of adult periodontitis by reducing bleeding.[49]

― Chapter 13 ―

ORAL HEALTHCARE INGREDIENTS

This chapter looking at oral hygiene delves into product ingredients including controversial ingredients, potentially toxic ingredients to avoid, as well as 'natural' ingredients that might be beneficially included in dentifrices and mouthwashes.

Some beneficial ingredients have previously been mentioned: oils for oil-pulling, salt for rinses, and the sweeteners stevia and xylitol. More are discussed below.

Information in this chapter is important because clients welcome product ingredient suggestions and practitioners can use this information as a starting point.

Overview

Oral care products are big business. The diversity of product type is expanding. Today, in addition to collapsible-tube toothpastes, there are stand-up tubes, pump delivery method and choice of paste or gel, as well as the option of tooth powder.

Included ingredients have different purposes – some of them relate to the overall intention of the product, which should be maintenance of healthy oral tissue and teeth, whilst others relate to the production or delivery of the product (e.g. humectants), or are added to entice the customer to purchase (e.g. colours). See Appendix 3.

Fluoride

Fluoride remains a controversial ingredient in oral health products. It is clear that caution should be exercised – for example, with adults for whom thyroid health is an issue (due to displacement of iodine, a mineral needed for function of salivary and mammary glands, gastric mucosa and the thyroid)[1] and for those wanting children (due to the effect on testosterone concentration[2] and male fertility,[3] association with Down syndrome births,[4] decreased birth rates[5] and impact on fetal brain development).[6] Approximately half of ingested fluoride is stored in bone, where it lowers compressive strength and resilience/toughness of bone.[7] Fluoride can accumulate in the body,[8] including the pineal gland,[9] and negatively impact IQ[10] and health in various ways,[11] being toxic at 1ppm with potential effects on the central nervous system.[12]

Fluoride can also confer some benefits, interfering with demineralization processes that occur in tooth decay and promoting remineralization.[13] Some believe fluoride inclusion in toothpastes designed for children under age eight is acceptable, even necessary, on the basis that the advantages outweigh the disadvantages. The critical period in terms of fluoride exposure and the risk of fluorosis is between the ages of 15 and 30 months, with the risk reducing by approximately age eight.[14] Under eights are also arguably the group for whom ensuring toothpaste is not swallowed is most difficult. Data indicates that the risk of dental fluorosis for children between 12 and 15 years in the USA has risen over recent years.[15]

FLUORIDE LABELLING AND ADVERTISING

Fluoride is a substance that warrants cautionary advice on packaging; the US Food and Drug Administration (FDA) requires specific wording or labelling on over-the-counter 'anti-caries drug products' such as toothpastes and mouth-washes, including strict warnings for children.[16] An example warning reads: 'Keep out of reach of children under 6 years of age. If more than used for brushing is accidentally swallowed, get medical help or contact a Poison Control Center right away.' It should be remembered that only a pea-sized amount of toothpaste is generally advised. And most toothpaste tubes are kept at bathroom sink level for convenience.

A 2014 research article looking at marketing strategies and warning labels on children's toothpastes found aggressive and misleading marketing strategies often used, as well as depiction of full swirls of toothpaste (which directly contradicts dentists' recommendations for young children)[17] rather than a pea-sized amount.

Chronic fluoride toxicity symptoms include many common complaints: chronic fatigue, throat dryness, frequent urination, urinary tract infections, muscle/bone aches/stiffness, and skin rash/itching.[18]

Decisions regarding the use of toothpastes containing fluoride, mouth rinses, dental floss and gel formulas applied by dental hygienists needs to be a personal call. When it comes to children, parents must be made aware of the issues to enable them to make an educated decision, taking account of local fluoride levels in water (naturally occurring and municipally added) and the individual health circumstances of their child.

Carrageenan

Carrageenan, from seaweed, is a common thickening agent found in toothpastes, including natural toothpastes. Whilst carrageenan is natural, it may not be totally safe for everyone. Carrageenan may trigger or magnify intestinal inflammatory responses, and, although unlikely to be determined as sole factor in IBD (inflammatory bowel disease) development, may contribute, especially in light of increasing use of carrageenan in a number of 'Western' foods.[19]

The inclusion of carrageenan in toothpastes is somewhat controversial. Other ingredients may be more beneficial. Individuals with existing inflammatory gut issues should probably avoid carrageenan in foods and oral care products.

Glycerine

Glycerine is controversially found in some natural oral care products. Glycerine (aka glycerol) is a sweet, colourless liquid and a component of triglycerides. It may help with the distribution of oil (including essential oils) in water emulsions.[20] In toothpastes, glycerine serves as a moisturizer and humectant, preventing the paste from drying out. Despite being controversial, glycerine is harmless to teeth.[21]

Glycerine/glycerol has the same caloric value as sucrose and only 40 per cent of the sweetness, with a mildly sweet taste. This by-product of soap manufacture is harmless to teeth but can have a mild laxative effect. It may not be suitable for vegetarians, depending on the source.[22]

To avoid the use of glycerine, demineralizing powders (which are, in effect, dehydrated toothpastes) may be a useful option.

Titanium dioxide: Unclear effects

Titanium dioxide (TiO_2) is a product whitener found in toothpastes and chewing gums as well as in cosmetics, foods and pharmaceuticals as TiO_2 nanoparticles. Titanium dioxide is also found in paints, providing maximum whiteness and opacity.

A 2016 study looked at the effects of titanium dioxide nanoparticles on the gastrointestinal tract, finding some particle sizes induced an inflammatory response.[23] Nano-TiO_2 is commonly used in food products, and over 93 per cent of TiO_2 in chewing gum is nano-TiO_2, which is easily swallowed when the product is chewed.[24] The full potential effect of this is still being investigated.

Triclosan

Triclosan, which is found in a wide range of products from soap, cosmetics and deodorant to kitchenware, clothes and children's toys, has a number of toxic characteristics according to a 2004 article which discusses both acute and chronic effects, the ability of triclosan to bioaccumulate in fatty tissues, its link with allergies and dioxin and the possibility that it may promote bacterial resistance.[25] Triclosan, like other endocrine-disrupting compounds (e.g. bisphenol A), may negatively affect human immune function.[26]

A pesticide used as an antibacterial agent in toothpastes, triclosan is the trade name for 5-Chloro-2-(2,4-dichlorophenoxy)phenol and it is manufactured from the same raw material as 2,4-D, a component of Agent Orange (the infamous defoliant used in the Vietnam War).[27]

Although triclosan was banned by the USA in 2016 from soaps, it is permitted in toothpaste. Since exposure is both longer than for soap, and internal for toothpaste rather than external for soap, the rationale for its continued status in oral care products is surprising.

Other toxic ingredients

The area under the tongue readily absorbs substances – both good and bad. Although toothpastes and mouthwashes are meant to be spat out, harmful chemicals from these products can enter the body, even when they are spat out.

Some of these synthetic ingredients found in toothpastes are well known for causing health problems as ingredients in other products. Sodium lauryl sulfate (SLS) and sodium laureth sulfate (SLES) are foaming agents. SLS and SLES are penetration enhancers and surfactants with the main purpose of providing a foaming lather.

SLS has been shown to be associated with mouth ulcers; the denaturing effect of SLS on the delicate oral mucin layer, with exposure of the underlying epithelium, induces increased incidence of recurrent mouth ulcers.[28]

Propylene glycol is a type of mineral oil used in anti-freeze. Its use in toothpaste is as surfactant; it has been shown to be an irritant to skin, eyes and lungs.[29]

DEA (diethanolamine) is considered by the EWG (Environmental Working Group)[30] to be high on its list of toxic cosmetic ingredients. This foaming agent and pH adjuster is considered by the California Environmental Protection Agency as a possible human carcinogen.[31]

Parabens are widely used preservatives. Research suggests that parabens have oestrogen-mimicking properties and may be associated with impaired fertility and fetal development, as well as having a potential association with increased risk of breast cancer.[32]

Another glycol, diethylene glycol, which appears harmless and tastes sweet, is extremely toxic and has been found in Chinese-made toothpastes exported world-wide; in the UK a counterfeit batch of Sensodyne toothpaste containing this was found on sale in Derbyshire in 2007.[33]

Microbeads and alcohol

Microbeads, tiny plastic pellets often found in facial scrubs, have been used in toothpastes, although the recognition that they might become trapped under the gums, potentially causing or contributing to gum disease, means microbeads use has been banned in some locations. In 2016, the UK government announced its intention to ban manufacture and sale of personal care products containing microbeads. Ingredients lists should be checked for polyethylene or polypropylene when outside the UK.

Alcohol (ethanol) is found in many over-the-counter mouthwashes but does not contribute to any therapeutic action. Since it is not an active ingredient in mouthwash, in some countries alcohol does not have to be listed, although it can cause a burning sensation (via activation of vanilloid receptor-1), may irritate xerostomia (dry mouth) and is an epithelium irritant.[34]

Artificial colours and sweeteners

Many conventional toothpastes include synthetic colours. Titanium dioxide may be added to whiten, whilst other colours may be added for interest – some toothpastes even have stripes. Many synthetic colours are derived from coal tar. In the USA, many colours have been banned and some are under review for links to hyperactivity, migraines, anxiety and more serious conditions.

Since toothpaste should be spat out, the question is raised: should it be sweetened?

Artificial sweeteners are included in many conventional and some 'alternative' toothpastes. In addition to sweetening the paste, making it more pleasing in taste to the user, some sweetening ingredients may have other functions. For example, sorbitol may also be added to prevent the toothpaste from drying out. With respect to fluoridated toothpastes, fluoride necessitates the addition of a sweetener since fluoride is bitter. Sweeteners are found in both fluoridated and non-fluoridated toothpastes.

CAUTION: ASPARTAME

Aspartame, which is composed of aspartic acid and phenylalanine, is sometimes found as a sweetener in toothpastes. The phenylalanine in aspartame is synthetically modified with a methyl group that often results in the formation of methanol, a harmful by-product that, unlike the methanol found in fruit and vegetables, which is bonded to pectin and easily passes through the digestive tract, is unbonded in aspartame.[35]

Because humans cannot break down methanol into harmless formic acid, methyl alcohol travels through the body, including to the brain, where it converts to formaldehyde, which damages the sensitive brain tissue.[36] A number of symptoms from methanol poisoning can occur.

Choose instead toothpastes that use stevia, erythritol or xylitol as sweeteners as these may have benefits to oral health.

'Natural' toothpaste ingredients

There are increasing numbers of toothpastes marketed as 'natural' and brands professing to be all natural. 'Natural' has even been defined by some brands as 'of plant source'. But natural should also mean unprocessed (more realistically, minimally processed). Careful read of packaging/labelling is needed to find products which most benefit and suit individual need (see Appendix 3).

Whilst natural, plant-based, unprocessed ingredients are desirable in toothpaste/tooth powder, alongside absence of potentially harmful/undesirable ingredients, each ingredient in oral care products must confer benefit.

Some commonly found oral care ingredients have already been discussed: clays, activated charcoal, sea salt, xylitol and stevia. A large number of other natural ingredients may be found in both conventional and 'alternative' oral care products. Many are herbs and spices. Some of those most commonly found are discussed below; this is not an exhaustive list.

Baking soda may provide numerous useful functions as part of oral care programmes, so is commonly found in dentifrices. Baking soda (sodium bicarbonate) may help remove stains as well as being both alkaline and mineral rich. It is also abrasive, so care is required to avoid damaging enamel. Baking soda does not kill bacteria, but dentifrices with this ingredient show enhanced plaque removal effectiveness.[37] Baking soda dentifrices are useful for occasional use.

Hydrated silica is used as a mineral abrasive in dentifrices because it provides gentle cleaning without damaging tooth enamel. It is sometimes added to whitening toothpastes. There are many grades of hydrated silica based on particle size; very fine, powder-like silicas are usually used as thickening agents and included even in non-whitening products. Hydrating the silica creates a smooth gel so it is abrasive enough to remove stains but not enough to damage tooth enamel.[38]

Hydrated silica was described as a 'high-performance abrasive' in an assessment of 41 toothpastes available to the European market (in 1995) which found that its inclusion is associated with reduced abrasiveness without loss of cleaning efficacy.[39]

L-arginine has been found to remove mature oral biofilm and may enhance efficacy of mouth rinses[40] and toothpaste.[41] Higher arginine deaminase system activity by oral bacteria (which increases local pH) is associated with fewer caries lesions.[42]

Mints

Peppermint typically has a higher percentage of menthol (40%) than spearmint (0.5%), which smells more delicate and is less pungent and tastes milder, its flavour coming more from carvone content.[43] Both are used in toothpastes, although peppermint is considered more medicinal and may be more frequently used.

Peppermint oil has shown antibacterial properties[44] as well as being antifungal and antibiofilm.[45]

The cooling sensation of mint can be soothing. Menthol in mints does not decrease surface temperature but evokes a perception of coolness via the TRPM8 ion channel. Binding to this receptor by menthol opens a pore, causing calcium influx into cells, generating action potentials that signal the brain. Since it is the same receptor that responds to cool temperature it sends the same message to the brain, which cannot distinguish between causes, so menthol gives a sensation of 'coolness'.[46]

Natural and synthetic menthol have different effects on the body. Although some toothpastes use synthetic mints, they are less refreshing and have about 25 per cent of the cooling power of natural versions.

Wintergreen (*Gaultheria procumbens*, not mint but has a mint-like flavour) has been used for hundreds of years in tooth powders and chewing gum. Native Americans used wintergreen for pain and as an anti-inflammatory; one of its active components is methyl salicylate (with similar action to salicylic acid, i.e. aspirin).[47] Wintergreen activates TRPA1 ion channels which are activated by noxious cold.[48,49]

Spices

Cloves, cinnamon, ginger and mustard oil also activate TRPA1 ion channels.[50] Cloves have been traditionally linked to oral health and used to soothe toothache since at least the 13th century.[51] Clove can be used as a natural antiseptic and has antimicrobial[52,53] properties as well as great taste.

Cinnamaldehyde (the main constituent of cinnamon oil) and mustard oil (an active ingredient of horseradish and wasabi) are robust TRPA1 activators.[54] Main volatile components of wasabi are isothiocyanates; these compounds are antimicrobial, showing anti-caries activity.[55] Wasabi has been used in toothpastes.

Pharmacological activities of *Cinnamomum cassia* (the form most used in the UK for cooking) include anti-inflammatory, anti-diabetic, antioxidant, liver-protecting, anti-ulcer, antimicrobial, antifungal, anti-gout, anti-cancer and anti-HIV activity.[56,57] Cassia cinnamon, however, is not 'true' cinnamon; *Cinnamomum zeylanicum* ('true' cinnamon) is well researched for antimicrobial effect in oral issues.

Volatile oils from *C.zeylanicum* bark, leaf and root vary in composition; essential oil from bark contains trans-cinnamaldehyde, eugenol and linalool. Cinnamaldehyde is the major constituent of this oil and, with respect to oral health, shows antimicrobial, antimutagenic and possible antiparasitic effect.[58] *Cinnamomum zeylanicum* also has antioxidant and free-radical scavenging properties, inhibitory effects on osteoclastogenesis, wound-healing properties, and anti-nociceptive and anti-inflammatory activity.[59]

Cinnamomum zeylanicum bark essential oil has antimicrobial activity against *C.albicans*,[60] antibacterial activity against cariogenic bacteria *S.mutans* and *S.sobrinus* strains,[61] ability to impair *P.gingivalis* membrane integrity by enhancing cell permeability,[62] and to control bad breath via inhibitory effect on production of H_2S by *Solobacterium moorei* (Gram-positive anaerobic bacterium specifically associated with halitosis).[63]

Although a relatively uncommon disorder, contact stomatitis (inflammation of mouth/lips) associated with consumption of cinnamon (unspecified form) flavouring agents has been documented;[64] such reactions may be caused by cinnamon 'mints'/sweets or chewing gum.[65] Hypersensitivity to cinnamon should be considered and ruled out in cases of burning sensation, ulceration or inflammation.

Some people react badly to cinnamon in contact with mucous membranes; it can sensitize and irritate the mouth and be highly caustic. Cautions around cinnamon do not suggest its exclusion from oral care products because there are also many potential benefits. However, for some individuals, cinnamon can be an irritant, and this should be noted in cases of symptoms that might suggest a reaction to this spice.

Essential oils

Several essential oils may be found in toothpastes; most commonly they include clove, oregano, peppermint, tea tree and cinnamon. Whilst these have useful antibacterial properties which may help fight oral infection (cinnamon being perhaps the strongest),[66] there is also potential for them to negatively impact the oral microbiome[67] and some have been shown to negatively impact periodontal tissue.[68] It may be wise to alternate use of highly antimicrobial dentifrices. Ingredients lists indicate the relative volume of antimicrobial ingredients.

Mouthwashes with antibacterial chamomile and calendula extracts were found to have a less damaging effect than essential oils such as salvia.[69] Not all essential oils are highly antibacterial – for example, aniseed (*Pimpinella anisum*) is a usefully included essential oil.[70]

Essential oils are highly concentrated and extremely potent. Many carry serious warnings for this reason. When compared to topical (skin) or internal use, essential oils for use in oral cavities and toothpastes have the lowest recommended dosage.[71] Some essential oils should be avoided during pregnancy.

Whilst reputable companies should provide safe dilutions and instructions for use, essential oils should be used internally only under the guidance of suitably qualified medical professionals (in the UK, aromatherapists are not trained on internal use).[72] Individuals should not attempt to make their own toothpastes or mouth rinses with essential oils without first discussing this with a suitably qualified professional.

Essential oils can, however, be used topically (diluted, on skin) and in diffusers for inhalation. Lavender oil is particularly recommended for its soothing, anti-anxiety effects and potential to aid relaxation and relieve stress. Dentists may use an essential oil during treatment or recommend its addition to water used in Waterpik® (or similar) devices.[73] Always check for how long the dentist recommends such use.

Like cinnamon oil, *Eucalyptus*, *Melaleuca alternifolia* (tea tree), lemon and lavender essential oils also show various antimicrobial actions with respect to oral health.[74]

Other natural oral healthcare ingredients

Salvadora persica, also known as the toothbrush tree, has been used most extensively for centuries as one of many plant species providing 'miswak', the chewing sticks used by various cultures to clean teeth. Chemical constituents of *S.persica* include fluorides, silica and flavonoids which may benefit oral health; research indicates antimicrobial and anti-cariogenic effects with use of this plant.[75]

Zanthoxylum armatum, also known as 'toothache tree' and as Indian prickly ash, has many traditional uses, particularly in the Indian system of medicine. North American natives also used this plant, applying crushed bark to gums for toothache relief. Studies indicate antifungal, antibacterial and many other properties.[76]

Other botanicals offering anti-inflammatory or soothing effect include German chamomile[77] and *Calendula officinalis*[78] which show improvement of gingival inflammation.

Myrrh, resin from stems of *Commiphora* plants, is one of the oldest known medicines and has been used for numerous oral health conditions including mouth ulcers, sore throat and gingivitis.[79] Myrrh has antiseptic properties as well as anti-inflammatory and antimicrobial action,[80] promoting healing and repair of damaged tissue when used short term (less than two weeks) in low-concentration suspension.[81] Use gentle and soothing myrrh to help keep gums strong and for anti-inflammatory and antiseptic properties.

Rhatany/ratanhia is the root of *Krameria triandra*, rich in oligomeric proanthocyanidins and tannins and with a powerfully astringent and significant antimicrobial action.[82] Ratanhia is considered a useful agent alone or with myrrh for addressing spongy and bleeding gums and for preserving teeth,[83] helping to strengthen gums. Ratanhia has also been studied for its beneficial effect in cases of oral mucositis in cancer chemotherapy patients.[84]

Horse chestnut (*Aesculus hippocastanum*) extracts and its active constituent saponins (collectively known as aescin) are potent anti-inflammatory and astringent compounds which may help tone gums.[85] Horse chestnut constituents may inhibit metalloproteinases (gelatinase, collagenase) which detach periodontal ligaments from the alveolar bone.[86]

The well-known Indian botanical, neem (*Azadirachta indica*), with more than 135 constituents including nimbin, quercetin and beta-sitosterol,[87] exhibits antimicrobial and anti-plaque activity;[88] neem-based mouth rinses are highly efficacious for periodontal disease treatment.[89]

Other useful botanicals for periodontitis include *Aloe vera*, chamomile, liquorice root (*Glycyrrhiza glabra*), pomegranate (*Punica granatum*) fruit and *Centella asiatica* (gotu kola).[90]

There are many other natural substances with potential benefits including sage, fennel, *Bambusa arundinacea*, barberry, papaya, bromelain and colloidal silver.

Propolis, which bees use to seal hives and provide an immune system, has been used as a tincture for ulcers, abscesses and inflammation, and as a mouthwash to freshen breath and provide antibacterial qualities.

Plantago tincture rubbed onto or around teeth may be useful for toothache or sensitivity.

Nutritional support implications
Familiarity with and understanding of possible negative effects of some ingredients used in oral healthcare products, as well as benefits of specific natural ingredients, may aid practitioners when advising clients to reduce exposure to toxins and synthetic ingredients and replace them with natural alternatives.

— Chapter 14 —

DENTAL AND ORAL OPTIMAL HEALTH: DIET

Since the connection of periodontal disease with many chronic health conditions appears to be bi-directional, it is important to consider health protocols which address both periodontal health and whole-body health. Inflammation may be an important link, and this should be discussed with clients.

Oral health is not routinely addressed in individuals with diabetes; patients often do not understand the significance of dental care even when they are advised to see a dentist. There's a bi-directional link with a host of other disease states and, in these conditions too, oral health should be considered and addressed where necessary.

Epidemiological evidence suggests that metabolic syndrome increases the risk for periodontitis; dietary counselling needs to be both orally and systemically focused.[1] Individuals with orally focused issues such as caries, gingivitis, periodontitis, xerostomia, loss of masticating function and need for oral surgery, as well as systemically focused issues such as diabetes, cardiovascular disease, stroke, certain cancers and eating disorders, all might benefit from dietary counselling.

The overall aim must be to encourage a healthy holobiont.[2] This may also involve prevention of unhealthy biofilm, reduction of inflammation, promotion of healthy salivary flow, and support for calcium homeostasis, barrier integrity and tissue repair.

In recognition of the bi-directional impact that oral cavity and dental health has on systemic health, this book proposes dietary and lifestyle options, outlined below and in the following three chapters. This is in bullet-point format as the rationale has been provided within the earlier chapters of this book. For specific oral health issues, including the loss of taste, the protocol implications may already have been discussed.

This chapter looks at dietary considerations.

Eating can be dangerous

It stands to reason that the gateway to the human body would have a disproportionately important influence on its overall health. What enters the oral cavity by way of food/drink choices impacts the environment (e.g. pH) of the oral cavity as much as dental hygiene. Both impact systemic health as well as oral health.

Without doubt, food and drink that passes the lips and enters the body through the oral cavity exposes the body to potential toxins, both natural and man-made. The quality and quantity of food and drink, chosen for hunger, thirst, tiredness or satiety, also impacts health, and obesity and other chronic health conditions potentially raise systemic inflammation levels.

Satisfaction of the innate and universal liking for sweetness may generate the brain circuitry seen in binge-eating disorders[3] and other addictive behaviours,[4] indicating another example of how eating can be dangerous.

These are additional considerations to the potential for toxin/poison exposure via substances consumed as food and drink, whether through food contamination, spoiling or misidentification. Without a doubt, eating can be dangerous.

Equally, mindful choices can provide the optimum potential for health.

Dietary considerations

Below are dietary considerations in promoting oral and systemic health – for use preventatively, alongside lifestyle and dental interventions and in conjunction with other health-focused protocols. Food choices are important; dietary supplements may be used as required.

- Choose a low-inflammatory diet with plenty of antioxidant-rich foods and healthy fats that also maintains steady blood sugar levels. The primary consideration must be to use a low-inflammatory diet alongside other means to reduce post-prandial effects (e.g. reducing the number of meals and intermittent fasting). Ingesting glucose increases reactive oxygen species (ROS) generation and raises circulating levels of inflammatory cytokines (e.g. TNF-α, IL-6 and IL-18).[5] High-fat diets and saturated fatty acid (SAFA) consumption modulate gut microbiota composition and low-grade systemic inflammation. Mechanisms linking dietary fat, gut microbiota and obesity are mediated by increased intestinal permeability, systemic endotoxaemia and activity of the endocannabinoid system; high-fat diets and SAFA consumption should be avoided and monounsaturated fatty acids (MUFA) and omega-3 polyunsaturated fats (PUFA) consumption encouraged to aid regulation of gut microbiota and inflammation.[6] A low-inflammatory diet (including olive oil, omega-3 PUFA) and limiting/avoiding sugar and refined carbohydrates, alongside high intake of antioxidant-rich vegetables/fruit and adequate protein, may help promote optimal systemic health and counter inflammatory processes when, as with periodontal conditions, these are initiated.

- Maintain optimal body mass index (BMI) to minimize inflammation and avoid storage of toxins in fat tissue.

- Include sufficient protein for tooth structure, connective tissue health and immune function.

- Avoid sugar (regarding acid production in the oral cavity and AGEs production), and make informed and cautious use of sweeteners. When decay-forming bacteria are forced to consume some sweeteners instead of glucose/fructose, they are unable to produce enamel-attacking acids and sticky mucopolysaccharides that encourage adhesion and biofilm. Note that stevia extracts are non-acidogenic, do not support the growth of *S.mutans* and reduce its biofilm formation.[7] Ethanol and acetone extracts of *Stevia rebaudiana* show the highest activity against *S.mutans*.[8] Other non-cariogenic sweeteners include monk fruit, lucuma and yacón syrup.

- Cautionary xylitol use may be beneficial. The critical daily dose for adults of 5g xylitol (when xylitol is consumed three to five times a day with a total daily dose of 5–10 grams)[9] can be achieved by using toothpastes, chewing gums, mouth sprays, etc. Research suggests that using xylitol gum during tooth eruption may give greater caries protection.[10] Non-GMO erythritol may be a better option.

- Limit foods high in dietary AGEs (foods high in proteins/sugars, processed at high temperature, including roasted, grilled, fried, broiled, barbequed meats, cereals, peanut butter and chocolate).[11] Marinating meats (and other high-protein foods) in lemon or vinegar may have an AGE-reducing effect by lowering the pH.[12] Vegetarians were found to have high plasma concentrations of AGEs (higher than omnivores), so excluding meat entirely is unlikely to reduce AGE formation.[13]

- Be cautious in using honey. Manuka honey, prized for its methylglyoxal content, may also contribute to increased AGEs formation.[14] High-fructose agave syrup also contains methylglyoxal in higher amounts than in some commercial honeys.[15,16]

- Exercise caution about starchy foods, which have the potential for a more negative effect on oral cavity environment than sugary foods. Findings suggest that higher sugar content foods are removed more rapidly and depress plaque pH for a shorter time than starchy foods containing less sugar, so that retention of food in the mouth may be as important an indicator of cariogenic potential as the pH level produced in plaque.[17]

- Maintain oral cavity pH.

- Snacking may worsen decay and dysbiosis as the time between eating/drinking enables the recovery of pH. Snacks, when needed, should not be high in sugar/simple carbohydrates.

- Steam cruciferous vegetables until just cooked, as consuming large amounts raw may affect iodine uptake/utilization.[18]

- Support immune function (and aid stress tolerance) by including vitamins C and D, zinc and other natural immune-boosting nutrients. Although cavitations and oral health conditions may not be a direct cause of systemic conditions, they may be factors in preventing recovery.[19]

- Avoid flavoured sparkling water and other fizzy drinks.

CARBONATED WATER

Links between obesity and consumption of carbonated beverages have commonly been considered to be due to sugar content. Today's carbonated beverages often contain artificial sweeteners instead of sugar and, notwithstanding the effects of artificial sweeteners on satiety and adiposity, scientists are also looking at the health effects of adding CO_2 to beverages.

Gastrointestinal effects of carbonated drinks occur in the oral cavity, oesophagus and the stomach. Studies of the properties of carbonated beverages consider three aspects: the CO_2, the sugar/sweeteners and the effect of other substances used in preparation, with carbonation itself being of most interest.

Since CO_2 is a waste product of cell respiration, it impacts body functions in a number of ways: acid-base balance, control of respiration and tonic influence on heart and peripheral circulation, according to Cuomo *et al.* who describe its actions as hormone-like since it is produced by every tissue and possibly acts on every organ.

Most of the CO_2 in carbonated beverages (actually carbonic acid H_2CO_3 – carbon dioxide in water) dissipates (decomposing back to H_2O+CO_2) when the beverage is opened (or is dispelled as belching when combined with swallowed air) and does not reach the stomach; the small amount that does is readily and rapidly absorbed through the GIT wall where it is most likely to have been converted and be present as carbonates and bicarbonates. The gas may influence the alimentary tract via the nervous system and by direct mechanical and chemical means.[20]

Carbonated drinks, like spices, can elicit oral irritation via thermal and textural sensations conveyed to the brain.[21] The carbonic acid stimulates lingual nociceptors, triggering neuron signalling and chemesthetic sensation, which is both stimulating and slightly sour in taste,[22] a 'biting' effect. This modifies mouthfeel of fizzy beverages and may alter the perception of digestive symptoms.[23]

Although this plays a minor role,[24] beverage carbonation causes tooth erosion, with additional ingredients and salivary pH potentially having an additive effect.[25] Flavoured sparkling waters, however, should be considered as potentially erosive[26] and are not generally advisable for a tooth-friendly diet.

No direct contributory effect has been found for carbonated beverages on gastroesophageal reflux. Larger quantities of carbonated beverages (i.e. greater than 300ml) may produce satiety and may slightly increase hydrochloric acid which might indirectly worsen acid-related conditions and may positively influence digestive processes.[27] However, studies also show that carbonated water decreases satiety, with an ability to improve dyspepsia, constipation and gallbladder emptying.[28]

Fizzy water is thirst-quenching due to anaesthetization of nerve endings in oral mucous membranes by CO_2, and, since fizzy water is generally bicarbonate-rich, facilitates digestion.[29] However, carbonated drinks have also been shown to induce weight gain and obesity onset via ghrelin release and stimulation of hunger response in male mammals.[30]

- Since quality of tap water varies, many use bottled water in plastic containers, which are often acidic and missing essential alkalizing minerals.[31]

MINERAL WATERS

Mineral waters can be classified according to ion composition (as bicarbonate waters, sulphurous waters, etc.) or based on biological activity: diuretic, cathartic or with antiphlogistic properties (reducing inflammation).[32] Mineral content may vary greatly. They are sometimes a good mineral source, especially where diets are low in these important nutrients. Italy is the main producer (and consumers) of bottled mineral water world-wide; a study of 186 bottled mineral waters from Italy for 69 elements showed a wide spread in composition, with differences of up to five orders of magnitude between the lowest and highest measured concentrations for some elements.[33]

The majority of mineral waters on the market are low in mineral content and may have a diuretic effect. Those that are rich in mineral salts may impact health and are defined as medicinal waters (e.g. bicarbonate waters may neutralize acid secretions, sulfate waters may aid constipation, magnesium-rich waters may prevent atherosclerosis, and calcium-rich waters may help prevent hypertension and contribute to calcium intake to counter osteopaenia/osteoporosis).[34]

- Alkaline water products, which contain alkaline minerals and have negative oxidation-reduction potential, are controversial. Some positive benefit has been shown (e.g. possible therapeutic benefit for acid-buffering capacity in connection with denaturing pepsin for those with reflux disease),[35] but there is insufficient proven scientific research as yet regarding the benefits and possible negative effects. Use products with a quality water source only, and then only occasionally because, although considered safe, they may affect stomach acidity and cause mineral deficiency.[36] There may also be an impact on digestion and gut reactivity to invading microbes.

- Support collagen production regarding gingival connective tissue fibres and dentine. Vitamin C deficiency has an impact on collagen and its building blocks. A number of skin and dental effects are seen in its severe deficiency state (scurvy). Essential for connective tissue (including gingiva), vitamin C acts as cofactor for three enzymes involved in collagen hydroxylation.[37] Subclinical vitamin C deficiency may be difficult to recognize since the first symptom is the non-specific and common complaint fatigue.[38]

- Ensure optimal vitamin C intake for antioxidant and immune support and connective tissue support; vitamin C deficiency is implicated in many chronic diseases. Vitamin C is also important for healing and the formation of new tissue after cavitation treatment. Camu-camu contains the most concentrated fruit source of vitamin C.[39]

- Consume bone broth, which is a rich source of nutrients (including collagen and gelatine) to support connective tissue. It is especially useful when there are mouth wounds (e.g. from cheek-biting or tooth extraction). Mouth wounds may heal quicker, and with less scarring, than those to external skin,[40] possibly due to salivary mucus which keeps the oral mucosa from becoming desiccated.[41] Salivary VEGF (vascular endothelial growth factor) may also have a role in mucosal wound healing and may be an essential stimulus for oral mucosal tissue repair.[42] Bone broth is rich in glycine, which is required for VEGF promotion.[43]

- Ensure optimal status of vitamin A which is important for tissue repair/wound healing and bone health.[44,45] Dry lips and reduced immunity may indicate a deficiency. Foods high in vitamin A/beta-carotene include orange-coloured vegetables/fruits, dried apricots, liver, kale and egg yolks. Note also that vitamin A toxicity symptoms can include gingivitis.[46]

- See Chapter 10 for other connective tissue support suggestions.

- Nutrient-rich foods and assessing nutrient status are important, especially in disease conditions. For example, the likelihood of gingival disease in rheumatoid arthritis patients was significantly decreased by increasing vitamin C intake and higher serum vitamin D levels.[47]

- Exercise caution with foods that may stain teeth: wine, curry, coffee, tea, blackberries, blueberries, soy sauce, artificial colours. Rinse afterwards.

- Some crunchy foods may act as natural stain removers: apples, celery, raw carrots, raw cauliflower.

- Oranges and fresh pineapple may encourage saliva production (for natural cleansing); exercise caution with lemons, which have high acid content.

- Dairy foods may benefit. Milk and casein protect against enamel dissolution in acids; including milk in a fermentable (caries-causing) food reduces destructiveness to dental enamel.[48] Casein may be the major protective factor.[49] The mechanism of action for reduced/reversed cariogenic effects conferred by milk and cheese involves buffering, reduced bacterial adhesion, salivary stimulation, reduced enamel demineralization and/or promotion of remineralization by casein, and ionizable calcium/phosphorus.[50,51] Whilst milk and yoghurt can be considered non-cariogenic and protect against periodontitis,[52] cheese has the highest anti-cariogenic capacity. Chewing may confer benefit. Avoid processed cheeses. Milk fermentation results in lactic acid production which may drop pH, inhibiting growth of pathogenic microorganisms;[53] yoghurt may confer benefit. Hard/semi-hard cheeses (e.g. Cheddar, Edam, Gruyère, Monterey, mozzarella, Muenster, Parmesan, provolone, Swiss) generally provide higher calcium content.[54]

- Ensure the optimal dietary ratio of calcium to phosphorus since enamel and dentine development is disturbed under high phosphorus diet and improper ratio.[55]

- Include probiotic-rich foods (e.g. fermented foods such as kefir, sauerkraut and yoghurt) and prebiotic-rich foods (e.g. chicory, leeks and bananas).

- Include bitter foods.

- Three important considerations about food choices:
    - Chewing: vegetables may help scrub tooth surfaces, hard cheeses may

remove other food particles; chewing can massage gums to stimulate blood flow.

- Saliva production: helps to cleanse teeth. Provides protection.
- Staining foods: rinse and brush to limit effects.[56]

- Although staining, red wine (which is rich in polyphenol) shows inhibitory effects in relation to *P.gingivalis*, *A.actinomycetemcomitans* and *F.nucleatum*.[57]

- Proanthocyanidin-rich foods (e.g. cranberries, blueberries, green tea) may help prevent attachment and colonization by pathogenic bacteria.

- Include glycan-rich foods and supplements. Consider food sources – e.g. chanterelle mushrooms,[58] *Aloe vera*, brans (brown rice, slow-cooked oatmeal), pectins (apples, citrus), arabinogalactans (corn, leeks, coconuts, curcumin, radishes)[59] and beta-glucans (oats, mushrooms). Supplement, if necessary, with reishi,[60] shiitake, maitake, *Coriolus versicolor*, inulin, oligofructose and glucosamine.[61]

- Curcumin has antimicrobial, antioxidant, astringent and other properties and has many uses for mouth health, including as a mouth rinse for instant relief (boil 5 grams of turmeric powder, two cloves and two dried guava leaves in 200 grams water) or apply a paste twice daily (one teaspoon of turmeric with half a teaspoon of salt and half a teaspoon of mustard oil to relieve gingivitis/periodontitis).[62]

- Garlic has a strong anti-bacterial effect, killing *P.gingivalis* almost immediately.[63] Chopped garlic held in the mouth for five minutes can sterilize the oral cavity; fresh garlic juice kills *S.pyogenes* in two to three minutes.[64]

- Drink high-EGCG (epigallocatechin-3-gallate) green teas. Gallotannin-rich extracts inhibit adherence of *S.mutans* to smooth surfaces.[65] Green tea polyphenols, especially EGCG, show an inhibitory effect on the growth and adherence of *Porphyromonas gingivalis* onto buccal epithelial cells.[66,67] The ability of EGCG to decrease MMP secretion suggests its benefit for periodontitis.[68] Theaflavins in black tea have also shown the ability to attenuate MMP-mediated inflammatory response by *P.gingivalis*.[69]

- Tannin-rich teas are best between meals.

- Exercise caution when drinking excessively hot beverages (e.g. tea, tea with milk, coffee with milk) as they are associated with an increased risk of oesophageal cancer.[70]

- Denture users should be aware that sensation may be altered; hot food/drinks and dangerous food components like fish bones may be more difficult to feel. Carbohydrate-rich diets and poor salivary flow may predispose denture-wearers to fungal infection.

- Oral health behaviours are associated with the risk of dementia in older adults;[71] older individuals (particularly men) who struggle with chewing are more likely to develop dementia – they may choose less healthy foods, or overcook them so that the nutrients are destroyed.

- Ensure optimal detoxification function: optimize bowel transit time. The need for specific detox regimens depends on the clinical response and adherence to the rest of the protocol.

- Minimize toxin exposure – consider organic foods.

- Avoid/minimize alcohol consumption.

- Ensure hydration.

- Chew well.

- Consider the significant association between osteoporosis and tooth loss.[72]

- Ensure adequate but not excessive intake of salt, preferably using sea salt or Himalayan salt, which contain more trace minerals, and without risking the over-consumption of iodine via table salt.

- A highly satiating diet with defined unrestricted eating alongside other features (with inclusion of red pepper and hot pepper flavour) may benefit in controlling weight in obesity.[73]

- Chewing gum (preferably with xylitol) may stimulate salivary flow in caries management and lubrication,[74] but use chewing gum cautiously and avoid over-use.

CHEWING GUM: ABSOLUTELY STICKY QUESTION[75]

Leaving aside the question of whether chewing gum is healthy, what about the ingredients themselves?

What makes chewing gum chewy is the gum base. The list of ingredients does not always state what has been used and today rubber may be used instead of natural bases. Chicle, a kind of natural latex sap from sapodilla trees or other tree saps, used to be used. And beeswax has been used in parts of the world.

Today 'gum-base' may be a blend of ingredients including plasticizers, resins, elastomers and fillers. As one well-known health writer has commented: the manufacturers may not want the chewers to know they are potentially chewing on 'petroleum-derived paraffin wax, polyvinyl acetate (carpenter's glue) and talc, all of which are linked to cancer'.[76]

Another possibility is the use of mastic gum (*Pistacia lentiscus*), a gummy tree resin which has added benefit in that it helps prevent periodontitis and gingivitis. The green sprigs of the tree were used to clean teeth for hundreds of years. Dioscorides, a Greek physician and botanist, described mastic as making 'unstable teeth firm'.[77,78] Even its name 'mastic', from the Greek *mastikhen* meaning 'to grind the teeth', indicates a use of this plant.

Other ingredients include softeners to retain moisture (often glycerine), sweeteners, flavourings and colours.

Benefits and disadvantages of sweeteners used are another whole topic. Xylitol, for example, has shown benefits for dental disease prevention[79] but the evidence is not conclusive.[80] And xylitol and other sugar alcohols may have negative side effects on gut health – causing abdominal pain, diarrhoea and aggravating IBS symptoms.

Leaving aside the sweetener issue, acid flavourings and preservatives in sugar-free gum may lead to dental erosion.[81]

There are lots of sugar-free chewing gums to choose from. Always check the ingredients list. Different countries have different permitted ingredients. Ingredients found in chewing gum may include titanium dioxide (whitener linked with various conditions), calcium casein peptone/calcium phosphate (highly processed whitener/texturizer), BHT (butylated hydroxytoluene, banned in some countries), aspartame and a variety of other artificial sweeteners.

Other more natural ingredients found in chewing gum may be beet juice, cinnamon or ginger.

Ingredients may be added to aid smokers to quit, prevent bad breath or fight nausea. Studies have shown that chewing gum with specific added natural ingredients may prevent and improve acid reflux.[82] Cinnamon chewing gum was found to improve memory, attention and reflexes.[83]

What is important to remember is that mostly these ingredients will bypass digestion as they enter the body through cells in the mouth – quickly and directly. It is therefore essential that these ingredients are natural and safe.

The relative safety of chewing gum is, absolutely, a sticky question – and complicated.

Chewing gum, the sugar-free sort, may help fight tooth decay. Studies show that chewing sugar-free gum after a meal reduces the acidity of dental plaque and so reduces damage to tooth enamel.[84] In fact, chewing sugar-free gum for 20 minutes after a sugary meal or snack enhances remineralization of the teeth,[85] stopping loss of minerals in tooth enamel caused by acid produced by bacteria in the mouth. The benefit appears to be for people who don't brush their teeth.

Non-brushing of teeth is not recommended.

Chewing gum may also release mercury from fillings.[86,87] That would make chewing gum potentially dangerous for anyone with amalgam fillings.

Chewing gum has been shown to reduce acid reflux and heartburn[88] if chewed post-meal. It increases saliva production and clears acid quickly. Caution is advised to avoid mint flavours which may increase acid and worsen heartburn.

Mint chewing gum, however, may be great for increasing alertness as it is thought to stimulate nerves. Chewing gum may also boost mental performance (chewing is thought to increase blood flow to the brain).

Chewing sends the body signals which activate enzymes and acids. However, with chewing gum, there is no food to digest, so chewing gum instead of chewing food may result in bloating and over-production of stomach acid. It may also affect the ability to produce enzymes and acids when food is eaten. As chewing means swallowing excess air, it may result in abdominal pain, bloating and IBS-type symptoms.

Similar symptoms affecting the gut – abdominal pain, diarrhoea and IBS symptom aggravation – are potential negative side effects with the use of xylitol and other sugar alcohols.

Some people believe chewing gum may ward off food cravings. There is no evidence that chewing gum reduces hunger or energy/calorie intake. Mint gum may even deter consumption of fruit and reduce diet quality[89] – in particular less fruit and more 'junk food' may be consumed – possibly due to the effect of minty gum which makes fruit and vegetables taste bitter.

Additionally, all sweeteners may cause weight gain by stimulating appetite, increasing cravings for carbohydrates and stimulating hormones like insulin and leptin that signal increased fat storage.[90]

The action of chewing (gum or otherwise) may help prevent or relieve ear pain during flying. However, the action of chewing may trigger TMJ as it can cause jaw muscle imbalance.[91]

Regular gum chewing is likely not healthy, although there is some indication that regular use of xylitol chewing gum may be caries-preventive.[92] If chewing is for a specific known health benefit and benefit is seen, then choose the product wisely, carefully checking the ingredients list. And use only as long as beneficial and necessary.

The content is reproduced by kind permission of Vitfinder.com and was originally published under the titles 'Chewing gum: a sticky question' and 'Is Chewing Gum Healthy?'

- Chewing gum with arginine may inhibit dental caries[93] and confer anti-inflammatory benefits in treating gingivitis.[94]
- Dietary L-arginine may increase the rate of orthodontic tooth movement,[95] reducing the treatment time required.
- Encourage trying new (especially bitter) foods repeatedly as taste perception can be 'learned'.[96]
- Set healthy eating patterns early in life.
- Enjoy healthy wholesome food. Add seasoning to flavour.

— Chapter 15 —

SUPPLEMENT CONSIDERATIONS

This chapter looks at supplement considerations when working towards optimal dental and oral health.

Supplement considerations

- Protect with adequate antioxidants. The evidence is still insufficient on the benefits of mono-antioxidant supplementation; use antioxidant complex.[1]

- Resveratrol may decrease production of pro-inflammatory cytokines in human periodontal ligament cells stimulated by *P.gingivalis* LPS,[2] and prevents alveolar bone loss by inhibiting inflammatory response and stimulating antioxidant defence systems.[3]

- Useful anti-inflammatories: omega-3, *Curcuma longa*, ginger, white willow bark, black pepper, berberine, clove, resveratrol, *Uncaria tomentosa*, *Cistus incanus*, pycnogenol, cinnamon, *Tabebuia impetiginosa*, noni (*Morinda citrifolia*).

- Useful analgesics: clove, peppermint, propolis, neem, ginger, *Aloe vera*,[4] white willow bark (*Salix alba*).[5]

- *Cistus incanus* may reduce bacterial adhesion in the oral cavity.[6]

- *Ceanothus americanus* shows growth inhibitory effect against *S.mutans*, *P.gingivalis* and other oral pathogens.[7]

- Antibacterial *Uncaria tomentosa* may help with infected root canal dentine[8,9] and in denture stomatitis.[10]

- Berberine may help address endotoxins and reduce cytokine (NF-κB) activation.[11] Berberine may also modulate gut microbiota and help ameliorate periodontal bone loss by beneficially affecting intestinal barriers in cases of oestrogen-deficient conditions (e.g. postmenopausal osteoporosis which is a risk factor for periodontitis).[12] Additionally, berberine spares bifidobacteria and lactobacilli.[13]

- Natural sialogogues include citric acid,[14] malic acid, ascorbic acid (which may negatively affect tooth enamel) and numerous botanicals (in decreasing potency) including: *Piper nigrum* (black pepper), horseradish, *Zingiber officinale* (ginger root), *Cinchona* bark, chamomile, *Gentiana lutea* root, orange peel, anise seed, caraway seed and cinnamon bark.[15] A ginger spray may increase saliva to address xerostomia in T2D.[16]

- Melatonin, an important antioxidant, is synthesized in the pineal gland and gastrointestinal tract from which it passes into the circulatory system.[17] Melatonin secreted into the blood can be detected in saliva (where it is found at levels between 15% and 33% of those in plasma). Melatonin contributes to oral cavity protection, regarding tissue damage, via the action of receptors, and helps to suppress oral diseases including periodontal disease, herpes and oral cancer.[18]

- Iodine has an important role in oral mucosa and salivary gland physiology as well as oral immune defence, aiding prevention of oral and salivary gland diseases.[19,20] Ensure adequate iodine uptake. This is especially important in pregnancy since iodine may affect mental and physical growth of the fetus. Iodine-rich foods include kelp, seaweed, miso soup, cod, cranberries and yoghurt. Note that iodized salt is often suggested (conventionally) to ensure adequate levels across populations. Chloride is a major component of iodized salt (with 30,000 times more chloride than iodide); research suggests only 10 per cent of iodide in iodized salt is bioavailable due to competition from chloride also in the salt.[21] Supplementing iodine can displace toxic halogens (fluorine, bromine, chlorine) already in cells and may cause unpleasant detoxification reactions;[22] start with low doses. Excess iodine also causes problems and it is important to check levels via testing (Thyroid Hormone Panel) to determine protocol before taking high levels of iodine or in cases of symptoms indicating possible deficiency (lethargy, skin problems, thinning hair, shortness of breath, poor concentration/memory retention, brain fog, muscle pains/weakness, undesired weight gain/loss, sensitivity to cold, mood changes, difficulty producing sufficient saliva/sweat). When doses of iodine higher than the recommended daily amount are indicated via testing, they should be accompanied by a 200mcg daily dose of selenium.

- Maintain optimal selenium levels; salivary levels may be associated with dental caries.[23]

- Maintain optimal magnesium levels, especially in areas of water fluoridation; fluoride in water/toothpaste can interfere with intestinal absorption of magnesium.[24]

- Ensure optimal status of calcium, vitamins D3, K2 and A/retinoic acid – especially if there is much root decay. Vitamin D has a role in calcium homeostasis and electrolyte and blood pressure regulation. Both vitamin D and the vitamin D receptor (VDR) have roles in immune function and are involved in T-cell antigen receptor signalling. Dysregulation of VDR may be associated with an exaggerated inflammatory response.[25] Exercise caution about excessive vitamin D supplementation in known cases of FDOJ (fatty degenerate osteolysis of jawbone).[26] Vitamin K2 may stimulate bone formation and suppress bone resorption;[27] this bone-mass-increasing effect may slow rates of tooth loss with age. Vitamin K2 also aids salivary buffering by impacting secretion/flow of calcium and inorganic phosphates. K2 can sustain hormone-induced dentinal fluid flow, boosting inflammatory responses.[28] Since vitamin K is used by *Porphyromonas gingivalis* as a nutrient for growth,[29] in cases of periodontal disease, it is perhaps best not used in liquid or lozenge formats. Increasing vitamin K2 intake may improve efficiency of (K2-dependent) osteocalcin[30] which pulls calcium from the bloodstream, depositing it in bones/teeth.[31] Osteocalcin and type 1 collagen have a role in dentine formation. Retinoic acid can induce secretions of these.[32] There is a synergistic effect between vitamins A and D3 on osteocalcin expression in human osteoblasts.[33] Retinoic acid is also essential for maintaining mucosal tissue integrity.[34] Calcium is best obtained via diet (exercise caution about supplementation).

- Silicon promotes bone and connective tissue health and may have a modulatory effect on inflammatory and immune responses; this may relate to effects on the formation and/or utilization of glycosaminoglycans, mucopolysaccharides and collagen in these tissues.[35] Silicon is found predominantly as orthosilicic acid in humans, especially in bone and tendons.[36] Silica (oxide of silicon) may aid calcium uptake and collagen synthesis (regarding connective tissue/bone).[37] Supplemented silicon can significantly upregulate mineralization of human dental pulp cells, and has shown a synergistic effect with calcium.[38]

- Arginine silicate inositol complex was shown to inhibit periodontal tissue loss and may benefit.[39]

- By supporting ligaments that secure teeth to the alveolar bone, hyaluronic acid (HA) may be beneficial regarding gingival health, periodontitis and especially in ageing. It may also be useful in dry mouth. Mucous membranes of the mouth absorb HA ideally.

- *Centella asiatica* and *Punica granatum* (pomegranate) extracts significantly improve clinical signs of chronic periodontitis.[40] *Centella asiatica* may stimulate HA production.[41]

- Myricetin, a naturally occurring (in vegetables, berries, teas and wines) phenolic compound with diverse biological activities and a similar structure to quercetin,[42] decreases the enzyme activity of MMPs in human gingival fibroblasts and inhibits osteoclastogenesis. It therefore has a potentially therapeutic effect on the bone-destructive processes of periodontal disease.[43]

- Lips are composed of surface epidermis, connective tissue and muscle layer.[44] Connective tissue health is therefore important. Glycosaminoglycans (the main constituent of connective tissue ground substance) include hyaluronic acid, levels of which change with age, impacting the appearance of lips in older individuals. Hyaluronic acid is sometimes used in lip fillers, can be topically applied and can be promoted through diet and supplementation.

- Oral and/or topical (oral spray) CoQ10 may benefit.

- Sea buckthorn (*Hippophae rhamnoides*) oil (rich in omega-7) may relieve dry mouth symptoms and improve oral mucosa.[45] Sea buckthorn mouthwash shows anti-biofilm activity against certain oral bacterial species.[46]

- EGCG-rich supplements may be beneficial in periodontal disease states.

- Clove (*Syzygium aromaticum*) and active component eugenol have considerable antifungal activity.[47] Studies also show *in vitro* anti-cancer activity of clove oil regarding oesophageal cancer cells, with cytotoxicity due to cell disruption and subsequent membrane rupture.[48] Clove seed extract may be useful in toothpaste due to its growth-inhibitory activity against *S.mutans*.[49] Clove has an analgesic effect and has been used traditionally for toothache[50] and gingivitis.[51]

- Myrrh (*Commiphora molmol*) has antiseptic properties as well as anti-inflammatory and antimicrobial action[52] and promotes healing/repair of damaged tissue when used short term (less than two weeks) in a low-concentration suspension.[53] It is useful for mouth ulcers, sore throat and gingivitis.[54] Caution: oil should not be swallowed.

SUPPLEMENT CONSIDERATIONS

- Liquorice (*Glycyrrhiza*) may be useful topically for mouth ulcers[55] and has antimicrobial properties.[56]

- *Aloe vera* is useful for addressing toothpick injuries, gum abscesses, periodontal surgery sites, mouth ulcers, burning mouth syndrome, infections and xerostomia.[57]

- Propolis may be useful for halitosis, lichen planus, abscesses, dentinal sensitivity and gingivitis.[58]

- Grape seed extract (*Vitis vinifera*), with antioxidant capacity, has demonstrated anti-plaque/anti-biofilm activity against *P.gingivalis*, *S.mutans*, *S.sobrinus*, *F.nucleatum*, *Actinomyces viscosus* and *L.rhamnosus*.[59]

- Potentially useful for mouth ulcers: coconut oil, clove, propolis, Manuka honey, sage, turmeric, hyaluronic acid, zinc/vitamin C lozenges and salt water rinses.

- Coconut water is useful storage media for an avulsed tooth.[60]

- Cranberry may inhibit dental plaque film formation and stop bacterial adhesion. However, cranberry juice is very acidic and can erode teeth.[61]

- Papaine has bactericidal characteristics and is effective against Gram-positive and Gram-negative organisms.[62]

- Colostrum supplements may provide immunoglobulin and lactoferrin[63] and be beneficial in numerous ways:[64,65] immune support, muscular–skeletal repair, growth capabilities and wound healing.[66]

- Collagen or gelatine may support gum healing.

- Vitamins E and D3 combined reverse the toxic effects of fluoride on male reproductive organs.[67] Amla (*Emblica officinalis*) may also aid mitigation of fluoride-induced toxicity.[68] *Moringa oleifera* fruit extract shows protective effects against experimental fluorosis.[69] Magnesium shows the potential to block NMDA glutamate receptors and decrease free radical production in fluoride neurotoxicity.[70]

- Fluoride toxicity – flavonoids demonstrate neuroprotectant properties and, in particular, quercetin sulfonate (a water-soluble form of quercetin) protects liver and kidney cells from ammonium fluoride suppression of mitochondrial energy production.[71] Curcumin may significantly reduce fluoride's neurotoxic effects.[72]

- Curcumin may be useful in caries, oral lichen planus, gingivitis and halitosis.[73]

- Modulation of the endocannabinoid system may help those with addictive behaviours related to the oral intake of food. CB_1 receptors, which are widely expressed in brain regions that control food intake, reward and energy balance,[74] may be influenced by substances that modulate the endocannabinoid system. Although it won't decrease food intake on its own, CBD can prevent hyperphagic effects of CB_1 and 5-HT1A (serotonin) receptor agonists, so may be useful for those with eating disorders.[75] Consider CBD oil use for this as well as for toothache. Cannabis has a history of use for pain relief, including mouth pain; early American president George Washington reportedly used cannabis for tooth pain.[76]

- Chromium picolinate may be effective generally to control sweet cravings.

- *Gymnema sylvestre* has a sugar-blocking effect and may be helpful in controlling blood sugar.

- Alpha-lipoic acid may help improve glucose utilization and prevent protein glycation and AGE formation.[77]

- Support the liver in relation to endotoxin clearance with chlorophyll-rich and hepatoprotective herbs.

- Supplement, if necessary, with reishi,[78] shiitake, maitake, *Coriolus versicolor*, inulin, oligofructose and glucosamine[79] to provide beneficial saccharides for salivary components and mucosal layer support.

- Zinc gluconate, 140mg/d for four months, may help in idiopathic dysgeusia.[80]

- Consider using colloidal silver spray (anti-inflammatory, antimicrobial, biofilm-reducing).

- Consider probiotics use, particularly oral-cavity specific probiotics.

ORAL-CAVITY PROBIOTICS

To encourage a healthy holobiont, oral-cavity probiotics may be useful alongside other diet and lifestyle measures. Oral-cavity probiotics might be particularly useful in disease conditions and in ageing (when there is an increased propensity for a dysbiotic environment with increased pathogens).

The oral cavity contains the second most diverse microbial community

SUPPLEMENT CONSIDERATIONS

in the body;[81] a growing body of research contributes to understanding this environment and the implications for oral, and whole-body, health. The species for oral health may be different from those for gut health.[82]

Oral-cavity probiotics may benefit in numerous ways: by providing colonization competition, genetic modification of microbiota[83] and immune stimulation.[84]

- *Streptococcus salivarius* strains particularly have been studied; this commensal is a pioneer oral-cavity colonizer that persists through life, and many produce bacteriocins (bacteria-suppressors) which function like antibiotics.[85]

- *Streptococcus salivarius* M18 kills harmful oral bacteria, readily colonizes the oral cavity and aids rebalance; it produces bacteriocins (specifically, powerful lantibiotics) and enzymes (dextranase and urease), which may reduce dental plaque accumulation and acidification.[86,87] *S.salivarius* M18-containing lozenges have reduced both moderate-to-severe gingivitis and moderate periodontitis.[88]

- *Streptococcus salivarius* BLIS K12 may be beneficial for throat infections in children, with a 96 per cent reduction in streptococcal pharyngotonsillitis incidence and 80 per cent reduction in viral infection incidence.[89]

- *Streptococcus salivarius* K12 may reduce oral volatile sulphur compound levels in halitosis,[90] and shows efficacy in relation to otitis media and upper respiratory tract viruses as well as activity against *S.pyogenes*.[91]

- In a randomized open-label clinical trial with 64 healthy volunteers randomly divided into four groups, *Lactobacillus salivarius* tablets increased resistance to caries risk factors – i.e. decreased the numbers of mutans streptococci.[92]

- *Lactobacillus rhamnosus* GG probiotic may benefit children's dental health according to a randomized, double-blind, placebo-controlled intervention study examining the effect of long-term consumption of *L.rhamnosus* GG in milk.[93]

- Heat-treated *L.plantarum* L-137 boosts the oral immune function, reduces inflammation and promotes healing; it significantly reduces periodontal pocket depth in periodontal diseases (64% improvement) and potently induces IL-12[94] (downregulated by *P.gingivalis*,[95,96] and naturally decreased in ageing).[97]

- *L.reuteri* ATCC PTA 5289 and *L.reuteri* Protectis® lozenges significantly reduced gingivitis, plaque index (in a randomized controlled trial to assess the impact of *L.reuteri* on pregnancy gingivitis in healthy women)[98] and prevalence of *Candida* (in a double-blind randomized placebo-controlled design with two parallel arms and 215 older adults aged 60 to 102 years).[99]

- In a 2007 Finnish study that investigated the effects of cheese containing mixed probiotics, on the growth of oral *Candida* in the elderly (aged 70–100 years in old people's homes and sheltered housing units), probiotic intervention reduced risk of high yeast counts by 75 per cent, also reducing risk of hyposalivation by 56 per cent.[100]

- In a study of 42 healthy institutionalized women, 65 years or older, in Brazil, a probiotic intervention (*L.casei* and *B.breve*) reduced *Candida* numbers in the elderly oral cavity and increased anti-*Candida* IgA levels.[101]

- Multispecies probiotic formulations containing *L.rhamnosus*, *L.acidophilus* and *B.bifidum* may help reduce *Candida* infections in elderly denture wearers, according to a double-blind, randomized study of 59 denture wearers asymptomatically harbouring *Candida* in their oral cavities.[102]

- *Lactobacillus casei* Shirota may help maintain salivary sIgA and reduce the frequency of upper respiratory tract infections in athletes, as determined by a double-blind, placebo-controlled, randomized study that examined the effects of probiotic supplement during four months of winter training in 84 highly active men and women.[103]

- *L.paracasei* SD1 may reduce levels of salivary mutans streptococci and *Lactobacilli* in adolescents with cleft lip and palate (which is associated with orthodontic appliances that facilitate the colonization of mutans streptococci), according to a double-blinded, randomized, placebo-controlled study of 30 orthodontically treated nonsyndromic cleft lip and palate patients.[104]

- *L.fermentum* CECT5716 and *L.salivarius* CECT5713, commonly found in human breast milk, enhance the natural and acquired immune response and induce a broad array of cytokines including TNF-α and IL-1β, according to an *in vitro* study.[105]

- *L.reuteri* may be beneficial in the treatment of chronic periodontitis, as determined by a systematic review and meta-analysis of randomized controlled trials.[106]

- *L.salivarius* WB21 reduced the numbers of five periodontopathic bacteria, including *Tannerella forsythia*, in a double-blinded, placebo-controlled, randomized clinical trial with 66 healthy volunteers without severe periodontitis.[107]

- Salivary bifidobacteria may help to suppress *P.gingivalis* via competition, as determined in a study looking at 65 *Bifidobacteria* strains obtained from the mouths of periodontally healthy subjects.[108]

- Multispecies probiotic formulations have been designed to promote good oral health by inhibiting oral pathogen growth, inhibiting biofilm and strengthening the immune system. One multispecies probiotic formulation contains *B.bifidum* W23, *B.breve* W25, *B.lactis* W51, *Enterococcus faecium* W54, *L.plantarum* W21, *L.rhamnosus* W71, *L.salivarius* W24, *L.salivarius* W57 and *S.thermophilus* W69 and may inhibit oral pathogen growth, inhibit biofilm and strengthen the immune system.[109]

- According to a clinical study, *Weissella cibaria* exhibits an inhibitory effect on the proliferation of *S.mutans* colonies/biofilm, potentially reducing the plaque index score and bad breath.[110]

- Probiotic-containing ice-cream (*B.lactis* BB-12, *L.acidophilus* LA-05) can reduce the *S.mutans* count, according to a randomized controlled, double-blind study (in children aged 6 to 12 years) with six months follow-up.[111]

- Three strains (*Lactobacillus fermentum* YIT, *Lactobacillus gasseri* YIT 12321 and *Streptococcus mitis* YIT 12322) were shown to have no cariogenic potential in an artificial mouth system and are 'expected as new probiotics with potential oral health benefits and no adverse effects on general health'.[112]

- Other strains that have been more recently researched, and are showing promise as new probiotics with potential oral health benefits, include *S.salivarius* strains ST3, 24SMB and T30.[113]

- Spore-formers (e.g. *Bacillus coagulans*) may also reduce mutans streptococci, according to a placebo-controlled study of 150 healthy children (aged 7 to 14 years).[114]

- Oral probiotics are generally recommended after meals/teeth cleaning and/or at bedtime.

- Oral microbiome balance may help disease resistance; oral microbiome dysbiosis may contribute to failing health, particularly in older age.

Antimicrobials and detox considerations

Generally speaking, detoxification should be something considered as part of the daily routine – by diet and lifestyle choices. Everyday detoxification considerations might include a chlorophyll-rich drink, plenty of water, exercise/sweating, organic choices, plenty of fresh vegetables and ensuring a minimum of one daily bowel movement (preferably more).

The body sometimes needs more detoxification support – for example, before, during and after mercury amalgam removal.

There can also be a need for greater detoxification support during fat loss because toxins are stored in fatty tissue and will be released with fat loss. Ensuring optimal detoxification beforehand and during fat loss can help.

There can also be a greater need for detoxification support when addressing known microbial infection (during which time lipopolysaccharide/endotoxin levels may be high, biofilms may form and toxins held in parasites might be released during die-off).

Herxheimer reactions may occur during antimicrobial protocols. They are an indication that the protocol is destroying microbes effectively, but result in worsening or additional negative symptoms. The client feels worse and may give up the protocol, believing it is worsening their health condition. Support clients by informing them of the likelihood of Herxheimer reactions, explaining that they are an indication of protocol effectiveness. Ensure clients understand what may help relieve unpleasant Herxheimer reaction symptoms.

Below are some further detoxification considerations.

- Ensure hydration with fresh pure water.

- If using sweat therapies, replace lost magnesium; ensure electrolyte balance.

- Use chlorophyll-rich sources: chlorella, barley grass, spirulina, parsley, broccoli.

- Use hepatoprotective herbs (milk thistle, dandelion, artichoke).

- Provide botanical detoxification support via milk thistle, *Desmodium molliculum*, cilantro (*Coriandrum sativum*) leaf, parsley (*Petroselinum crispum*), *Pimpinella anisum* and (for sulfites/sulfates) *Asparagus officinalis*.

- Citrus pectin (found in peel/pith of citrus fruit – use organic, unwaxed) may aid detoxification and help lower inflammation (by suppressing pro-inflammatory responses induced by lipopolysaccharides);[115] citrus pectin may also exert an immunomodulatory effect.[116]

- Support glutathione production with glutathione-rich foods (spinach, asparagus, avocado, okra),[117] sulphur-rich foods (protein-rich foods, brassicas, *Allium* vegetables), vitamin C,[118,119] vitamin E,[120] selenium,[121,122] glycine,[123,124] L-cysteine (e.g. via pressurized whey protein),[125] N-acetyl-cysteine,[126] SAMe (S-adenosyl-L-methionine),[127] curcumin,[128] milk thistle (silymarin),[129,130] and a number of other substances,[131] including alpha lipoic acid which has been shown to increase cellular glutathione level and support mobilization and excretion of mercury.[132]

- Other useful detoxifying natural substances and binders are important for transporting the toxins out of the body, including activated charcoal, clays and zeolite.

Antimicrobials are best rotated, with a break incorporated. This can help ensure resistance doesn't develop, as well as to allow a break in microbial cycles (e.g. parasitic egg-hatching). The cooperation between microbes necessitates consideration of the full spectrum of microbial types where periodontitis is concerned. This highlights the need to always ensure optimal immune function. Some nutrients and natural substances that may support immune function have been previously discussed.

- Useful antifungals include *Tabebuia impetiginosa* (pau d'arco), monolaurin, olive leaf extract, caprylic acid, grapefruit seed extract, berberine (e.g. *Mahonia aquifolium* or *Berberis vulgaris*).

- Useful antivirals include zinc, L-lysine, medicinal mushrooms, monolaurin, humic/fulvic acid, *Cecropia strigosa*, *Houttuynia cordata*, *Uncaria tomentosa*, *Polygonum cuspiatum* (Japanese knotweed), *Aloe vera*, *Hypericum perforatum*, *Melissa officinalis*, *Echinacea*, *Sambucus nigra*, olive leaf extract, *Andrographis*, *Scutellaria baicalensis*.

- Useful antiparasitics include *Achillea millefolium*, artemisinin, *Cinchona calisaya*, *Juglans nigra*, *Artemisia absinthium*.

- Useful antibacterials include myrrh (*Commiphora molmol*),[133] goldenseal (*Hydrastis canadensis*), *Uncaria tomentosa*, *Usnea barbata*, cinnamon. Also, *Rosmarinus officinalis*, *Salvia sclarea*, *Origanum vulgare*, *Thymus longicaulis*.[134]

- Useful biofilm-busters include *Stevia rebaudiana*, serrapeptase, L-cysteine. Also, curcumin,[135] N-acetylcysteine,[136] L-arginine solution,[137] grape seed extract (*Vitis vinifera*),[138] and *Cistus* spp, *Rosmarinus officinalis* and *Salvia sclarea*.[139]

- Useful broad-spectrum antimicrobials include oregano, *Otoba parvifolia*, *Triplaris peruviana*, *Quassia amara*, *Tabebuia impetiginosa*, garlic, neem (*Azadirachta indica*).

— Chapter 16 —

ORAL HYGIENE CONSIDERATIONS

This chapter looks at oral hygiene considerations. Below are some protocol considerations, some of which are outside the scope of nutritional therapy practice but are conversations for the client to potentially hold with a holistic dentist.

Dental/oral considerations

- Assess and address, as necessary: caries, gum infection, inflammation, cavitations, dental implants, potentially toxic dental materials (mercury, nickel).
- Assess/correct dental misalignment if determined to be a contributory factor.
- Good oral hygiene/toothbrushing may be associated with a lower risk of gastrointestinal cancer.[1]
- IBDs (especially Crohn's disease) are associated with an increased risk of oral health problems.[2]
- Don't ignore lumps or blisters on gingiva. These may be the result of an infection and therefore inflammation. Other signs of inflammation may include cracks in teeth, decay, dry mouth, fungal infections and bleeding.
- Smoking is associated with oral inflammation. Vaping may be associated with gingivitis.[3]
- Remember that periodontitis is a contagious infection.[4]
- Galvanic reactions, which can be caused by dissimilar metals placed in the mouth, are thought to contribute to metallic taste, jaw tension, temporal headache and tinnitus.

METALLIC TASTE

Galvanic reactions (due to amalgam dental fillings and other metallic restorations) are thought to be involved in metallic mouth-taste.[5,6,7,8,9,10] Reactions from dental material randomly or unpredictably conducted through anatomical structures/spaces can overwhelm normal neuronal control. The effect may manifest as localized pain, inappropriate muscle tone (e.g. jaw tension, TMJ), temporal headache, or skin pallor due to low-level vasoconstriction.[11]

An article by the IABDM (International Academy of Biological Dentistry and Medicine) registered holistic dentist, Dr Michael G. Rehme, compares this galvanic current to the electric current of a battery. He describes how two adjacent teeth restored with dissimilar metals allow a current to flow through dentine, bone and tissue fluids causing discomfort and tooth sensitivity. When the electric current passes through pulp, pain may be experienced.[12] Galvanism may also cause a metallic or salty taste in the mouth, increase salivary secretion and result in a burning/tingling sensation in the tongue.

Dr Rehme also explains that CNS effects may occur due to the proximity of teeth to the brain (upper teeth are less than 2 inches from the brain); potential currents from oral cavity metals may be a thousand times stronger than those on which the brain works, potentially enabling excess electrical activity to misdirect impulses in the brain. He cautions that having had numerous dentists over the years may increase an individual's risk of having several dissimilar metals in the mouth, thus increasing a propensity for these galvanic reactions and symptoms.

Dr Rehme also relates a case study of tinnitus being resolved with amalgam removal and reduction of galvanic current.[13]

- Chewing may release mercury vapour from amalgams.[14] High levels of mercury vapour exposure are associated with adverse effects in the brain and kidneys, where bio-accumulation occurs.[15] Mercury exposure may cause some of the same biochemical effects seen in Alzheimer's-diseased brains, as well as disrupting the immune system by potently inhibiting phagocytosis.[16]

- Mercury toxicity should be evaluated in all patients with hypertension, cardiovascular disease, stroke and vascular diseases.[17]

- If mercury amalgams are present, research and seek advice about these. Note that mercury amalgam removal may not always be necessary, particularly if fillings appear to be in sound condition, since removal may result in unnecessary loss of healthy tooth structure and result in exposure to additional mercury vapour released in the removal process.[18] Removal may be contraindicated in some cancer patients, although removal of devitalized teeth and cavitation surgery might still be indicated and beneficial.[19] Ensure mercury-safe dental care and safe removal of mercury amalgam. See Dr Dana Colson's article 'A safe protocol for amalgam removal' for an excellent description of the process.[20]

- For those who decide to remove dental amalgams, the IAOMT recommend the Safe Mercury Amalgam Removal Technique (SMART) for which there are licensed practitioners and guidelines for safeguarding both patient and dental professionals/staff involved. Nutrition professionals may want to investigate local provision, and may suggest a detoxification protocol before, during and after SMART procedures.

- Dr John Roberts, integrative medicine doctor and holistic dentist, advises removing mercury from the body by binding mercury in saliva and gut to prevent it from entering the body. He advises using a zeolite product (most effective is clinoptilolite) to bind mercury and other harmful substances. Clinoptilolite naturally absorbs mercury, functioning like a magnet to attract and transport mercury out of the body, avoiding reabsorption, and without burdening the body's detoxification system or affecting metabolism. Stored toxins (in muscle, fat, bone) can then be released through detoxification systems and be removed via the bowel.[21] Leo Cashman, from DAMS, recommends vitamin C, B complex (including methylcobalamin), magnesium, zinc picolinate and seleno-methionine, vitamin D (if needed), chlorella, and liposomal glutathione.[22,23]

- Support all detoxification pathways as part of dealing with microbial infections, mercury amalgam exposure/removal, and indications of cavitation, etc. In all cases, consider the possibility of a Herxheimer reaction and re-toxification. Recommend a protocol accordingly.

- Advice from Dr Weston Price (1870–1948), who looked for causes of dental decay and physical degeneration, still holds today: most biological dentists find that patients in otherwise excellent health can handle the stress of root canal teeth (with monitoring) but that those suffering chronic illness may need to extract a devitalized tooth. And in cases of grave diagnosis (e.g. breast cancer), removal of all root canal teeth should be considered, according to this dentist.[24] Consider discussion with a holistic dentist.

- With regard to cavitations, once suspected, high-quality X-rays are essential to diagnosis and evaluation. A 3-D cone beam CT (computed tomography) scanner which uses digital technology to record images reveals much more information than simple two-dimensional X-rays. A dental 3-D cone beam CT produces a three-dimensional image of teeth, soft tissues, nerve pathways and bone in a single scan. Although radiation from this type of image is lower than from conventional computer tomography, it is higher than for conventional 2-D X-ray images; the advantage of a 3-D cone beam CT is that the information it provides allows for more precise treatment planning. This technology is used to evaluate diseases of the jaw, dentition, bony structures of the face, nasal cavity and sinuses. It is commonly used for accurate placement of dental implants, assessing TMJ, detecting, measuring and treating jaw tumours, determining bone structure/tooth orientation, reconstructive surgery and locating the origin of pain or pathology.[25]

- Cavitation can be a source of low- or high-level stress on the entire body and may interfere with the energy flow of the body's meridians, usually without a localized symptom. Consider adrenal support and/or TCM therapies that look at energy flow through body meridians.

- Those receiving anti-oestrogen therapy (for breast cancer) may require support in relation to increased gingival inflammation, gingival bleeding, periodontal pocketing, xerostomia and burning issues.[26] According to a 2014 award-winning paper, more education to improve dental care for those undergoing breast cancer treatment is needed.[27]

- Chronic tonsil infection may indicate an infected tooth or root canal.

- Use of homeopathy may be beneficial prior to dental surgery, particularly for very ill individuals – to optimize immune, nervous and metabolic system functioning.[28]

- Prior to dental surgery (a minimum of one to two months), ensure the individual has a sufficiency of protein – especially vegans and lacto-ovo-vegetarians who typically consume insufficient protein.[29]

- Following cavitation surgery, rest and recover for a period including four days post-surgery. Avoid physical activity and extensive car/plane travel. This is to avoid formation of a 'dry socket' (loss of the blood clot) from bacterial invasion in the area between the blood clot and the bone. Symptoms of dry socket are significant pain in the surgical site or ipsilateral ear and typically a foul odour. Nutrient-dense bone broths (pureed vegetables can be added) are useful for the first two days post-surgery until the surgical incision has closed; this may help to avoid food particles lodging.[30]

- For tooth extractions, use hot (not cold) compresses because cooling the site may reduce the number of white blood cells to attack bacteria that have invaded socket and bone.[31] Other considerations: acupressure, salt water rinse and arnica.

- Use of an aromatherapy oil diffuser, particularly lavender essential oil, is thought to reduce anxiety about dental treatment.

- For helping bone to grow following dental surgery consider homeopathic remedies and ensure optimal nutrients: protein, vitamin D3, calcium, magnesium, zinc, strontium, boron and vitamin C. B vitamin complex may help prevent and reduce post-surgical pain.[32] Avoid fluoride during periods when new bone growth is encouraged. See Appendix 1 for ways to avoid fluoride.

- Consider new dental procedures from an informed perspective regarding both the procedure and materials used.

- Periodontal disease may have a negative effect on the ability to conceive; meticulous oral hygiene is recommended during fertility treatments (both men and women) and during pregnancy.[33] Resolve oral issues before commencing fertility treatment and wait a few weeks after periodontal therapy before initiating fertility treatments (because of fluctuating inflammatory cytokines).

- Consider oral microbiome testing as an investigative and preventative tool to inform the protocol and lifestyle measures. See Appendix 4.

Everyday mouth and dental hygiene

For the most part, the term 'oral hygiene' today refers primarily to the use of toothpaste to brush/clean teeth. However, tooth powders are a much earlier version, recently making a comeback.

Oral hygiene protocols can include use of mouth rinses/mouthwashes, tongue cleaning, flossing, interdental brushes, oil-pulling, chewing gums, water-flossing (Waterpik®) and tooth whitening products as well as use of toothpaste/toothpowder on a toothbrush.

A useful summary of information on the history of oral hygiene is presented in a 2013 article on toothpaste, discussing the purpose, history and ingredients.[34]

- Toothbrushes:
    - After brushing, remove any remaining toothpaste/debris from the

toothbrush using water. Then store it upright so that moisture can drain away. Consider having several toothbrushes so that you can allow the bristles to dry between cleaning.

- Keep the brushes from touching each other when stored. This prevents migration of germs from one toothbrush to the next.

- Avoid sharing toothbrushes. Shared toothbrushes can result in an exchange of body fluids and microorganisms, highly increasing the risk of contracting infections.

- Avoid storing toothbrushes in moist containers. Moist environments are ideal for breeding bacteria.

- Get new toothbrushes every three to four months. Always replace after herpes simplex virus (and other viral) infections.

- Keep toothbrushes away from the vicinity of the toilet. *E.coli* was found on toothbrushes kept in bathrooms with an attached toilet.[35]

- Consider use of UV toothbrush cleaners. UV light destroys nucleic acids in bacteria, disrupting their DNA so periodontopathogens are unable to reproduce or function properly.

- Manual toothbrushing may be as effective as powered brushes, although powered brushes with rotation oscillation significantly reduce plaque and gingivitis in both the short and long term.[36] Mouthpiece electric toothbrushes have had mixed reviews.

- Those with limited mobility of arm/hand may find using an electric toothbrush easier.

- Microwave irradiation is an effective means for disinfecting bacteria and fungi from toothbrushes.[37] Dishwashers have also been suggested for cleaning toothbrushes and toothbrush holders. Soaking toothbrushes in mouthwash or white vinegar may help.

• Tongue cleaning, either by scraping or brushing, has been shown to benefit oral health by reducing the mutans streptococci level[38] and reducing the production of volatile sulphur compounds implicated in halitosis.[39] Consider using a tongue scraper, especially in cases of tongue coating. Care should be taken to use the tongue cleaner only as directed; inappropriate or overzealous use may cause damage to the taste buds[40] or tonsils.[41]

• Consider oil-pulling for cleaning/whitening.

- Consider using oral irrigators which direct a stream of water into the oral cavity for removal of food particles and plaque from around and between teeth. They are also referred to as water flossers and by their brand names, the best known of which is Waterpik®, a device that uses high-pressure pulsating water. Used alongside a toothbrush, it can reduce plaque, gingival inflammation and bleeding.[42] Oral irrigators are not a substitute for toothbrushing but offer a useful additional method of cleansing the oral cavity, thought to be particularly helpful for those with dental braces. Their use is associated with decreased levels of potent pro-inflammatory cytokine IL-1β alongside increased levels of anti-inflammatory cytokine IL-10.[43] Assessment of the effect of oral irrigation on people with both periodontal disease and diabetes (T1D/T2DM) found reduction of pro-inflammatory cytokines (IL-1β and prostaglandin E_2) and ROS – tissue destructive pathways implicated in the pathogenesis of many conditions; dental water jet combined with routine oral hygiene was 44 per cent more effective at reducing gingival bleeding and 41 per cent more effective in reducing gingival inflammation in diabetic patients, compared with routine oral hygiene alone.[44]

- Check the relative dentine abrasivity (RDA) of toothpastes – this can be found online for some brands. Do not use overly gritty toothpastes which can wear away the enamel. See Appendix 4 for a link to a list of RDA values for toothpastes in the USA.

- Tooth powders are a much earlier version of toothpaste. Dental powders, which often mostly contain natural ingredients, can be more effective at plaque removal than toothpaste,[45] and, because powders do not contain SLS or fluoride, may be a safer option. Creating a bespoke dental powder is easier than for toothpaste. However, dental powders can be less convenient to use than a paste and ingredients may leave a different texture in the mouth.

- Mouthguards should be cleaned regularly. Clean teeth before and after use, don't chew it and never share.

- Oral hygiene starts with healthy saliva. One of the many roles of saliva is, more or less, to constantly flush the oral cavity, remove food debris and keep the mouth relatively clean. Salivary flow diminishes considerably during sleep[46] and may allow bacterial populations to build up in the mouth overnight. Lysozyme in saliva can help to prevent the overgrowth of microbial populations by lysing bacteria. Low salivary flow during sleep means pre-bedtime tooth cleaning is very important.[47,48] In the daytime, acid formed in plaque is neutralized by saliva.[49] Encourage healthy salivary flow, especially where pharmaceutical products have a xerostomic effect.

- For good oral health it is necessary to remove fermentable carbohydrates (e.g. sucrose, glucose and acidic foods/drinks) as soon as possible after intake.[50] This is facilitated by salivary flow. It is especially important not to consume such foods/drinks before bedtime since salivary flow diminishes during sleep.[51]

- Whilst advice generally is to clean teeth before food, there is a suggestion that this might train the brain to associate teeth cleaning with an empty stomach/hunger, whereas brushing after eating may train the brain to associate teeth cleaning with a full stomach,[52] making teeth cleaning a potentially useful means to quash hunger at other times of the day. Individuals who seek hunger control might rinse with water after food, delaying teeth cleaning for an hour if possible after eating.

- Mouthwash is not a replacement for brushing and flossing. Although mouthwash may provide a 'quick fix' for bad breath, it just masks the problem. Tongue cleaning is a better option as it removes the cause. Salt rinses are an alternative option.

- To help keep teeth from staining, rinse the mouth with water after eating and drinking as well as after flossing and brushing. Consider using a straw when drinking beverages that are staining.

STRAWS: PROS AND CONS

The use of straws for drinking beverages has reported advantages and disadvantages with respect to health.

Reported advantages have focused on delivery location of staining and caries-causing beverages (straws deliver to the back of the oral cavity, reducing exposure to teeth). However, since beverages likely do make contact with teeth, straws may not confer this benefit. If delivery to the mouth is consistently behind the front teeth, straw-use may increase propensity for tooth decay/caries.

Additionally, straw-use may result in excessive air swallowing which may cause belching, bloating or flatulence.[53] For frequent-users of straws, repeated use of the orbicularis oris muscle around the mouth for the puckering of lips around the straw may result, in time, in deep lines around the mouth,[54] similar to those seen in smokers.[55]

- Avoid brushing teeth immediately after using inhaled corticosteroids (inhalers for asthma/COPD).[56] These and beta-2 agonist use are associated with the increased prevalence of dental caries,[57] and asthmatic children show a significant increase in caries.[58] Inhalation therapy may affect saliva (causing xerostomia), increasing the risk of dental caries, altering the mucosal environment (encouraging candidiasis, dysphagia, ulceration, etc.), and causing halitosis, gingivitis, periodontitis and taste disturbances. Gastrointestinal reflux due to beta-2 agonist use may increase the likelihood of dental erosions.[59] Xerostomia and impaired saliva secretion may be caused by use of beta-adrenergic agonists.[60] In a study of 30 children (aged 6 to 14 years) that looked at the effect of inhaler corticosteroids on saliva and plaque pH as well as the effect of chewing gum following its use, inhaler use caused a significant decrease in salivary pH after 30 minutes following use; chewing a xylitol-based (or similar) chewing gum for at least one minute may neutralize plaque pH.[61] Sugar-based inhalers have been observed to cause the most substantial pH drop.[62] Inhaler-users could rinse their mouth with a neutral or basic pH mouth rinse (e.g. milk, water) immediately after inhaler-use, especially before bedtime, to counteract the acidic pH of dry powder inhalers.[63]

- A spacer device is recommended for use with inhalers to reduce deposits of medication in the oral cavity and direct them toward the lungs.[64]

- Interdental brushing represents an important and essential part of oral hygiene according to the ADA[65] and is an excellent means of shifting food stuck between teeth as well as gently brushing the interdental surfaces. Flossing and interdental cleaning is important. Learn correct technique. Use dental floss/tape and/or interdental brushes at least once daily (preferably more frequently). Water-flossing may also help, although some dentists find this less effective and recommend it in addition to flossing, rather than instead of flossing.

- Brush and floss the teeth daily, twice (or more frequently), to remove biofilm in gingival crevices as biofilm/plaque presence stimulates an inflammatory response. For those who haven't been doing this, the initial response may be increased inflammation.

- With gingivitis, oral hygiene once resumed can quickly restore a healthier environment if plaque accumulation around the gingival margin is removed.[66]

- Use age-appropriate dentifrice, an appropriate level of fluoride (where advisable) and an appropriate amount (a small pea-sized amount, not a 'ribbon' of toothpaste). Spit out after brushing. Some suggest the mouth should not be rinsed with water after tooth-brushing to enhance the effectiveness of toothpaste[67] but since mouth contents may have a mixture of toothpaste and undesirable substances, it is probably best spat out rather than swallowed. Supervise children to minimize the risk of swallowing toothpaste.

- Do not brush directly after eating as this may damage the enamel.
- Brushing teeth three times daily has been shown to lower the abundance of *Candida albicans* in stool 10-fold to 100-fold.[68]

Dental products

Oral hygiene products are big business, and trend analysis shows that market size has increased with continued projected growth in the period 2021 to 2028.[69]

The high incidence of dental caries drives the market and the delivery means for dentifrices have been the focus of development and innovation. All age groups are served by market forces but the older and youngest populations are common target populations for this market.

The desire for whiter teeth is not a new phenomenon. Pearly white teeth were a symbol of wealth in ancient times. Then, and now, they are a symbol of beauty. Rising awareness of available aesthetic/cosmetic dental treatments may drive this market going forward.

Consumers need to be able to make informed choices; some ingredients (and procedures) may have negative health implications and/or impact systemic health.

Today, as with toothpastes, commercial mouthwashes have diversified in type, and formulas are available for sensitive teeth and whitening. Hydrogen peroxide and sodium hexametaphosphate are now common ingredients included for lifting and preventing future tooth-staining.[70] Sodium hexametaphosphate is known to have a corrosive nature and cause skin irritation,[71] but is included in mouthwashes and whitening chewing gum.[72] The pros and cons of hydrogen peroxide, found in whitening products, are discussed below.

Some mouthwashes (and other oral products – e.g. chewing gum, toothpaste) contain the active ingredient chlorhexidine, an antiseptic and disinfectant. The pros and cons are discussed below.

Consider the following:

- When choosing dental products with antimicrobial ingredients, opt for those where the ingredient is not too high on the ingredients list. Ensure use of an oral probiotic (at a different time of the day).

- Cetylpyridinium chloride (CPC) is a synthetic ingredient often found in mouthwashes. CPC use can cause tooth discolouration in some individuals[73] – 3 per cent of users it is claimed.[74]

- Observe caution when using products containing chlorhexidine and other toxic and controversial ingredients such as triclosan, microbeads, alcohol, aspartame and SLS.

- Understand the risks and limitations of products for tooth-whitening (removing surface staining to restore natural shade) and tooth-bleaching (typically to lighten tooth colour, using ingredients such as hydrogen peroxide or carbamide peroxide). These ingredients may be used in at-home 'whitening' kits as well as in mouthwashes.

- Consider using topical ozonated oil for oral lesions and conditions.[75] Ozonated oils have useful antiseptic properties and have been found to have an antimicrobial effect against bacterial strains including the opportunistic *Staphylococcus aureus* and the periodontopathogenic *Porphyromonas gingivalis*.[76] Ozonated oil has been shown to be effective in maintaining and improving gingival health. In addition to the potential antimicrobial effect, massaging gingiva with ozonated oil may mechanically disrupt dental biofilm and stimulate blood circulation to gingival tissues, strengthening the immune response.[77]

- See Appendix 3 for a list of ingredient types found in toothpastes.

Tooth bleaching

The safety of tooth bleaching (and tooth-bleaching ingredients) is called into question by a number of studies. Using tooth-whitening products should be an informed decision, recognizing the contraindications and potential side effects. There has been some suggestion that bleaching with chemicals should be in the sole control of dental surgeons and not, as at present, available as cosmetic over-the-counter products.[78]

Before dental bleaching is performed, external cleaning processes should be used to remove saliva and tannins on tooth surfaces, which can inactivate ROS.[79] After dental bleaching treatment, avoiding eating/drinking dark-coloured foods (e.g. red wine) and avoiding smoking are recommended as teeth may stain considerably straight after bleaching treatments.

Note that there are other, likely safer, oxidizing agents that can cause bleaching reactions, such as ozone.[80]

Appendix 4 includes a link for a referenced article on the safety of home bleaching techniques, including potential major long-term/systemic risks.[81]

HYDROGEN PEROXIDE

Even low concentrations of hydrogen peroxide are cytotoxic and can trigger molecular mechanisms in human dental pulp cells which activate apoptosis.[82] The potential for hydrogen peroxide to cause long-term tooth damage is unknown and possibly underestimated.

Since the effects of daily use of hydrogen peroxide mouthwashes have not been evaluated, daily use of a mouthwash with this ingredient is possibly not a safe option.

If hydrogen peroxide is to be used in a mouthwash product, swish, don't gargle and never swallow. Note that sensitivity may occur.

CHLORINE DIOXIDE

Chlorine dioxide gels for tooth bleaching may be available in beauty spas and on cruise ships (for delivery by beauty therapists and hair dressers) where, under maritime legislation, the treatments are not officially in the UK (where use of whitening treatment can only be by registered dentists). The safety of chlorine dioxide whitening gel has not been proven. The American Dental Association states that there is no evidence that chlorine dioxide products are safer than peroxide-based products.[83] Damaging effects on teeth have been seen including etching of teeth, loss of tooth lustre, teeth appearing more discoloured, teeth absorbing more stains than before, teeth feeling rough, teeth more sensitive and sometimes permanently sensitive.[84] Systemic effects have also been reported with the use of chlorine dioxide including inhalation and breathing difficulties, heart irregularities, eyes watering, exacerbation of asthmatic condition, increased heart rate and palpitations, even admission to A&E/emergency room.[85]

Carbopol and glycerine, two compounds added as thickeners to these products to improve adherence of the bleaching agent to teeth, may also cause alterations in the microhardness of enamel and dentine.[86]

CHLORHEXIDINE

Although the World Health Organization considers chlorhexidine to be one of the safest and most effective medicines,[87] it should be used with informed consideration.

Chlorhexidine molecules have positive charges at both ends. Interaction with bacteria and yeast cells, which tend to have negatively charged areas on their exteriors, causes damage to the cell membranes of microbes, thus slowing their reproduction and even destroying their cell membrane, thus killing the microbe.[88]

Chlorhexidine, also known as chlorhexidine gluconate (CHG), is used in a number of ways for its antiseptic and disinfectant properties: skin and instrument sterilization pre-surgery, cleaning wounds, preventing dental plaque and other situations. It is found in toothpastes, deodorants and as a preservative in eye drops, as well as its use in mouthwashes.

CHG is active against many types of microorganism – both Gram-positive and Gram-negative bacteria, fungi and some viruses.[89] Its inclusion in mouthwashes may help reduce plaque build-up and improve gingivitis.[90] Chlorhexidine mouthwash is sometimes prescribed by dentists to help control and kill oral bacteria and its powerful antibacterial properties may help maintain a healthy oral cavity after some dental procedures.

However, CHG also has a number of potential adverse effects: tooth discolouration, impaired taste, damage to the mouth lining, and tartar build-up[91] – what it is meant to reduce. Additionally, chlorhexidine mouthwashes may cause burning, tingling, a numb sensation on the tongue, dry mouth, peeling of the inside of the mouth, temporary staining of the tongue and swelling of the salivary glands.[92]

Chlorhexidine is incompatible with some ingredients of conventional toothpastes; either use the mouthwash at a different time of day than the toothpaste or, after using toothpaste, rinse the mouth with water and wait before using chlorhexidine mouthwashes.[93] The recommended interval between toothbrushing and rinsing with chlorhexidine mouth rinse is more than 30 minutes and, cautiously, close to two hours after brushing.[94]

Since rinsing with chlorhexidine for four weeks or longer causes extrinsic tooth-staining,[95] if products with this ingredient are used, they should be used short term. Avoid foods and beverages for at least an hour after using a chlorhexidine mouthwash to help prevent staining the teeth.[96]

Dental sealants and varnish

Dental sealants, intended to prevent tooth decay by using materials on pits and fissures of teeth thereby creating a smooth, easier to clean surface, are offered mainly for children although sometimes for adults. One such material used is the viscous resin bisphenol-a-glycidyl dimethacrylate (BIS-GMA; see below). Glass ionomer cement fissure sealants are also available and, because they release fluoride across an extended period, are considered by some to be advantageous.[97] Information in this section is provided for reader awareness of possibilities that can be raised with a holistic dentist or suitably qualified dental professional.

SEALANT INGREDIENTS

Concerns have been raised over BIS-GMA regarding an association with xenoestrogen bisphenol-A (BPA); dental sealants and composites ('white' fillings) contain compounds that turn into BPA on contact with saliva,[98] and the use of BIS-GMA-based resins in dental sealants and composites, particularly in children, appears to contribute to human exposure to xenoestrogens.[99]

BIS-GMA sealants leach varying amounts of BPA.[100] Small amounts of BPA may leach from dental sealants immediately after application but BPA was not detected in blood samples in one study indicating no detectable systemic exposure from the dental sealant.[101]

A systematic review found BPA forms in the mouth after application of some dental sealants and 'white' fillings and can be found in saliva up to three hours after completion of a dental intervention. Cleaning and rinsing surfaces of sealants/composites immediately after placement can reduce BPA exposure, and, overall, the proven benefits of these interventions alongside the brevity of BPA exposure suggest that, as long as precautionary application techniques are strictly adhered to, use should be continued.[102]

Manufacturers do not have to disclose all the product ingredients, and it should be noted that other little-studied compounds (e.g. triethylene glycol dimethacrylate and urethane dimethacrylate) may also pose risks.[103]

BPA exposure may not be a potential consequence of BIS-GMA-based resins in dental sealants (and 'white' fillings). Endocrine-disrupting compounds such as BPA may negatively affect human immune function.[104] This may represent a potential risk to patients and needs to be considered alongside the potential functional benefits of the sealant.

Disclosure of ingredients in sealants and composites should be required. For some clients, such ingredients may hamper the effectiveness of the protocol.

Dental fluoride varnishes are sometimes used in conjunction with dental sealants. There is some evidence that sealants may be more advantageous than fluoride varnishes.[105]

A Cochrane Review of fluoride varnishes for preventing dental caries in children and adolescents found a substantial caries-inhibiting effect (as much as 43% reduction average in decayed, missing and filled tooth surfaces) in both permanent and primary teeth, although the quality of evidence was assessed as moderate due to issues with trial designs.[106] These are important considerations in light of the prevalence of dental issues in young people, since periodontal health is known to be associated with systemic health.

Whilst prevention of periodontal issues is an important aim and potential advantage of fluoride varnish, risks from fluoride exposure must also be considered.

'Tooth or consequences'

Without doubt the aim should be to avoid having 'toxic teeth' – from mercury (which focuses its toxins on the CNS), from bacterial endotoxins in cavitations and via oral hygiene products/procedures.

The moral of the story 'Tooth or consequences' is avoid all need for tooth replacement and restoration by practising informed, good oral hygiene. Dental interventions for cosmetic reasons may not be the best health choice. Good dental health is important to whole-body health.

— Chapter 17 —

LIFESTYLE OPTIONS

This final protocol chapter outlines other lifestyle considerations for dental and oral optimal health. Complementary therapies are also included. Dietary supplements may be used as required but have mostly been discussed earlier in the book.

Other considerations

- Ensure optimal detoxification function – exercise to the point of sweating (or consider sweat therapies); consider massage therapies and saunas.

- Resolve infections in the mouth, tonsils and elsewhere (e.g. herpes virus) and eliminate reasons for contracting new infections.

- Address sleep issues including sleep apnoea.

- Mouth-breathing (which is generally normal only during exercise, and abnormal when it occurs during rest) alters the salivary flow rate and buffering capacity[1] and significantly increases levels of free sialic acid, suggesting higher bacterial retention.[2] Excessive mouth-breathing has been linked to a wide range of oral conditions (e.g. halitosis, caries) as well as medical conditions (e.g. asthma, altered posture).[3] Explore the Buteyko breathing method.

- Address blocked olfaction, which may result in reduced gustation.

- Protect the lips generally, especially from sun exposure. As no melanin is produced in the lips, there is a higher risk of sunburn; lip cancer is not uncommon. The vermillion of lips has no sebaceous glands, sweat glands or facial hair.[4] The skin overlying the soft tissue of the vermillion (the red part of the lips) is less thick than that on the face – approximately three to five cellular layers compared with up to 16 layers on typical facial skin. The lips dry out faster than facial skin, becoming chapped because, without sebaceous and sweat glands, there is no protective, moisturizing layer of sweat/body oils to keep lip-skin smooth and inhibit pathogens.[5] The pink-red tone of the vermillion zone of lips is due to the underlying blood vessels; lips bleed easily when injured.

- Heal cracked lips with *Aloe vera* or cucumber. Avoid salty/spicy foods.

- Address hormone imbalance (e.g. oestrogen, testosterone, thyroid hormone) and monitor; an imbalance may negatively impact body cells, calcium metabolism and bone metabolism. Adjust gradually.

- Address neurotransmitter imbalance if necessary – particularly re satiety.

- Regulate stress, which may significantly decrease the salivary secretion rate of sIgA[6] and alter immune function.[7]

- Salivary IgA and IgM concentrations decline immediately after a bout of intense exercise and usually recover within 24 hours;[8] habitual intense exercise may suppress mucosal immunity. An increased risk of respiratory illness is associated with low levels of salivary IgM and IgA. Support immune health if an individual regularly does intense exercise.

- Consider alternative/holistic therapies as appropriate: homeopathy, tissue/cell salts, acupuncture, tongue diagnosis. Lymphatic drainage, especially of the oral and nasal cavities, may benefit.

- Clients using prescription medications should understand the potential side effects on salivary flow. In all cases of xerostomia, stomatitis, dysgeusia and perhaps with some other oral cavity issues, pharmaceutical prescription medications should be investigated first as the cause.

- Anticoagulant natural substances (garlic, high-dose vitamin E, omega-3 fatty acids, *Ginkgo biloba*, ginger) may increase bleeding during dental treatment[9] and gingivitis.

- Guaraná and yerba maté may enhance the effects of numbing substances used by dentists.[10]

- Bisphosphonates may impact healing in the oral cavity.[11] Aim to address periodontal health before using these medications.

- Bisphosphonate use should be revealed to the dentist and considered in treatment plans; ensuring the patient is dentally healthy prior to or at the early stages of bisphosphonate administration is advisable. Extractions and implants may carry a risk for such individuals; where aggressive surgical salvage procedures are needed, a bisphosphonate drug holiday should be discussed as a possibility with the treating medical practitioner.[12]

- Use of Teflon™ and other non-stick pans may impact health by increasing exposure to fluorine. Polytetrafluoroethylene (PTFE), marketed as the non-stick surface Teflon™, as well as for cable insulation, for plumber's tape, and as the basis of Gore-Tex® (used in waterproof shoes and clothing)[13] as well as for other water/soil-repellent finishes (e.g. Scotchgard by 3M Corporation),[14] is shown to break down into PFOS (perfluorooctane sulfonate), a man-made perfluorochemical that doesn't decompose in nature.[15] PFOA (perfluorooctanoic acid) which is/has been used in association with PTFE manufacture is an emerging health concern and subject of regulatory action and voluntary industrial phase-outs. PFOAs have been detected in industrial waste, house dust, water, food, Teflon™ cookware, carpet cleaning liquids and microwave popcorn bags. See the discussion of iodine in Chapter 15.

- Modern pharmaceuticals that contain 'organofluorines' (chemical compounds containing carbon and fluorine), for example Prozac/Fluoxetine, may impact health by increasing exposure to fluorine. Not all organofluorine-containing pharmaceuticals increase fluorine exposure as this depends on the strength of the bond between fluorine and the carbon.[16] Some of these drugs do, however, metabolize into fluoride (e.g. Cipro,[17] fluorinated anaesthetics such as Isoflurane[18] and Sevoflurane[19]).

- Whilst an alkaline diet is generally recommended (for caries prevention and overall systemic health), individuals with generalized chronic gingivitis (but not generalized chronic periodontitis) have been found to have more alkaline salivary pH.[20] Rinsing the mouth with water after food/drink may help neutralize salivary pH and should be encouraged. Be aware that strongly alkaline substances may also damage teeth, destroying parts of the organic content of the tooth, increasing the vulnerability of its enamel. Exposure to highly alkaline solutions (e.g. alkaline degreaser used in the car industry) can degrade tooth enamel surfaces (flaking, increasing porosity), potentially increasing profoundly the risk for caries from acidic foods/beverages.[21,22] Other highly alkaline substances that may cause similar damage to teeth are used in the food industry, and in substances to remove graffiti.

- Use of illicit drugs may be associated with oral health complications including caries, periodontal diseases, xerostomia, bruxism, tooth wear, tooth loss, mucosal dysplasia, burns/sores on lips/inside mouths and, in relation to cocaine snorting, with perforation of the palate.[23] Use of methamphetamine ('meth'/'speed') is associated with blackened, crumbling and rotting teeth. Xerostomia is common. Hydration, sialogogue use, pain management and dental treatment, including for bruxism, may be needed.[24]

- Those for whom fluoride exposure through water fluoridation may be a particularly problematic health factor include bottle-fed infants who may be receiving excessive doses,[25] children with fluorosis, dialysis patients and those with poor kidney function, and individuals with arthritis and conditions associated with thyroid function. Individuals with iodine deficiency may suffer amplified neurological damage from even low levels of fluoride exposure. Individuals with deficiencies of vitamin C, vitamin D and/or calcium may suffer amplified toxic effects on bone tissue.[26] Individuals who drink large quantities of tap water (including athletes) may also be affected.

- Know if water is fluoridated in order to make educated choices. Whilst fluoride may have potential benefits for teeth in relation to prevention of caries, it may also negatively impact teeth, act as a neurotoxin, displace iodine and can negatively impact many life processes, including fertility. Fluoride, chlorine and bromine can displace iodine. See Appendix 1 for discussion on how to reduce exposure to fluoride. See Appendix 4 for further information and resources about fluoride.

- To minimize exposure to chlorine, use bottled water or a quality water filter. Alternatively, to remove most of the chlorine from tap water, fill glass bottles with tap water and allow it to sit uncovered in the refrigerator for 24 hours. Or boil the water.

- Tobacco smoke contains thiocyanate which has an inhibitory effect on iodine uptake.[27]

- Smoking diminishes taste sensation.[28] Additionally, smoking disrupts oral microbiome homeostasis and has shown an association, during gingival inflammation, with lower activity/output of cystatin C[29] (which has a protective role in the neuronal health of the brain).[30]

- Smoking may cause noticeable upper-lip wrinkles,[31] referred to as 'smoker's lips' or 'smoker's lines' caused by the repetitive activity of the circular orbicularis oris muscle. The overall effect of altered muscle use may cause a sad facial expression.[32]

- Management of candidiasis might include cessation of smoking, improved oral hygiene, addressing xerostomia, using antifungals and general immune support.

- Vomiting (including from excess alcohol, food poisoning and purging associated with disordered eating) affects oral health, altering pH and disrupting the mouth environment.

- Dental, oral mucosal and saliva abnormalities are typically observed from the early stages of eating disorders; oral manifestation of anorexia nervosa and bulimia nervosa include dental lesions, mucosal lesions, periodontal lesions, salivary manifestations, dysgeusia and oral pain. The reason for the presence of ghrelin (often dysregulated in eating disorders) in saliva has yet to be determined[33] but it appears to play a regulatory role in the innate immune response to inflammatory infection in the oral cavity.[34]

- Bariatric surgery may increase the risk for periodontal disease.[35]

- Consider the impact of psychogenic pain, referred pain and neurological and vascular disorders on oral health and address as necessary. Mood-boosting and other therapies may be indicated.

- Antibiotics use can impact oral microbiome health. If used, recommend suitable probiotics for protection.

— Chapter 18 —

RESEARCH DIRECTIONS

This chapter summarizes evolutionary and genetic research as well as existing and likely future research directions. These may inform protocol suggestions going forward.

Sialochemistry

Saliva may be seen as 'key to the pathological and disease biomarker library hidden inside our bodies';[1] saliva assessment/testing will likely be used more frequently in the future for diagnosis/prevention.

Saliva is 'the most available and non-invasive biofluid of the human body', offering a 'diagnostic window to the body', having been used diagnostically for more than two thousand years and considered as the 'brother' of blood in TCM.[2] Ancient people had a high regard for body fluids as important indicators of health; they also recognized the antimicrobial properties of external body fluids and used the topical application of saliva, colostrum and urine as a prophylactic or cure.[3]

Saliva has been referred to as 'one of the most complex, versatile and important body fluids'. This is probably partly in recognition of its ability to reflect normal internal characteristics and disease states. Saliva exchanges with substances from plasma due to the thin layer of epithelial cells which separate salivary ducts from systemic circulation.[4] Although there is this exchange from blood to saliva, qualitative and quantitative variety seen in saliva composition (which reflects food/drink, circadian and psychological factors) is a major difference from serum (in which concentrations of various constituents can only vary between narrow border values).[5]

Whilst blood tests are still the most commonly used type of body fluid test, saliva testing is increasingly used and valued. Proteins in both fluids show comparable functional diversity and disease linkage, although for some diseases saliva may have greater diagnostic potential. Nearly 40 per cent of proteins suggested as biomarkers for diseases such as cancer, cardiovascular disease and stroke are found in saliva. Saliva may have diagnostic potential for these as well as for gastrointestinal, inflammatory, infectious and respiratory diseases where saliva has higher numbers of implicated proteins than plasma.[6] In addition to these health conditions, saliva can be used for hormonal analysis and to investigate use of pharmaceutical drugs (e.g. lithium, barbiturates, cyclosporine), legal drugs (e.g. alcohol, tobacco) and illicit drugs (e.g. marijuana, cocaine, amphetamines).[7]

Endocrine function is effectively assessed via salivary hormone levels/patterns, which reflect circulating hormone levels and are considered the best way to evaluate diurnal patterns of cortisol and melatonin.[8] Insulin, aldosterone, oestradiol/oestriol, progesterone, testosterone and dehydroepiandrosterone (DHEA) can all be accurately assessed via saliva.[9]

Systemic diseases for which determination of salivary composition may be useful include cystic fibrosis, Sjögren's syndrome, cancer and cardiovascular disease.[10]

Infectious viral diseases are effectively assessed via salivary testing, including HIV, herpes virus, Epstein-Barr, cytomegalovirus and hepatitis. Saliva is also a useful tool to assess *Helicobacter pylori* infection and other bacterial disease conditions – dental caries, gingivitis and periodontal disease.[11]

Oral disease biomarkers are discussed in Greabu *et al.* (2009) who suggest that, 'as we enter the era of genomic medicine, sialochemistry will play an increasingly important role in early detection, monitoring and progression of systemic and oral diseases'.[12]

Saliva tests are non-invasive and are easy to do.

Genetics

Although there are genes known to associate with both caries and periodontal disease, there is currently no identified gene with effect greater than that of environmental factors according to the American Dental Association (ADA), which discusses genetics and oral health on its website and emphasizes the environmental effects of diet, oral hygiene, oral health literacy and socioeconomic status.[13]

Genes associated with caries include several involved in enamel matrix, and others which associate with saliva or MMPs (some of which are possibly protective).[14] Genetic variants of amelogenin (involved in tooth mineralization) have been the most consistently found associations with caries.[15]

Regarding periodontal disease, which has been hypothesized as a two-step process involving genetic propensity followed by 'bacterial challenge',[16] genes involved in inflammatory response and several associated with MMPs are widely believed to play a role.[17] A 2017 genome-wide association study looked at gene variants associated with periodontitis and with caries, finding no genetic variants associated with both, but found several which showed moderate to strong evidence of an association with periodontitis; particularly, SNPs (single nucleotide polymorphisms) in vitamin D receptor (*VDR*), *Fc-γRIIA* (platelet receptor) and Interleukin-10 (*IL10*) genes showed strong evidence of association, with moderate evidence of association shown for interleukin-1 (*IL1-alpha* and *IL1-beta*) genes.[18]

Genetic testing may prove useful in the future with respect to clinical application in oral care protocols. For individuals with raw genetic data, relevant gene information might be found in studies referenced in the ADA online article about this subject (see Appendix 4).

Evolutionary changes

Research on evolutionary changes in the human diet/culture has shown that oral microbiota composition shifted to a more disease-associated configuration when our human ancestors transitioned from being hunter–gatherers to adopt carbohydrate-rich Neolithic (farming) diets. This remained relatively stable until the Industrial Revolution when industrially processed flour and sugar began to be used, after which cariogenic bacteria became dominant.[19] Although DNA sequences in ancient calcified dental plaque used in these research studies may not be representative of loose plaque biofilm,[20] caries and periodontal disease were rare in pre-Neolithic hunter–gatherer societies.[21]

Overall, modern Europeans have much lower phylogenetically diverse microbiomes than our pre-Industrial Revolution ancestors;[22] it has been hypothesized[23] that, since greater phylogenetic diversity associates with greater ecosystem resilience,[24] such a decline in diversity may be associated with less resilience to disturbances[25] of diet and greater susceptibility to invasion by pathogenic species.[26] Phylogenetic diversity, rather than species richness, may be associated with greater stability because the more distantly related two species are, the greater the likelihood that they differ ecologically in terms of form and function.[27]

It is important to note that caries and periodontal disease (like many other diseases in a growing list)[28] are polymicrobial[29,30] with disease initiation associated with increased microbial diversity rather than low diversity and richness, which is associated with oral health.[31]

This knowledge continues to inform research, and suggests that the most promising means to discourage caries and periodontal disease may be to encourage the 'exclusive nature of the healthy oral microbiome [using] probiotics derived from the dental plaque of healthy individuals [which] sharply antagonize cariogenic species, [alongside use of] targeted antimicrobials for the killing of specific pathogens'.[32] Rather than adding to the oral microbial community, targeted removal of problematic species might be a more effective approach.[33] 'Proactive management of oral health through an ecological approach to the holobiont' has been suggested as future clinical practice.[34]

Human microbiome project

The human microbiome project (HMP) research, initiated in 2008 to aid understanding of microbial involvement in human health and disease, has shown that microbiota are associated with a multitude of diseases including diabetes, obesity, Crohn's disease and periodontitis, and that microbial population alterations associated with disease can vary from patient to patient. Whilst differences exist between patients regarding microbial species involved with oral cavity disease, microbial communities (as functional units) have been shown to have 'highly conserved metabolic gene expression profiles,'[35] so, whilst species may vary within a plaque population, a metabolic function – enzyme expression, for example – may be well conserved and different species with capacity to perform an enzymatic function may instead be present.

Turnbaugh *et al.* (2007) discuss the HMP in terms of 'core' microbiome and 'variable' microbiome. 'Core' microbiome is comprised of predominant species found in healthy conditions in the majority of humans at varying body sites.[36] 'Variable' microbiome is unique to the specific individual (perhaps as 'unique as a fingerprint')[37] and occurs as a result of a combination of factors including host genotype, host physiological status (including properties of innate and adaptive immune systems), host disease status, host environment and host lifestyle (including diet).[38]

Each microbiome in an individual – gut, skin, oral, etc. – maintains its unique ecosystem that provides an intra-active environment (between microorganisms within that ecosystem) and interactive environment with the host.[39] Whilst each individual maintains its own unique set of microbiomic ecosystems, microbiomes of the same body location are more similar among individuals than microbiomes from different locations on the same individual.[40]

A database of the taxa present in the oral cavity, the Human Oral Microbiome Database (HOMD; www.homd.org), stores cloned sequences representing healthy and diseased oral cavity sites across the wide variety of intraoral sites. In 2010, 772 microbial species were included, 57 per cent of which were officially named.[41] Included in this abundant mix are species of the following genera: *Streptococcus, Actinomyces, Prevotella, Capnocytophaga, Fusobacterium, Corynebacterium, Veillonella, Neisseria, Selonomas, Porphyromonas, Treponema, Campylobacter, Haemophilus, Gemella* and others.[42]

The genera prevalent in either health or disease are likely to depend on nutrient availability. The primary source of nutrients for oral bacteria is found in saliva and GCF rather than the human diet itself since food is generally quickly swallowed, though it stimulates saliva production.[43] Dietary fermentable carbohydrates, however, are an exception as some bacteria can ferment sugars to produce acid which may result in dental caries; high, frequent intake of dietary fermentable carbohydrates may therefore alter microbiota, encouraging acid-tolerant species[44] with the potential to damage tooth enamel.

HMP data continues to inform research and suggest future directions.

Oral health research

Greater understanding of the systemic (as well as oral) effects of oral care ingredients and therapies may help inform protocols with the most benefits and fewest side effects/least toxicity. Therapies using ozone and ozonated oil/water, for example, are the subject of recent and ongoing research and discussion.[45,46,47,48,49]

Whilst much is known about oral (and other) microbiomes, there are a number of challenging factors related to periodontal microbiology research: samples must be obtained from periodontal pockets – small spaces that contain large numbers of pathogens including opportunistic as well as pathogenic species; some of the organisms collected are difficult to cultivate. New methods for identifying uncultivated bacteria in the oral cavity include DNA-based detection methods such as ribosomal-16S cloning and sequencing.[50]

Glycanbiology

Glycanbiology is not a new concept but is a rapidly growing science, looking at the structure, function and biology of glycans.

Glycans play a 'pivotal role' in microbial interactions in the oral cavity according to a 2018 review of oral glycobiology and glycoimmunology,[51] which discusses glycan-mediated oral cavity host defence mechanisms, including how these support systemic human health. The authors discuss how salivary mucin glycans interact with oral microbes, and how glycan recognition contributes to both colonization and clearance of oral microbes, being involved in microbial attachment, pellicle formation, microbial coaggregation and other microbial interactions.

A better understanding of the role(s) of glycans may reveal potential therapies for supporting periodontal and systemic health. Glycan-rich supplements may be usefully included in protocols.

Ongoing RANTES research

Recently, an association was found between the pro-inflammatory mediator RANTES (with a known association to cancer and other health conditions) and periodontal conditions. Future research may reveal much to inform oral health and systemic disease protocols.

How many basic tastes are there?

Although scientists have determined our three macronutrients to be fat, protein and carbohydrate, these macronutrients are not fully represented in the current five primary tastes model, which has led to speculation and investigation of fat as another (sixth) primary taste. Water, essential to our survival, has also not been recognized as either a macronutrient or a primary taste.

Scientists continue to seek explanations and find receptors and biochemical pathways to validate other tastes – water, starchiness, calcium, heartiness and alkalinity.

Although only five basic tastes have been defined in Western tradition, other cultures define basic taste sensation differently. In traditional Chinese medicine (TCM) there are five defined flavours: salty, spicy, sour, sweet and bitter. The harmony of these flavours is important in TCM, which considers the function of this harmony with respect to promoting health. Regional cuisine varies, with each area tending to have one or two of the five flavours dominating popular dishes.

According to Ayurvedic tradition, there are six tastes: *Madhura* (sweet), *Amla* (sour), *Lavana* (salty), *Tikta* (bitter), *Katu* (pungent) and *Kashaya* (astringent).[52] Each of these tastes is predominantly composed of two of five Ayurvedic elements: earth, fire, air, water and ether/space. Each of these tastes has a role, according to Ayurvedic principles, in physiology, health and well-being.

Taste research may provide a better understanding of behaviours and mechanisms in conditions that impact oral and systemic health.

Fat perception

Lipid taste detection may be determined as the sixth primary taste. Recent research has looked at the possible relationship between saliva and fat, finding that the composition of saliva may have a role in fat perception and liking.[53] Since oral hypersensitivity to fatty acids (FAs) may be associated with lower energy and fat intakes (and BMI), fat perception may be a factor in body-fat consumption,[54] and thus a propensity for obesity. With increasing numbers of clinically obese individuals, research to determine the science behind fat perception and fat intake might provide a novel means to address this unhealthy trend.

If being effective at tasting fats in food is associated with lower consumption of high-fat foods, this might also impact consumption of essential FAs (e.g. oily fish). If this is so, there may be detrimental as well as beneficial health effects of being hypersensitive to FAs. The extent to which a taste or flavour is liked plays an important role in whether the voluntary act of placing that food into the mouth is chosen, so that it can ultimately be digested and its component parts impact the body's state of health – both negatively and positively.

Experiments suggest that free FAs stimulate the perception of foods containing fat. Lipids in food are mainly triglycerides (FAs esterified with glycerol) requiring breakdown into free FAs for orosensory perception. Although there is some discussion about the extent of its effectiveness, it is thought that lingual lipase released from glands into saliva facilitates this important feature, enabling lingual lipolysis and thus orosensory perception of fats/lipids.[55] Lingual lipase may hydrolyse triglycerides, releasing free FAs in the oral cavity where they may impact taste receptor cell function.[56]

Fat perception is linked to genetic and anatomical differences (higher density of fungiform papillae, more trigeminal innervation in supertasters) between individuals[57] which potentially has implications for dietary behaviour. Keast and Costanzo found a functional significance in the oral chemosensing of fats, with an association between increased sensitivity to fat taste and increased fat consumption as well as maximization of the capacity for fat absorption in a high-fat diet (thus encouraging obesity). The authors conclude that the likely mechanism linking insensitivity to FA taste with being overweight/obesity relates to the development of satiety after consuming foods.[58]

Other contenders for a sixth taste

Water homeostasis, crucial for survival, is associated with sodium balance, and is regulated by thirst. Taste detection of water is also known to activate the gustatory system but has been comparatively less researched than the five primary tastes. Aquaporins expressed in taste receptor cells may account for water taste transduction.[59]

An article in the *New Scientist* in 2016 hailed 'starchiness' as the newest contender for a 'sixth taste',[60] citing a study that demonstrated an ability to detect the starchiness of glucose oligomers as distinct from sugars.[61]

Since starchy foods like rice, bread, pasta, potato, maize, cassava, yam and plantain are staple foods, considered by some to be a necessary component of most meals, it would make sense that humans would have an ability to taste starchiness, as distinct from sweetness. Although studies show that starchiness can be perceived as distinct from sweetness, the receptor has not yet been determined.

Since calcium and magnesium are essential for survival, they have been investigated in relation to taste perception. Calcium 'taste' does not seem appetitive, although humans may have a calcium 'appetite' when intake is dangerously low – for example in pregnancy or dialysis, since such individuals tend to have strong cravings for chalky, calcium-rich cheeses.[62] Scientists are particularly interested in calcium taste perception to investigate ways of making calcium-rich foods more palatable, thus increasing intake to prevent osteoporosis and improve intake for those at risk of health conditions exacerbated by low intake. Therapeutic agents that activate or inhibit calcium receptors may benefit in neurological diseases, hepatic diseases, cardiovascular diseases, digestive system conditions and others.[63] Calcium-rich dairy products may be palatable because calcium is bound to fats and proteins.[64]

T1R3, also involved in perceiving sweet and umami tastes, was the first receptor to be implicated in calcium–magnesium taste reception.[65] Humans were determined to detect calcium by taste via this receptor.[66]

GPCR calcium-sensing receptor (CaSR) was found to sense calcium and L-amino acids within the gastrointestinal tract.[67,68] CaSR has roles in breast and colorectal cancer, Alzheimer's disease, pancreatitis, diabetes mellitus, hypertension, and bone and gastrointestinal disorders.[69] Developments suggest that CaSR is involved in modulating appetite, controlling satiety and anti-diabetic hormone secretion in response to amino acids/dietary calcium. It may therefore have potential benefits in relation to obesity and osteoporosis and related disorders.[70]

CaSR has also been implicated in the 'kokumi' taste, a heartiness or 'mouthfulness' sensation termed by the Japanese; kokumi enhances the five basic tastes and other marginal tastes such as thickness.[71]

Kokumi appears to relate to a number of γ-glutamyl peptides (e.g. in mature Gouda cheese) and sulphur-containing amino acids (e.g. in onions and garlic).[72] Glutathione is a known *kokumi*-imparting substance.[73] *Kokumi* taste is thought to be perceived through a CaSR in humans.[74]

Alkalinity has also been researched as a taste sensation. Alkalinity would be in opposition to acidity, which is experienced as a sour taste. Sodium bicarbonate ($NaHCO_3$, baking soda) is a commonly found alkaline substance in kitchens; egg whites are also naturally alkaline.

Whilst the acid–alkaline balance of the human body is important for its function and survival (see the earlier discussion of pH), as yet no evidence has been found that humans recognize alkalinity as a 'taste'.

Research continues in this area of oral taste receptors and extra-oral taste receptors. A paper in 2015 looked at taste receptors, suggesting that oral sensing mainly influences food discrimination and nutrient appetite, while post-oral chemosensors may relate to nutrient utilization and inhibition of appetite.[75]

Foods rich in free nutrients (soup stocks, aged meats and cheese) that have clear gustatory and odorant cues may allow for 'more robust information to the brain, stronger learned anticipatory responses and better handling of nutrients in the body', suggesting that this is a key factor in more efficient food intake regulation with the potential to support weight management and treatment of metabolic diseases.[76]

Taste integration and flavour creation

In the mind, the perceived taste of food is intricately connected with its flavour, which is the distinctive taste or essential character of food and drink, is experienced in combination with olfaction and stimulation of the trigeminal nerve and is a unified sense.

In *Neurogastronomy*, Gordon M Shepherd describes how the brain creates flavour and why it matters; the concept of flavour is not due to taste and does not reside in food since the brain creates the flavour sensation. Shepherd explains that volatile molecules in foods are assessed quickly at the brain's highest level, indicating its importance, and describes how human physiology processes the information via olfactory pathways and nerves in proximity to the brain's highest cognitive centres.[77] Smell involves both orthonasal smell (the common understanding of smell, evoked on sniffing) and retronasal smell (experienced when breathing out – see the retronasal smell experiment below), and is experienced in conjunction with taste, touch, tongue movement and more.

Flavour perception involves both multi-sensory experience (smell, taste, mouth-sense, sight, sound) and behavioural response. Brain processing in the olfactory pathway is impacted by behavioural state (hungry/satiated, awake/asleep, angry/sad), thus affecting the perception of food smells and potentially modulating appetite. The role of neocortex, hippocampus, limbic and hypothalamus on emotional and motivational response, and the impact of memory, craving and language on flavour experience, may each have an impact.

Shepherd explains that understanding the human brain flavour system may inform protocols to treat the loss of smell (e.g. in Alzheimer's) and failure to thrive, including in aged individuals.

RETRONASAL SMELL

The mouth takes the credit, but the nose knows flavour according to the neuroscientist GM Shepherd.[78]

Try this experiment that Shepherd describes in *Neurogastronomy*. Using a small amount of something tasty (e.g. lemon candy), hold the breath, pinch the nose and place the food on the tongue. Preventing exhaled air from going through the nose, experience the food. Sweetness, softness and temperature, for example, may be experienced but flavour will not until the nose is unpinched, allowing stimulation of smell receptors in the nasal cavity. If there is no exhalation, no smell or flavour is experienced.

New sweeteners

There always seems to be a potential market opportunity for new or novel sweetening substances. Research continues – for example, lucuma, a natural caloric sweetener from a popular Peruvian fruit, has recently become popular. A new zero-calorie natural sweetener from the Oubli climbing plant is exciting interest.

Why taste research is important

The five basic tastes of Western tradition are well researched, although there is still much to learn. There is the potential for findings to be applied in the food and pharmaceutical industries and in therapy (e.g. dysgeusia, satiety) to benefit systemic and oral health. The number of tastes (as distinct from flavours) is also still a matter for research and there is the potential here too to contribute to therapeutic applications. In particular, research on fat taste receptors may help determine new protocols for weight management.

Greater understanding of the physiological and sensorial processes involved in taste/flavour perception, and the neurogastronomic experience of food, may also give insights that could provide commercial and therapeutic benefits.

— Chapter 19 —

ORAL HEALTH: A MISSING LINK IN FUNCTIONAL MEDICINE

Mouth and taste conditions and periodontal health are important factors in overall health and well-being, but often their contribution to health/disease states is not given proper consideration. This final chapter looks generally at why periodontal health should be given greater consideration by healthcare practitioners.

Prevalence and potential impact

Periodontal disease is the most prevalent infectious oral condition and has implications world-wide – in both developed and developing countries. Data suggests that there is a high incidence of periodontal disease in the UK, Germany, the USA and other countries in adults aged 35–44 and 65–74. Many countries, for example Germany, also have a high incidence of periodontal disease in the 15–19 years age group.[1] Although periodontitis is thought to affect 20–50 per cent of the global population,[2] it is largely preventable and treatable.

In addition to genetics, risk factors associated with periodontal disease include microorganisms (including *Porphyromonas gingivalis*), smoking, diabetes mellitus and neutrophil defects.[3] Studies indicate that risk indicators include age, osteoporosis (related to hormonal changes in women and alveolar bone density loss), drugs (e.g. calcium channel blockers associated with gingival overgrowth[4] and numerous pharmaceuticals that reduce saliva flow) and tooth-related/anatomical factors that predispose periodontium to disease. Risk markers which might predict the course of periodontal disease include nutrition, obesity, alcohol, psychosocial factors (stress and adaptation) and systemic factors (e.g.

immune suppression).[5] Poor oral hygiene is an important risk factor. Many of these factors can be addressed with suitable interventions.

Inflammation has been shown to be associated with poor oral health and a propensity for chronic illness. Environmental factors may also impact; stress, smoking, diet and a variety of lifestyle and social factors may affect host inflammatory and immune responses,[6] which also impact the oral microbiome. By addressing inflammation in the oral cavity and providing diet and lifestyle recommendations for improved/optimal oral health, health practitioners may also improve other health outcomes.

A fuller understanding of taste perception as it relates to health, including satiety and obesity, may suggest protocols to improve whole-body health.

The impact of oral health and mouth/dental conditions on mood, emotional health and self-esteem is another important consideration. Everyone likes a smiling face – the smiler and the receiver. Greater oral health literacy may positively impact these health parameters too.

Oral health protocols must be applied throughout life. The cumulative effects of inflammation, which can occur at any age, may become more problematic in older age and in states of overweight and obesity.

Healthcare practitioners, through basic understanding of the potential impact and contributory effects of compromised oral health, may recognize the benefits of addressing these and other inflammatory, oxidative and immune issues for many clients.

Concluding remarks

Oral cavity health, for which dental health is only a component, is an important consideration in whole-body health. Tooth decay and periodontal diseases are prevalent and largely preventable. Perio-systemically associated conditions (e.g. diabetes, obesity, cardiovascular disease, neurological disease and infertility) are also prevalent.

Mounting evidence shows the systemic impact of periodontal disease, including from factors such as elevated RANTES and cavitations, and the long-known impact of mercury amalgams. Addressing periodontal issues may positively impact whole-body health. As research improves our understanding – for example, of taste perception as it relates to factors such as satiety and obesity, and the role of ghrelin in saliva – it may suggest further natural means to improve both oral and whole-body health.

These chapters have covered a range of topics on oral health and its relationship with whole-body health. They include anatomical information and processes, along with discussion of the oral microbiome, important functions of saliva and the role of inflammation. They also outline oral cavity conditions, and explore oral hygiene, biological dentistry and controversial aspects of oral health. And they provide suggestions about foods, supplements and lifestyle choices for optimal oral health. Deeper recognition, understanding and appreciation of the role the oral cavity may play in inflammation and overall individual health status, greater awareness of links between oral health and systemic health and increased knowledge of biological dentistry practices would enable health practitioners to address more comprehensively the whole-body health of clients.

— Appendix 1 —

Reducing Fluoride Exposure

The addition of fluoride to municipal water supplies in some areas of the world where there are low naturally occurring levels is generally supported by their government bodies. See, for example, the NHS England website, which includes links to six scientific reviews on fluoridation of water from across the world and concludes that 'there is no credible scientific evidence that water fluoridation is harmful to health.'[1]

Other referenced evidence outlining some of the potential risks fluoride and water fluoridation may have to whole-body health has been included within the chapters of this book. The use of fluoride in toothpastes (where it should be directly applied to teeth but not swallowed) or in gels applied by dentists (often at higher ppm level), would seem to make more sense than practices such as water fluoridation schemes that daily, indiscriminately dose entire populations, raising issues of medical ethics.

Reducing exposure to fluoride in tap water (at home/work, in restaurants, on holiday, via crops irrigated with fluoridated water, in processed foods from factories using fluoridated water, etc.) may be a desired aim. To avoid fluoride in tap water, consider using spring water, water filtration (see more info below on water filters) and consider the general advice below. The Fluoride Action Network also provides a grocery store guide to avoid fluoride in beverages and food (www.fluoridealert.org).

Much of the below-listed general advice is from the Fluoride Action Network.[2]

- Reduce black and green tea consumption (and/or drink tea with younger leaves). Instant and bottled varieties are worst. Tea plants accumulate high levels of fluoride. Antioxidant levels in tea are highest in younger leaves which also have lower levels of fluoride.

- Avoid Teflon™ pans.

- Buy organic grape juice and wine because in the USA many vineyards use a fluoride pesticide called cryolite.

- Medications that contain fluoride include antidepressants, antibiotics, antihistamines, antifungals, anaesthesia, chemotherapy drugs and cholesterol-lowering drugs. Ask about any pharmaceuticals used. Avoid use of Cipro and other fluorinated pharmaceuticals (e.g. Niflumic acid, Flecainide, Voriconazole, and the anaesthetics Isofluorane and Sevoflurane). Some fluorinated drugs have been found to metabolize into fluoride within the body.

- Minimize consumption of mechanically deboned chicken (e.g. chicken fingers, chicken nuggets) as it increases the quantity of bone particles in the meat (fluoride accumulates in bone).

- Avoid processed foods, especially processed beverages.

- Don't swallow fluoride toothpaste.

- Be cautious about using fluoride gel treatments at the dentist (not suitable for all patients).

- Spring water: check levels in popular brands of water online at www.fluoridealert.org/faq and look for brands with less than 0.2ppm, ideally less than 0.1ppm.

- Not all water filters remove fluoride. Three types can remove fluoride: deionizers (using ion-exchange resins), reverse osmosis and activated alumina. These can remove about 90 per cent of fluoride.

- Brita® and Pur® filters using activated carbon filters do *not* remove fluoride.

- Water distillation will remove most (or all) fluoride.

Some additional suggestions and information to note:

- Avoid fluoridated salt (produced in Austria, the Czech Republic, France, Germany, Slovakia, Spain and Switzerland).[3]

- Distilled water does not contain fluoride as the distillation process effectively removes this (and other) contaminants.[4] Note that whilst the process of distilling water removes contaminants, distilled water tends to draw minerals from contact surfaces such as plastic containers and teeth.[5]

- Reverse osmosis strips everything out of water and makes it more acidic.[6]

- Note that boiling water concentrates fluoride[7] (a different effect to that on chlorine in water).

- Where water is fluoridated, the body is also exposed when bathing/showering.[8]
- Pastes used by dentists during teeth cleaning can be more than 20 times higher in fluoride than commercial toothpastes.[9]
- Fluoridated dental floss can release high amounts of fluoride.[10]
- Many types of dental restorative material (e.g. used for fillings and orthodontics) contain fluoride.[11]

— Appendix 2 —

Periodontitis

Warning signs of gingivitis or periodontitis according to the CDC (Centers for Disease Control in the USA)[1] are:

- halitosis or bad taste that won't go away
- red, sore or swollen gums
- tender or bleeding gums. Bleeding is a sign of inflammation. Smoking decreases blood flow to gingiva and can mask bleeding, and thus gingivitis. Uncontrolled diabetes will cause gums to bleed more than expected.
- receding gums that have pulled away from teeth, causing teeth to look longer
- painful chewing
- loose teeth or teeth that have moved/separated
- food that gets stuck between teeth more often than previously
- sensitive teeth. Tooth sensitivity can also be a sign of tooth decay, fractures or other damage. It can be caused by sensitivity to pulp, dentine or both and usually involves pain in response to pressure or temperature extremes.
- any change in the way teeth fit together when biting down
- any change in the fit of partial dentures
- a history of periodontal abscesses.

Risk factors for periodontitis according to the CDC are:[2]

- smoking
- diabetes

- poor oral hygiene
- stress
- heredity
- crooked teeth
- underlying immunodeficiencies (e.g. AIDS)
- fillings that have become defective
- taking medications that cause dry mouth
- bridges that no longer fit properly
- female hormonal changes (e.g. pregnancy, oral contraceptives).

— Appendix 3 —

Oral Healthcare Products

Ingredient types

Ingredients in oral healthcare products have different purposes as summarized below by Lippert (2013):[1]

- fluorides (ingredients indicated with 'fluor' in its name) – various fluoride compounds are found (note that toothpastes must contain fluoride to obtain the ADA Seal of Acceptance)[2]

- anti-malodor agents (e.g. zinc salts): typically rely on chemical reaction with volatile sulfur compounds

- anti-tartar/anti-calculus agents (e.g. condensed inorganic and organic phosphates) – anti-tartar formulations often include high-flavour contents to mask the taste of condensed phosphate

- whitening agents (e.g. condensed phosphates, papain, peroxides, abrasives)

- relief of dentine hypersensitivity either via nerve desensitization (e.g. by potassium salts such as citrate and nitrate) or physical blockage of dentinal tubules (e.g. by strontium salts, stannous fluoride, calcium sodium phosphosilicate, and arginine bicarbonate in combination with calcium carbonate)

- erosion prevention agents

- other active ingredients (e.g. xylitol, re-mineralizing agents)

- excipients:
    - abrasives (e.g. hydrated silica, calcium carbonate, dicalcium phosphate dihydrate, calcium pyrophosphate, sodium metaphosphate, alumina, perlite, nano-hydroxyapatite, sodium bicarbonate) to remove stains
    - surfactants (e.g. SLS, sodium lauroyl sarcosinate, sodium cocoyl

sarcosinate, cocmidopropyl betain): responsible for foaming action and aid intraoral dispersion of toothpaste

- viscosity and rheology modifiers (e.g. carboxymethylcellulose, hydroxy-ethylcellulose, carrageenan, xanthan gum, cellulose gum): to produce gel phase containing homogenous distribution of all ingredients and prevent components from separating during storage

- humectants (e.g. glycerine and sorbitol most common, also propylene glycol, xylitol, isomalt, erythritol): to avoid water separation and evaporation and provide smooth, glossy appearance

- flavours (e.g. mint, cinnamon, lemon): for palatability

- sweeteners (e.g. xylitol, sodium saccharin, sucralose rarely): to improve taste

- colouring/sometimes stripes

- preservatives (e.g. sodium benzoate, ethyl and methyl paraben): to prevent bacterial growth during storage

- water (purified to remove calcium and trace elements)

- other

  mica – for sparkle and polishing ability

  sodium hydroxide – for pH adjustment

  ethanol as solvent

  polyethylene and prolypropylene glycols – humectants, dispersants to keep xanthan gum uniformly dispersed in toothpastes

- actives (considered by Lippert, 2013, as excipients):

  - enzymes (e.g. glucose oxidase, lactoferrin, lactoperoxidase, lysozyme): for prevention of plaque growth

  - herbal extracts for antimicrobial properties.

What to look for on oral care products labels

Each brand has its own ethical stance and marketing strategies with regard to toothpastes. Below is a list of 'Free-From' ingredients to look for:

- SLS/SLES

- foaming agents
- triclosan
- DEA
- artificial preservatives
- artificial colours (including titanium dioxide*, used for whitening toothpastes)
- artificial flavours
- artificial sweeteners, especially aspartame
- propylene glycol
- parabens
- alcohol
- microbeads
- fluoride*
- carrageenan*
- glycerine*.

*denotes ingredients which should be considered on an individual basis, by personal choice

Some features to look for in oral care products (depending on personal requirement):

- organic
- cruelty-free
- vegan or vegan-friendly
- gluten-free
- if sweetened, use of natural sweeteners such as stevia, erythritol and xylitol. Note that sorbitol is a lot less effective at controlling caries, but its less expensive cost makes it more appealing as an ingredient in toothpastes.[3]

As a general rule, if the name of the ingredient looks like a chemical name, it is often synthetic. However, basic ingredients are sometimes listed by technical names. Some acceptable, and potentially useful, ingredients which might be listed in this way are:

- sodium hydrogen carbonate: baking soda
- aqua: water
- sodium chloride: salt.

— Appendix 4 —

Information and Resources

Organizations

ADA (American Dental Association): www.ada.org/en. Seeks to power the dentistry profession and assist members in advancing overall oral health of patients.

AAEM (American Academy of Environmental Medicine): www.aaemonline.org. Founded in 1965, international association of physicians and other professionals interested in clinical aspects of humans and their environment, providing research and education in recognition, treatment and prevention of illnesses induced by exposure to biological and chemical agents encountered in air, food and water.

BDA (British Dental Association): https://bda.org. Professional association and trade union for UK dentists.

DAMS (Dental Amalgam Mercury Solutions): www.dams.cc and www.amalgam.org. Educational non-profit group founded in 1990 to provide information on amalgam and other dental health problems.

HDA (Holistic Dental Association): www.holisticdental.org. Established in 1978 to provide support and guidance to practitioners of holistic and alternative dentistry.

IABDM (International Academy of Biological Dentistry and Medicine): www.iabdm.org. Founded in 1985, an international network of dentists, physicians and allied health professionals committed to integrating body, mind, spirit and mouth in caring for the whole person. Non-profit organization 'dedicated to advancing excellence in the art and science of biological dentistry...[and] encourage[ing] the highest standards of ethical conduct and responsible patient care'.

IAOMT (International Academy of Oral Medicine and Toxicology): www.iaomt.org. For information about sources of fluoride exposure, SMART (Safe Mercury Amalgam Removal Technique), dental mercury facts, mercury poisoning symptoms, fluoride information and articles on a variety of associated topics. IAOMT is a 'trusted academy of allied professionals providing scientific resources to support new levels of integrity and safety in healthcare'. Patient resources are available online.

ICIM (International College of Integrative Medicine): https://icimed.com. Not-for-profit medical organization seeking to teach latest research in preventative, alternative and innovative treatments. Members are physicians.

IFM (The Institute for Functional Medicine): www.ifm.org. Advocate of functional medicine.

NIDR/NIDCR (National Institute of Dental and Craniofacial Research): www.nidcr.nih.gov. Branch of US National Institutes of Health, whose aim is to 'advance the nation's oral health through research and innovation'.

Oral Health Foundation: www.dentalhealth.org. Independent charity dedicated to improving oral health and well-being around the world, 'providing expert, independent and impartial advice' on all aspects of oral health.

SMART (Safe Mercury Amalgam Removal Technique): https://thesmartchoice.com. Developed by IAOMT, SMART is a set of recommendations based on scientific research. Licensed practitioners must exercise own judgement concerning specific treatment options to utilize in their practices.

Background information/discussions

Authors Hal A Huggins DDS, MS (considered the world's most controversial dentist because he tried to convince dentistry to stop using mercury in dental fillings) and Thomas E Levy (medical doctor) discuss the hidden dangers in dental care including root canals: Huggins HA, Levy TE (1999) *Uninformed Consent: The Hidden Dangers in Dental Care*. Charlottesville, VA: Hampton Roads Publishing Company. Also see Hal Huggins' website www.hugginsappliedhealing.com.

Chris Bryson's book about connections between commercial/military influences and historic government public health reassurances of fluoride safety: Bryson C (2004) *The Fluoride Deception*. New York: Seven Stories Press.

Book about science and politics of fluoride: Connett P, Beck J, Micklem HS (2010) *The Case against Fluoride*. White River Junction, VT: Chelsea Green Publishing.

Fluoride Action Network, www.fluoridealert.org. International coalition seeking to broaden public awareness about toxicity of fluoride compounds and health impacts of current fluoride exposures. Many journal articles can be accessed at their website.

Dr Joseph M Mercola interview about fluoride with Dr Bill Osmunson: https://articles.mercola.com/sites/articles/archive/2011/10/11/dr-bill-osmunson-on-fluoride.aspx

Other information sources

Books on oral cavity anatomy: Shannon JB (2012) *Dental Care and Oral Health Sourcebook* (4th edn). Detroit, MI: Omnigraphics; Tortora GJ, Derrickson B (2007) *Tortora's Principles of Anatomy and Physiology* (11th edn). Hoboken, NJ: John Wiley & Sons.

Dr Marilyn Glenville's book about natural alternatives to sugar: Glenville M (2016) *Natural Alternatives to Sugar*. Tunbridge Wells, Kent: Lifestyle Press.

Professor of Neurobiology Gordon M Shepherd's book about how the brain creates flavour and why it matters, in which he discusses 'neurogastronomy': Shepherd GM (2012) *Neurogastronomy: How the Brain Creates Flavor and Why It Matters*. New York: Columbia University Press.

Book about the eight 'beneficial saccharides' and glyconutrients: Mondoa EI, Kitei M (2001) *Sugars That Heal: The New Healing Science of Glyconutrients*. New York: Ballantine Books.

Arthur McCooey's website about sugars with stated aim of providing basic, accurate and up-to-date information on sweeteners: www.sugar-and-sweetener-guide.com/glycemic-index-for-sweeteners.html

Toothpaste Abrasiveness Ranked by RDA (Relative Dentin Abrasion) Value by Mike Williamson DDS, MS (Austin, TX, USA): www.williamsonperio.com/wp-content/uploads/2014/07/Toothpaste-Abrasiveness-Ranked-by-RDA.pdf

Referenced article on safety of home bleaching techniques, including potential major long-term/systemic risks: Tam L (1999) The safety of home bleaching techniques. *J Can Dent Assoc* 65: 453–455, www.cda-adc.ca/jcda/vol-65/issue-8/453.html

Buteyko breathing method: www.buteyko.co.uk

Article by Dr Dana Colson describing the process of safe removal of mercury amalgam: Colson DG (2012) A safe protocol for amalgam removal. *Journal of Environmental and Public Health*, https://dx.doi.org/10.1155%2F2012%2F517391

List of localized and systemic diseases and pathophysiological processes associated with ischaemic osteonecrosis (cavitations): Bouquot JE, McMahon RE (2000) Neuropathic pain in maxillofacial osteonecrosis. *J Oral Maxillofac Surg 58*: 1003–1020.

Information about the association between RANTES and cavitations: numerous studies by Dr Johann Lechner can be accessed via databases including GoogleScholar and PubMed.

Discussion of genetics and oral health, including list of associated genes, on ADA website: www.ada.org/en/member-center/oral-health-topics/genetics-and-oral-health?source=VanityURL

Information on homeopathy in dentistry: Wander P (2010) *Dental Homeopathy*, www.britishhomeopathic.org/charity/how-we-can-help/articles/conditions/d/top-5-reasons-we-visit-the-dentist, and Newadkar UR, Chaudhari L, Khalekar YK (2016) Homeopathy in dentistry: is there a role? *Phamacognosy Res 8*, 3, 217.

Information on tissue salts and dentistry: Gilbert P (1989) *Thorsons Complete Guide to Homeopathically Prepared Mineral Tissue Salts.* Wellingborough, Northamptonshire: Thorsons Publishing Group.

List of pharmaceuticals impacting oral health: Aps JKM, Martens LC (2005) Review: the physiology of saliva and transfer of drugs into saliva. *Forensic Science International 150*: 119–131.

Photographs, articles and PowerPoint presentations on various subjects related to oral cavity health, especially NICO and ischaemic bone disease: Dr JE Bouquot's informative DropBox at www.dropbox.com/sh/umu7o3jce1p5vz6/AABhfYreRJu165xBU1yKUdzta?dl=0

Short articles and blogs on oral health by the author, available at https://roseholmes.info/oral-health-systemic-disease-book:

- Anatomy for Those Who Don't Know What Gleeking Is (extended version)
- Sugars 101 (extended version, including The Not So Sweet History of Sugars)
- Are Teeth Bone?
- What Lips Can Tell Us
- Two Tastes Humans Share with Penguins
- Gram-Negative vs Gram-Positive Bacteria

- 'Delicious' History: The Discovery of Umami
- Miswak, Snail Shells and Crushed Bones: History of Oral Hygiene Products

Products/product ranges focussing on periodontal health

The list includes varying product types, ingredient types and naturalness. Not all products by these companies will be relevant or natural. Inclusion in this list does not suggest endorsement, nor is this list definitive.

Dentalcidin™ Broad-Spectrum Toothpaste and Dentalcidin™ LS Liposomal Oral Care Solution with Biocidin® from Bio-Botanical Research®: www.biocidin.com

Toothpastes: Green People®: www.greenpeople.co.uk/shop/by-product/natural-toothpaste

Toothpastes, mouth rinses: Jāsön®: www.jason-personalcare.com/en/category/oral/show-all

Toothpastes, mouth rinses: Weleda: www.weleda.co.uk/shop/dental-care

Toothpastes, tooth powders: Uncle Harry's Natural Products: www.uncleharrys.com

Tooth powders: Jeanie Botanicals: https://www.jeaniebotanicals.com/botanical-tooth-powder

Toothpastes: Dr. Bronner's: https://shop.drbronner.com/body-care

Tooth powders, toothbrushes, tongue scrapers: Dirty Mouth® by Primal Life Organics®: www.primallifeorganics.com/collections/dental

Toothpastes, mouth rinses: Tom's of Maine®: www.tomsofmaine.com/products/oral-care

Toothpastes, mouth rinses: Desert Essence®: www.desertessence.com/dental-care

Toothpastes: LeBon: www.lebontoothpaste.co.uk

Toothpastes: Kiss My Face®: www.kissmyface.com/collections/personal-care

Toothpastes: Himalaya®: www.himalayaherbals.com/products/oralcare/index.htm, available in UK from Rio Health: https://riohealth.co.uk

Viridian Oral Care Complex: www.viridian-nutrition.com/Shop/Oral-Care-Complex-P582.aspx

OralBiotic® Lozenges by Now®: www.nowfoods.com/supplements/oralbiotic-lozenges

BioGaia® Prodentis lozenges: www.biogaia.com/product/biogaia-prodentis-lozenges

Jarro-Dophilus® Oral Probiotic by Jarrow Formulas®: www.jarrow.com/product/669/Jarro-Dophilus_Oral_Probiotic

Oral probiotics, toothpaste: Hyperbiotics®: www.hyperbiotics.com/collections/dental-ent

Toothpaste, supplements for oral health: Designs for Health®: www.designsforhealth.com

Biogena Coenzym Q10 Active Spray Ubiquinol: www.biogena.com/en/products/product.coenzym-q10-active-spray-ubiquinol-30-ml.html

Best Choice® Oral Spray Co-enzyme Q10: https://riohealth.co.uk/products/best-choice-co-enzyme-q10-oral-spray

Zymbion® Q10 Toothpaste, oral health supplements: Pharma Nord: www.pharmanord.co.uk/all-products/oral-health

Dentavital range of dental nutrients: Cytoplan: www.cytoplan.co.uk/dental-nutrients

Oral probiotic, Bio.Me™ Oral by Invivo®: https://invivohealthcare.com/products/therapeutics/bio-me-oral-60g

Liquid Stevia Extract and other South American botanicals (including anti-microbial and detoxification support) in the UK: Rio Health: https://riohealth.co.uk

Articles and do-it-yourself oral hygiene: Wellness Mama®: https://wellnessmama.com

Testing: Oral EcologiX™ Oral Health and Microbiome Profile by Invivo®: https://invivohealthcare.com/products/diagnostics/oral-ecologix

Glossary and Abbreviations

3-D cone beam scanner	A three-dimensional cone beam computed tomography scanner uses digital technology to record images of teeth, soft tissue, nerve pathways and bone in three dimensions in a single scan, revealing much more information than simple two-dimensional X-rays
Acesulfame potassium (acesulfame K)	Artificial sweetener commonly mixed with aspartame
Acidogenic	Producing acids
Aciduric	Refers to species which are highly tolerant of acidic conditions/environment, able to withstand an acid environment
Acinus	Flask-like (or sac-like), blind-ended cavities in secretory salivary ducts. Acini is the plural; acinar is the adjective
Actinobacillus actinomycetemcomitans	Gram-negative, facultative anaerobe bacteria associated with periodontitis; aka *Aggretatibacter actinomycetemcomitans*
Adhesins	Proteins on the surface of cells that mediate adherence, thus aiding colonization. Adhesins consist of polysaccharides, lipoteichoic acids, glucosyltransferases and lectins
Adsorption	Process by which adhesion to a surface occurs. Negatively charged particles (e.g. in bentonite clay) can bind with positively charged particles (such as toxins and impurities like viruses, bacteria, fungi and parasites)
AGEs	Advanced glycation end-products; proteins or lipids that become glycated due to sugars
Ageusia	Complete loss of taste perception. Hypogeusia is diminished sensory perception of taste. Dysgeusia is distorted taste

Agglutinin	Protein that protects oral cavity tissues; a substance in blood that causes particles to aggregate and coagulate
Alveolar processes (aka alveolar bone)	The thickened ridge of bone that contains the tooth sockets on the jawbones. The alveolar processes hold teeth
Amalgams	Dental amalgams commonly consist of mercury and metal alloy mixture; used to repair decayed teeth
Ameloblasts	Cells that produce enamel for teeth
Approximal surface	Contact point between teeth
Aspartame	Artificial sweetener, aka E951, made of two amino acids (excitatory aspartic acid and synthetically modified phenylalanine) and methanol
Astringency	Puckering sensation of the oral mucous membrane such as from rhubarb, red wine, tea, nuts and unripe bananas
ATP	Adenosine triphosphate; provides energy for living cells
Ayurveda (or Ayurvedic medicine)	One of the world's oldest holistic healing systems, developed in the Indian subcontinent more than 3000 years ago, based on the belief that health and wellness depend on a delicate balance between body, mind and spirit
Bacterial co-aggregation	A process by which genetically distinct bacteria become attached to one another, contributing to the formation of multi-species biofilms[1]
Bacteriocins	Bacteria-suppressors which function like antibiotics
BDA	British Dental Association
Bifidobacterium	Gram-positive, non-motile, anaerobic bacteria that ubiquitously inhabit the gastrointestinal tract, vagina and mouth in humans; prime cariogenic bacteria
Bisphosphonates	Prescription medication used to treat osteoporosis/osteopaenia. Bisphosphonates powerfully inhibit bone resorption
BMD	Bone mineral density; the amount of bone mineral in bone tissue. BMD measurements are used as a measure of osteoporosis risk
BMP1	Bone morphogenetic protein 1 with a role in maintaining homeostasis of periodontal formation; a metalloprotease which induces bone and cartilage development
Bruxism	Clenching and grinding of teeth
Buccal surface	Cheek-contacting

Burning mouth syndrome	Disputedly defined as burning pain in tongue or oral mucous membranes without accompanying clinical and laboratory findings; aka glossodynia
Calculus (or tartar)	Hardened dental plaque which firmly attaches to the tooth; calculus can be removed by dental hygienist via periodontal scaler or ultrasonic tools
Calprotectin	Inflammation-related protein; calprotectin is secreted in the mouth during inflammation of the gingiva, found in saliva and gingival crevicular fluid; functions as a salivary defence protein, inhibits bacterial growth
cAMP	Cyclic AMP, or 3'5'-cyclic adenosine monophosphate; second messenger, along with DAG and IP_3
Capnophilic	Capnophiles are microorganisms that thrive in the presence of high concentrations of carbon dioxide
Carbonic anhydrase VI	Enzyme (aka gastrin) that causes carbon dioxide and water to form carbonic acid; has a role in bicarbonate buffering system
Caries	Hole in a tooth caused by decay
CaSR	The calcium receptor, an extracellular GPCR calcium-sensing receptor that responds to calcium and magnesium cations, in gustatory tissue[2]
Cathelicidins	A class of antimicrobial peptides found in saliva
Cavitation	A hole in bone, often where a tooth has been removed and the bone has not filled in properly
Cavity	Defined as an empty space within a solid object. In this book the term oral cavity refers to the mouth space, the space between the lips and the pharynx/oesophagus through which food passes on its route toward the stomach and intestines. The oral cavity (or buccal cavity) includes the cheeks, tongue and hard and soft palates. In this book, the term 'caries' relates to a hole (from decay) in the tooth
CCK	Cholecystokinin, a neuropeptide, a peptide hormone of the gastrointestinal system responsible for stimulating digestion of protein and fat that plays a key role in facilitating digestion in the small intestine
Cementoblasts	Cells that produce cementum; found in the periodontal ligament
Cementum	One of four tissues of teeth, with similar composition to bone; attaches the root to the periodontal ligament and holds the tooth in place within the jawbone

Chaperokines	A term coined to reflect the cytokine and chaperone functions of heat shock proteins[3]
Chemesthesis	Refers to the chemical sensibility of the skin and mucous membranes (e.g. relating to the perceived 'coolness' or 'hotness'/pungency of substances)
Chemokine	Chemotactic cytokine
CIBD	Chronic ischaemic bone disease, one of many alternative names for ischaemic osteonecrosis
Circumvallate papillae	One of four types of lingual papillae. There are approximately 12 very large circular vallate papillae that form an inverted V-shaped row at the back of the tongue. Each contains a large number of taste buds
CMV	Cytomegalovirus, a herpes virus
CNS	Central nervous system
Coaggregation	Attachment between genetically distinct bacteria
Collagen	Triple helical structure with high content of glycine, proline and hydroxyproline
Commensal	Refers to microorganism that co-exists without harming (human) host
COPD	Chronic obstructive pulmonary disease
Crown	Part of the tooth; visible portion above the dental gums
CRP	C-reactive protein; an acute phase reactant
CT	Chorda tympani, the nerve on the tongue tip, a branch of the facial nerve, directly involved in transferring taste information from fungiform papillae on the tongue. Susceptible to damage, particularly via middle ear infection, dental anaesthesia and procedures, herpes zoster infection, stroke and head trauma
Curettage	Tissue removal with a curette, a small surgical instrument which is used to scrape or debride biological tissue
Cystatin	One of four major salivary proteins; a defence factor. A cysteine-containing phosphoprotein which can inhibit cysteine protease and block the action of endogenous and parasitic protozoan proteases
DAG	Diacylglycerol; a prolific second messenger
DALT	Duct-associated lymphoid tissue
DDS	Doctor of Dental Surgery, qualification

GLOSSARY AND ABBREVIATIONS

Deciduous teeth	Primary teeth, aka milk teeth or baby teeth
Defensins	Type of cationic peptide in saliva; defence factor; antimicrobial peptides with broad antibacterial activity, and antifungal and antiviral properties
Deglutition	The act of swallowing
Dental pellicle	A thin, protein-rich biofilm that forms on the surface enamel of teeth seconds after the teeth are cleaned and is involved in regulating reactions between the tooth surface, saliva and erosive acids[4]
Dentilisin	Protease used by *Treponema denticola* to damage the host
Dentine (American dentin)	One of four tissues of teeth; calcified connective tissue, forms the inside the tooth, giving shape and rigidity. Dentine contains collagen
DHEA	Dehydroepiandrosterone; endogenous steroid hormone produced in adrenal glands, gonads and brain and abundantly circulating in humans. It is a weak oestrogen and weak androgen, functioning as a precursor to more potent androgens (testosterone and DHT), and with the capacity to bind to and activate oestrogen receptors. Levels vary with age
Diphyodont	Having two sets of teeth; humans are diphyodont because they have deciduous (baby) teeth, then adult teeth
DMFT	Decayed, missing or filled teeth
DMP1	Dentine matrix protein 1
DPSCs	Dental pulp stem cells; odontoblasts are an example of DPSCs
DRK channel	Delayed rectifying potassium channels; implicated in the regulation of cell excitability regarding taste cells[5]
Dysgeusia	Distorted taste. Ageusia is complete loss of taste perception. Hypogeusia is diminished sensory perception of taste
EBV	Epstein-Barr virus, a herpes virus
ECM	Extracellular matrix; ECM consists primarily of extracellular polymeric substance (EPS)
Ecological community	Referring to the living organisms and relationships/interactions with other organisms, and with the surrounding environment
Edentulous	Lacking teeth

EGCG	Epigallocatechin gallate, aka epigallocatechin-3-gallate, a type of condensed tannin found in green tea
EGF	Epidermal growth factor; protective component secreted in saliva
EMF	Electromagnetic field
ENaC	Epithelial sodium ion channels – these modulate salty taste
Enamel	One of four tissues of teeth. Enamel is the hardest substance in the human body. It protects teeth from wear and tear (from chewing) and from acids that can easily dissolve dentine
Endocannabinoids	Orexigenic mediators that act via cannabinoid CB_1 receptors in the hypothalamus, limbic forebrain and brainstem to induce appetite[6] and stimulate food intake
Endodontic(s)/ endodontist	Endodontic means relating to soft tissues inside a tooth (the dental pulp). Endodontics is a dental specialty and branch of dentistry concerned with prevention, diagnosis and treatment of diseases that affect the pulp, root, periodontal ligament and alveolar bone.[7] Endodontists are dentists that specialize in treatments such as root canal treatment
Entamoeba gingivalis	One-celled protozoan parasite detected in periodontal pockets
Epiglottis	A flap in the throat made of elastic cartilage covered with mucous membrane, attached to the entrance of the larynx and keeps food from entering the windpipe and lungs
EPS	Extracellular polymeric substance. An exopolysaccharide-rich material which helps to create biofilm. Natural polymers (of sugar residues) of high molecular weight secreted by microorganisms into their environment.[8] Formerly EPS was used for the term extracellular polysaccharides but was altered to extracellular polymeric substances when it was realized the matrix also contains proteins, lipids and other substances.[9] The term exopolysaccharide is used to indicate the polysaccharide component. EPS can be described as a protective slime layer and is an important construction material of biofilms. Extracellular matrix (ECM) consists primarily of EPS
Eruption (of tooth)	The developmental process responsible for moving a tooth from its crypt position through the alveolar process into the oral cavity to its final position[10]

Facultative	Used as descriptive regarding bacteria, meaning occurring optionally in response to circumstances rather than by nature, capable of but not restricted to a particular mode of life. So, a facultative anaerobe is an organism that normally survives in aerobic (oxygenated) conditions but is capable of switching if oxygen is not present (anaerobic conditions) to facilitate survival
Fauces	Passages. The opening between the oral cavity and the pharynx (throat) between the soft palate and the base of the tongue, sometimes defined with reference to the two pillars formed by the muscles covered with mucous membrane
FDA	US Food and Drug Administration, federal agency in the United States responsible for health and human services
FDOJ	Fatty degenerative osteolysis of jawbone
Filiform papillae	One of four types of lingual papillae. Filiform papillae are pointed, threadlike structures that contain tactile receptors but no taste buds
Fluorosis	A chronic condition caused by the excessive intake of fluorine compounds causing increased porosity of dental enamel
Foliate papillae	One of four types of lingual papillae. Foliate papillae are leaf-shaped and located in small trenches on the lateral margins of the tongue and mouth lining and provide the sense of taste
Fungiform papillae	One of four types of lingual papillae. Fungiform papillae are mushroom-shaped and scattered over the entire surface of the tongue
GALT	Gut-associated lymphoid tissue
Galvanic current	Created when two or more dissimilar metals or alloys make contact, resulting in corrosion of metallic object due to electrolytic action (in the oral cavity, saliva serves as the electrolyte)
GCF	Gingival crevicular fluid; inflammatory exudate derived from periodontal tissues
GDP and GTP	Guanosine diphosphate and guanosine triphosphate; when G-proteins are bound to GTP they are 'on' and when bound to GDP they are 'off'
Ghrelin	Hunger hormone which regulates appetite, including strong hunger contractions and accelerating gastric emptying. Levels dictate meal timing, increasing before meals and decreasing thereafter

Gingipains	Cysteine proteinases used by *Porphyromonas gingivalis* as a virulence factor
Gingivitis	Common form of gum disease; inflammation of gingiva
Gleeking	The eruption of saliva whilst talking, yawning, eating or cleaning teeth
Glossitis	Inflammation of the tongue
Glossopharyngeal nerve	Ninth cranial nerve. Injury to this nerve may result in difficulty swallowing, reduced secretion of saliva, loss of sensation in the throat and loss of taste sensation
Glossopyrosis or glossodynia	Oral dysaesthesia, aka 'burning mouth'
GLP-1	Glucagon-like peptide 1; potent incretin hormone. Can decrease blood sugar levels by enhancing insulin secretion
Glucans	Polysaccharides derived from glucose monomers which are linked by glycosidic bonds. Alpha-glucan and beta-glucan are 'second generation glyconutrients'
GLUT4	Glucose transporter type 4; insulin-regulated glucose transporter
Glycans	Refers to the carbohydrate portion of glycoproteins, consisting of a large number of monosaccharides linked glycosidically, either by N-linkage or O-linkage; a polysaccharide also containing sugars other than glucose. Glycans are generally attached on the exterior surface of cells and are essential to virtually every biological process in the body
Glycation	Non-enzymatic attachment of reducing sugars (e.g. glucose, fructose, galactose and others) and proteins/amino acids, lipids or nucleic acids
Glycerol	Simple polyol, aka glycerine
Glyconutrients	Foods that provide glycoforms and the eight 'essential saccharides': mannose, galactose, fucose, glucose, xylose, N-acetyl-neuraminic acid, N-acetylglucosamine, N-acetylgalactosamine
Glycoproteins	Protein with attached oligosaccharide chains via glycosidic bonds. Glycoproteins protect oral cavity tissues
Glycosaminoglycans	Long linear (unbranched) polysaccharides consisting of repeating disaccharide units. Glycosaminoglycans are also known as mucopolysaccharides
Glycosylation	Modifications via glycosidic bonds. An enzymatic process

GLOSSARY AND ABBREVIATIONS

GPCR	G-protein coupled receptors. These are involved in taste and regulation of bitter, sweet and umami tastes
G-proteins	Guanine nucleotide-binding proteins. These function as molecular switches inside cells and participate in signal transmission from outside-the-cell stimuli to the cell interior
Gram-negative bacteria	A class of bacteria which have a second membrane
Gram-positive bacteria	A class of bacteria that lack the second membrane but have a substantially thicker cell wall
Gustation and gustatory	Gustation is sense of taste; gustatory means concerned with tasting or the sense of taste
Gustatory cortex (GC)	The GC is located in the cerebral cortex (outer part of the brain) and is responsible for the perception of taste and integration of the taste experience
Gustatory hair	A single long microvillus on each gustatory receptor cell that projects to the external surface through the taste pore
Gustducin	A G-protein found in some taste receptor cells, with a role in transduction of sweet, bitter and umami stimuli. Also expressed in gastric and pancreatic cells. Gustducin is a taste-cell-specific G-protein, closely related to transducins[11]
Gutta percha	Wax material used in root canals
HA (hyaluronic acid)	Hyaluronic acid (aka hyaluronan/hyaluronate) is a large, naturally occurring glycosaminoglycan (composed of glucuronic acid and N-acetylglucosamine, with a linear, rope-like structure) which holds a thousand times its weight in water, impacting the extracellular matrix of connective tissue including the gingivae
Halitosis	Medical term for bad breath
Halogen	Meaning salt-producing, refers to a group of elements (including fluorine, chlorine, bromine and iodine) in the periodic table that are chemically related. When halogens react with metals, they produce a wide range of salts
Hard palate	The anterior portion of the roof of the mouth
HDA	Holistic Dental Association
HFCS	High fructose corn syrup – aka glucose-fructose, isoglucose and glucose-fructose syrup – a modified sugar made from corn starch. Can contain up to 90 per cent fructose

Histadine-rich proteins	Proteins that play a role in non-immune defence mechanisms
Histatin	One of four major salivary proteins, secreted by Ebner's glands; a salivary protein and defence factor
HIV	Human immunodeficiency virus – a retrovirus
HSP	Heat shock proteins are produced in response to stressful conditions; HSPs are described as chaperokines
Hyaluronidase	Enzyme that catalyses the degradation of hyaluronic acid
Hydrofluorosilicic acid	Used for fluoridation of municipal water supplies, often not pharmaceutical grade but rather a toxic waste product from phosphate fertilizer industries
Hydrogen sulfide (H_2S)/ hydrogen sulphide	Produced from cysteine by anaerobic periodontopathogenic bacteria; may contribute to bad breath in periodontal disease
Hydroxyapatite	Naturally occurring mineral form of calcium apatite, found in teeth and bone and gives rigidity
Hydroxyproline	A proline derivative and one of the components (with glycine and proline) of collagen
Hypogeusia	Diminished sensory perception of taste. Ageusia is the complete loss of taste perception. Dysgeusia is distorted taste
IABDM	International Academy of Biological Dentistry and Medicine, promotes biological dentistry
IAOMT	International Academy of Oral Medicine and Toxicology
IBS	Irritable bowel syndrome
IgA1 and IgA2	IgA1 is one of two subclasses of IgA, predominates in salivary glands, spleen, tonsils and NALT, generated mainly in response to protein antigens. IgA2 is one of two subclasses of IgA, predominates in the GI tract, generated mainly in response to carbohydrate or lipid antigens
Impacted teeth	Teeth prevented from erupting by some physical barrier in their path[12]
IP3 (IP_3)	Inositol triphosphate, or Inositol 1,4,5-triphosphate, is abbreviated IP_3. IP_3 is a second messenger molecule involved in the release of intracellular stores of Ca^{2+}
Isothiocyanate	Pungent compounds in cruciferous plants including cabbage, horseradish, mustard oil and wasabi. They are responsible for bitterness in these plants and activate TRPA1

GLOSSARY AND ABBREVIATIONS

JON	Human jawbone osteonecrosis, now usually referred to as 'cavitation'
Lactobacilli	Genus of Gram-positive bacteria that convert sugars to lactic acid and are prime cariogenic bacteria
Lactoferrin	A component of saliva, a glycoprotein that inhibits microbial growth and protects oral cavity tissues
Lactoperoxidase	A constituent of saliva and a component of the salivary peroxidase system
Lamina propria	The thin connective tissue layer of a mucosa
Lantibiotics	Powerful bacteriocins
Leptin	Sometimes known as the 'satiety hormone', leptin lets the body know when it is full, inhibiting hunger
Lingual frenulum	The midline mucous membrane on the under-surface of the tongue. The lingual frenulum is attached to the floor of the mouth and limits the movement of the tongue
Lingual lipase	A digestive enzyme released in the oral cavity with saliva, and acts on triglycerides
Lipoproteins	Substance containing both lipid and protein. Lipoproteins are membrane proteins modified by the attachment of lipids which anchor the protein to a membrane[13]
LPS	Lipopolysaccharides, also known as endotoxins, LPS or lipoglycans. LPS are present in the outer wall of Gram-negative bacteria, and released mainly when bacteria die, inducing a strong immune response
Lysozyme	A protein and bacteriolytic enzyme, and component of saliva and gingival crevicular fluid that protects oral cavity tissues. Lysozyme is also known as muramidase and N-acetylmuramide glycanhydrolase
Malocclusion	Misalignment of teeth such that the upper and lower teeth do not properly meet when the jaw is closed
MALT	Mucosa-associate lymphoid tissue. The wider term, with GALT being its largest and best-defined part; MALT also includes BALT (bronchial/tracheal-associated lymphoid tissue), NALT (nasopharynx-associated lymphoid tissue), and VALT (vulvovaginal-associated lymphoid tissue)
Mandible, mandibular	The mandible is the lower jawbone
Maxillae, maxillary	The upper jawbone; 'maxillary' means of or attached to the upper jawbone
Mercury sulfide (HgS)	A relatively stable form of mercury compound that is toxic

Metagenome	The metagenome includes the genomic contribution of the microorganisms to those of the human body itself
Methyl thiol (CH$_3$SH)	Produced from methionine by anaerobic periodontopathogenic bacteria. May contribute to bad breath in periodontal disease. Also known as methanethiol or methylmercaptan
Methylglyoxal (MG)	Methylglyoxal is found in Manuka honey and is thought to give it antibacterial properties. The MGO level indicates amount of methylglyoxal in honey
Methylmercury	One of three forms of mercury. Abbreviated MeHg, an example of an organomercury compound, generated via biomethylation, the form of mercury found in fish. Other forms of mercury are elemental mercury (Hg), aka hydrargyrum or quicksilver, meaning 'water silver', and inorganic mercury (I-Hg)
MG1 MG2	MG1 is a high-molecular-weight mucin. MG2 is a low-molecular-weight mucin
mGluR4 and mGluR1	mGluR4 is one of three umami taste receptors; mGluR1 is another of the three umami taste receptors
Microbiome	The collection of genomes from all the microorganisms found in a particular environment; refers to microbial community, the genetic makeup of all microbiota collectively
Microbiota	The community of pathogenic, commensals and symbiotic microorganisms found within a specific environment, including bacteria, fungi, archaea and viruses
MMPs	Matrix metalloproteinase, calcium-dependent zinc-containing endopeptidases. MMPs are important extracellular matrix enzymes in collagen degradation. Collagenases and gelatinases are MMPs
MSG	Monosodium glutamate (aka sodium glutamate), the purest form of umami flavour
MUC5B and MUC7	MUC5B is one of two main mucins in saliva. MUC5B has high molecular weight. MUC7 is the other of the two main mucins in saliva. MUC7 has low molecular weight compared with MUC5B
Mucins	A glycoprotein constituent of mucus. Mucins are heavily glycosylated glycoproteins which form a slimy coating and act as lubricant.[14] Mucins have a role in protecting oral cavity tissue against pathogens and dehydration[15]
Mutualism	Ecological interaction between two (or more) species from which both species gain benefit

NALT	Nasopharynx-associated lymphoid tissue (i.e. adenoids and palantine tonsils)
NF-κB	Nuclear factor kappa-light-chain-enhancer of activated B cells, a protein complex which controls DNA transcription cell production and survival and has a key role in regulation of immune response to infection
NICO	Neuralgia inducing cavitational osteonecrosis, jawbone version of ischaemic osteonecrosis which commonly affects bone. NICO involves pain
NIDR/NIDCR	National Institute of Dental Research, renamed National Institute of Dental and Craniofacial Research
Nidus	A place where bacteria have multiplied or can multiply
NIH	National Institute of Health, part of the US Department of Health and Human Services; the largest biomedical research agency in the world
NMD	Doctorate in Naturopathic Medicine
Non-vital teeth	A 'dead' tooth, the nerves are damaged
Nrf2	Nuclear factor erythroid 2-related factor, a transcription factor; a protein that regulates expression of antioxidant proteins that protect against oxidative damage
Occlusal surface	Chewing surface of the tooth
Odontoclasts	Form of osteoclast involved in dental root resorption
Olfaction	Sense of smell
Orbicularis oris	Principal muscle of the lips which facilitates lip mobility
Oropharynx	Part of the pharynx that lies between the soft palate and the hyoid bone (horseshoe-shaped bone in the anterior midline of the neck between the chin and thyroid cartilage)
Orosomucoid	An acute-phase protein that is inflammation sensitive and found to be a biomarker in the association between obesity and periodontitis; aka alpha 1-acid glycoprotein (AGP)
Orthodontics	Branch of dentistry concerned with prevention and correction of abnormally aligned teeth[16]
Osteonecrosis	Degeneration of bone in cavitation areas; death of tissue due to poor blood supply. Also referred to as inflammatory liquefaction or gangrene
P.g (P.gingivalis)	See *Porphyromonas gingivalis*

Palate	The roof of the mouth
Papillae	Projections of the lamina propria covered with keratinized epithelium. Papillae increase the surface area of the tongue and increase friction between food and the tongue, enabling easier movement of food in the oral cavity. There are four types of papillae on the tongue
Parotid gland and parotid duct	One of three pairs of major salivary glands, the parotid gland pierces the buccinator muscle and opens opposite the second maxillary (upper) molar tooth. Parotid glands are the largest of the salivary glands and secrete saliva into the oral cavity. The parotid duct is also referred to as Stenson's duct
Pathobiont	Potentially highly destructive organism that, under normal circumstances, is a non-harming symbiont
Periodontal ligament/ membrane	Dense fibrous connective tissue that lines the sockets and anchors teeth to the socket walls
Periodontics	Branch of dentistry concerned with the treatment of abnormal conditions of the tissues immediately surrounding the teeth, such as gingivitis (gum disease)[17]
Periodontitis	Inflammation of tissue around the teeth; involves destruction of connective tissue attachment and adjacent alveolar bone
Periodontium	Specialized tissues surrounding and supporting teeth
Periosteum	Connective tissue membrane covering bone; a membrane that contains osteoblasts that can help manufacture new bone growth
PFCs	Perfluorochemicals. These are chemicals capable of repelling water, oil and other liquids that cause stains. PFC molecules have a carbon backbone, fully surrounded by fluorine[18]
Pharynx	Part of the throat behind the mouth and nasal cavity. The oropharynx is located behind the oral cavity, extending from the uvula to the level of the hyoid bone. The nasopharynx is the upper portion of the pharynx extending from the base of the skull to the upper surface of the soft palate
Photobiomodulation	A non-thermal light therapy that uses non-ionizing forms of lights including lasers, LEDs and broadband light in the visible and near-infrared spectrum[19] therapeutically for pain relief and wound healing
PIP	Prolactin inducible protein, a bacteria and LPS binding protein, which functions as a salivary defence protein

PKD2L1	Polycystic kidney disease-like ion channel is a candidate sour taste sensor, expressed in all taste papillae and palate taste buds
Plaque	Biofilm that forms on oral surfaces; plaque can harden, forming tartar/calculus
PLC	Phospholipase C is a signalling effector enzyme that cleaves phospholipids just before the phosphate group, generating DAG and IP_3
Polyol	Sugar alcohol, but neither a sugar nor alcohol; naturally occurring carbohydrates which cannot be fully metabolized so typically contain fewer calories per gram than sugar. Sugar alcohols do not cause tooth decay but excessive consumption can cause digestive effects. Examples include xylitol
Porphyromonas gingivalis	*Porphyromonas gingivalis* is a Gram-negative, black-pigmented, strictly anaerobic bacterium involved in the pathogenesis of periodontitis. A major periodontopathogen and part of the 'red complex'. Previously known as *Bacteroides gingivalis*, this invasive and evasive opportunistic pathogen can trigger periodontitis even at low numbers
ppm	Parts per million, a measure of concentration (used for measurement of fluoride in drinking water). One part per million = 1 mg/L (which is a dose, measured in mg/day[20])
Premolar	Tooth (having two cusps or points); premolars (aka bicuspids) are transitional teeth, located between the canine and molar teeth in humans
Proline	Non-essential amino acid synthesized from glutamic acid, with highest concentrations found in connective tissue where it participates in collagen synthesis
PRPs	Proline-rich proteins; one of four major salivary proteins. PRPs are a group of innate defence salivary proteins that together form a major fraction of salivary proteins
Ptyalin	An alpha-amylase in saliva that initiates carbohydrate digestion in the oral cavity; it is identical to pancreatic amylase
Pulp	One of four tissues of teeth; soft, loose connective tissue containing blood vessels, nerves and lymphatic vessels
PYY	Peptide YY; hormone involved in hunger and satiety. PYY is secreted into the blood soon after eating; release begins before nutrients arrive in the lower small intestine and colon[21]

Quorum sensing	System correlate to population density which enables bacteria to restrict the expression of specific genes in a way that enables the bacterial colony to function as one unit and increase to its benefit
RANTES	Regulated on activation, normal T-cell expressed and secreted; a chemokine encoded by CCL5 gene. Routes immune cells to sites of inflammation and infection.[22] RANTES is found at high levels in cavitational tissues and is implicated in many serious health conditions, causing inflammation and immune dysregulation
Rebaudioside A	Steviol glycoside with 200 times the sweetness of sugar
Retronasal	Relating to or situated at the back part of the nose. Retronasal smell/retronasal olfaction (aka mouth smell) refers to the ability to perceive the flavour of foods and drinks. Retronasal smell is crucial for experiencing food flavours rather than food tastes (salty, sour, sweet, bitter and umami)
Rivinus duct	Collective term for the ducts of the sublingual salivary glands. The ducts open into the floor of the mouth
Root canal (therapy)	Narrow extensions of pulp cavity that run through the root of the tooth; each root canal has an opening at its base through which blood vessels, nerves, etc. enter the pulp chamber. Root canal therapy is removal of the pulp tissue from the pulp cavity and root canals of a badly diseased tooth
Saccharin	Artificial sweetener, sodium saccharin (benzoic sulfimide); petroleum-based product with 300–400 times the sweetness of sucrose
Salivary amylase	A digestive enzyme that acts on dietary starch
SALT	Salivary-associated lymphoid tissue (sometimes SALT can be used to refer to skin-associated lymphoid tissue)
SCC	Solitary chemosensory cells; cells in respiratory epithelium which share similarities with cells in taste buds of tongue. SCCs express sweet and bitter receptors
Seromucous	Refers to salivary glands that produce both serous secretions and mucous secretions
Serous glands	One of two types of salivary glands in relation to secretions. Serous glands produce a watery secretion that contains a lot of proteins, including the enzyme ptyalin. Differentiated from mucous glands which provide mucus, secreting a thick viscous secretion containing mucus

GLOSSARY AND ABBREVIATIONS

Sialogogue	Descriptive term for substance that stimulates flow of saliva
Sialochemistry	The chemistry of saliva
Sialorrhoea	Excessive salivation (aka ptyalism or hypersalivation) caused either by excessive production or decreased clearance of saliva
Sialothiasis	Blockage of salivary ducts caused by salivary calculus/stone
sIgA	Secretory immunoglobulin A; the principal specific defence factor in saliva
Sjögren's syndrome (SS)	An autoimmune disorder affecting the body's moisture-producing glands. The mucous membranes and moisture-secreting glands of the eyes and mouth are usually first affected causing a decrease in tears and saliva[23]
SLPI	Secretory leukocyte protease inhibitor; cationic peptide in saliva
SMART	Safe Mercury Amalgam Removal Technique; a technique developed by the IAOMT based on scientific research, for which there are licensed practitioners and guidelines for safeguarding both the patient and the dental professionals/staff involved
Smectite	A clay mineral group which includes bentonite, montmorillonite and saponite
SNPs	Single nucleotide polymorphisms; gene variation with a substitution of a single nucleotide at a specific position in the genome
Soft palate	Tissue that forms the posterior portion of the roof of the mouth
spp	Abbreviation for species
Staphylococcus aureus	Gram-positive, round-shaped bacteria frequently found on the skin and upper respiratory tract, and involved in MRSA
Statherin	One of four major salivary proteins; salivary glycoprotein is thought to protect teeth by helping to maintain salivary levels of calcium (for tooth enamel remineralization) and phosphate (for buffering)
Stevia rebaudiana	Natural zero-calorie sweetener from South American plant
Stomatitis	Inflammation of mouth/lips

Streptococcus mutans	Gram-positive, facultatively anaerobic bacteria; prime cariogenic bacteria
Sublingual glands	Smallest of the three major pairs of salivary glands. Sublingual glands are found beneath the tongue and superior to the submandibular glands. Their ducts are collectively termed the Rivinus duct
Submandibular glands	One of three pairs of major salivary glands. Located in the floor of the mouth. Their ducts are known as Wharton's ducts. The submandibular glands were previously known as submaxillary glands
Subnucleus caudalis (Vc)	The trigeminal subnucleus caudalis (Vc) is a region in the medulla of the brain which receives information about touch, pain and temperature. The excitement of neurons in the Vc elicits an oral tingling sensation (e.g. in response to carbonated water)
Sucralose	Artificial sweetener, aka E955, created by inserting chlorine molecules into sucrose molecules
Sulcus	Latin word for groove. Plural is sulci. Gingival sulcus is an area of potential space between a tooth and the surrounding gingival tissue. Healthy sulcular depth is 3mm or less – this allows oral hygiene, aids easy access for cleansing. If the sulcular depth is chronically deeper than this, there may be a risk to the periodontal ligament, including destruction of soft tissue and potentially tooth loss
Supertasters	Person who can taste certain flavours more strongly than other people
Supragingival surface	Refers to the surface of the tooth above the gingiva
T1R1	Taste receptor type 1 member 1 – involved in umami taste. T1R1 is also known as TAS1R1
T1R2	Taste receptor type 1 member 2 – involved in tasting sweetness. T1R2 is also known as TAS1R2
T1R3	Taste receptor type 1 member 3 – involved in tasting both sweet and umami. T1R3 is also known as TAS1R3
T2DM	Type 2 diabetes mellitus
T2Rs	Bitter taste receptors, also known as taste 2 receptors (TAS2Rs)
Tannerella forsythia	Gram-negative, anaerobic, rod bacteria, previously known as *Tannerella forsythensis* and as *Bacteroides forsythus*. Part of the 'red complex'

GLOSSARY AND ABBREVIATIONS

Tannins	Water-soluble polyphenolic flavonoid compounds in plant foods that serve as a natural defence mechanism against microbial infections. Tannins are astringent and create a drying sensation
Tartar	Encrustation on teeth consisting of plaque that has become hardened by deposition of mineral salts.[24] Tartar is calculus (see Calculus)
TAS1R1	Taste receptor type 1 member 1 – involved in umami taste. TAS1R1 is also known as T1R1
TAS1R2	Taste receptor type 1 member 2 – involved in tasting sweetness. TAS1R2 is also known as T1R2
TAS1R3	Taste receptor type 1 member 3 – involved in tasting both sweet and umami. TAS1R3 is also known as T1R3
TAS2R	The gene symbol for the G-protein-coupled receptors of the taste receptor 2 family that mediate bitter taste
TAS2R38	Taste gene involved in sensitivity to bitterness. This gene can be affected by functional SNPs
Tastants	Taste-provoking chemical molecules dissolved in saliva or ingested liquids
Taste bud	Bulbous nerve endings on the tongue. Also known as taste receptor cells
Taste pore	An opening in the taste bud via which parts of food dissolved in saliva come into contact with taste receptors
TCM	Traditional Chinese medicine
TFF-3	One of three kinds of TFF (trefoil factor family) peptides, the role of which may be to alter the rheological properties of saliva (its ability to flow). Research indicates a contradiction between the tumour-suppressing and tumour-promoting functions of these peptides in various carcinomas[25]
The 'red complex'	Consortium of periodontopathogenic microorganisms: *Porphyromonas gingivalis*, *Tannerella forsythia* and *Treponema denticola*
TIMPs	Tissue inhibitors of metalloproteinases; multifunctional protein in salivary secretions. TIMPs potently inhibit MMPs
TMJ	Temporomandibular joint; also known as TMD or TMJD. TMJ is a disorder relating to pain (and clicking) on movement of the jaw

Transducin	Rod and cone photoreceptor G-proteins involved in nerve impulses for vision
TRCs	Taste receptor cells; aka taste bud or gustatory cells
Treponema denticola	Gram-negative, obligate anaerobic, motile, highly proteolytic, spirochaetal bacteria; part of the 'red complex'
Trigeminal nerve	Responsible for conveying impulses for touch, pain and temperature sensation and proprioception. Also responsible for chewing. Damage may result in neuralgia
Trigeminal neuralgia	Condition characterized by inappropriately intense or spontaneously generated facial pain[26]
Trigeminality	Sensation of heat and pressure, e.g. pungency, irritation; also known as chemesthesis
TRP	Transient receptor potential; TRPs are cation channels involved in taste perception
TRPA1	Transient receptor potential cation channel subfamily A member 1 – involved in perception of pungency, pain, cold and itch; an excitatory ion channel involved in pain pathway, activation of which is accompanied by vasodilation.[27] Activated also by cinnamon, ginger, clove and constituents in garlic
TRPM5	Transient receptor potential cation channel subfamily M member 5 – a taste ion channel; temperature-sensitive protein required for transducing sweet, bitter and umami tastes
TRPM8	Transient receptor potential cation channel subfamily M member 8 – associates with coolness sensation of mint and is also known as the cold and menthol receptor 1; an ion channel involved in the perception of coolness sensation, for example when exposed to menthol
TRPV1	Transient receptor potential cation channel subfamily V member 1 – activated by capsaicin and piperine and also known as the human vanilloid receptor 1 or capsaicin receptor; provides nociception regarding heat and is activated by physical heat above 43°C, which allows calcium ion flow through the ion channels in the lipid membranes of cells
Umami	A savoury or meaty taste reported by Japanese scientists in 1908. Stimulated by monosodium glutamate. Umami is the Japanese word for delicious. Various amino acids account for this savoury taste
Urea	Main breakdown product of protein (amino acids) metabolism in mammals, excreted in urine

Uric acid	Chemical created when the body breaks down purines or DNA. Food sources of high purine content include alcohol, some meats, some fish/seafood
Uvula	A conical muscular process that hangs from the soft palate, helping to close off the nasopharynx during swallowing, preventing swallowed liquids and foods from entering the nasal cavity. Translates to 'little grape'
Vagus nerve	Tenth cranial nerve. Involved in swallowing, coughing and voice production as well as smooth muscle contraction and relaxation in organs of the gastrointestinal tract, slowing of heart rate and secretion of digestive fluids. Injury may interrupt sensations from many organs and interfere with swallowing, paralyse vocal cords and cause increased heart rate
Vanilloid receptor	See TRPV1
VEGF	Vascular endothelial growth factor; plays a role in early wound healing
VEGh	Von Ebner glands protein, a cysteine proteinase inhibitor
Vermillion (of the lips)	Refers to the red part of the lips. The vermillion of the lips is often referred to as the lips, which, in fact, encompass the entirety of the pliable, mobile, muscular folds that encircle the oral cavity opening
Vestibular	The oral vestibule is the area between the lips/cheeks and the teeth. The oral cavity proper is the rest of the mouth which is bounded by the isthmus of the fauces at the back and the alveolar process (and teeth) at the sides and front
Virulence factors	Molecules produced by bacteria, viruses, fungi and parasites which contribute to their ability to colonize, avoid and/or inhibit host immune response, enter and/or exit cells of the host, and obtain nourishment from the host
Von Ebner's glands	Minor salivary glands, located on surface of the tongue
Wharton's ducts	Salivary gland ducts which empty the submandibular (submaxillary) salivary glands; these ducts of the submandibular glands run under the mucosa on either side of the floor of the mouth and enter the oral cavity next to the lingual frenulum
WHO	World Health Organization
Wisdom teeth	Also known as third molars, wisdom teeth usually erupt after age 17 and can remain embedded in the alveolar bone as impacted teeth if there is insufficient room to accommodate them

Xerogenic	Means causing the oral cavity to be unusually dry
Xerostomia	Dry mouth, also known as salivary hypofunction
Xylitol	A polyol (sugar alcohol) which is made from a naturally occurring substance in plant fibre which is refined for use as a sweetener
YKL-40	A new acute-phase protein which may have a role in cancer cell proliferation, survival and invasiveness[28]

Endnotes

PREFACE

1. Nazir MA (2017) Prevalence of periodontal disease, its association with systemic diseases and prevention. *International Journal of Health Sciences 1*(2): 72–80.
2. Peres MA, Macpherson LMD, Weyant RJ, Daly B, *et al.* (2019) Oral health 1: Oral diseases: a global public health challenge. *Lancet 394*: 249–260.

CHAPTER 1

1. Wolff MS, Larson C (2009) The cariogenic dental biofilm: good, bad or just something to control? *Braz Oral Res 23*(Special Issue 1): 31–38.
2. Rickard AH, Gilbert P, High NJ, Kolenbrander PE, Handley PS (2003) Bacterial coaggregation: an integral process in the development of multi-species biofilms. *Trends Microbiol 11*(2): 94–100.
3. Kolenbrander PE, Palmer RJ Jr, Rickard AH, Jakubovics NS, Chalmers Nl, Diaz Pl (2006) Bacterial interactions and successions during plaque development. *Periodontology 2000 42*: 47–79.
4. Wolff MS, Larson C (2009) The cariogenic dental biofilm: good, bad or just something to control? *Braz Oral Res 23*(Special Issue 1): 31–38.
5. Ibid.
6. Soares RV, Lin T, Siqueira CC, Bruno LS, *et al.* (2004) Salivary micelles: identification of complexes containing MG2, sIgA, lactoferrin, amylase, glycosylated proline-rich protein and lysozyme. *Archives of Oral Biology 49*: 337–343.
7. Maciocia G (1987) *Tongue Diagnosis in Chinese Medicine*, revised edition. Seattle, WA: Eastland Press.
8. Hsu P-Y, Yang S-H, Tsang N-M, Fan K-H, *et al.* (2016) Efficacy of traditional Chinese medicine in xerostomia and quality of life during radiotherapy for head and neck cancer: a prospective pilot study. *Evidence-Based Complementary and Alternative Medicine 2016*: 8359251.
9. Guan X-b, Bain J-p, Fu J, Zhang H-n, Wang L-h, Li P (2011) Clinical evaluation on treatment of oral lichen planus with yiqiyangyin mixture and its mechanism. *Electronic Journal of Biology 7*(2): 20–25.
10. Barrett S (undated) *Meridian Tooth Charts Signify Poor Judgment*. Available at www.dentalwatch.org/questionable/toothcharts.html, accessed 21 September 2019.
11. Smithsonian National Museum of Natural History (2009) Activity: Can You Identify the Age? In: Smithsonian's *The Secret in the Cellar Webcomic*, educational resource from the Written in Bone exhibition, February 2009–2014. Available at https://anthropology.si.edu/writteninbone/comic/activity/pdf/1dentify_the_age.pdf, accessed 20 May 2018.
12. McKenna CJ, James H, Taylor JA, Townsend GC (2002) Tooth development standards for South Australia. *Australian Dental Journal 47*(3): 223–227.
13. Priyadarshini C, Puranik MP, Uma SR (2015) Dental age estimation methods: a review. *International Journal of Advanced Health Sciences 1*(12): 19–25.
14. Smith DJ, Joshipura K, Kent R, Taubman MA (1992) Effect of age on immunoglobulin content and volume of human labial gland saliva. *J Dent Res 71*: 1891–1894.
15. Miletic ID, Schiffman SS, Miletic VD, Sattely-Miller EA (1996) Salivary IgA secretion rate in young and elderly persons. *Physiol Behav 60*: 243–248.

16. Evans P, Der G, Ford G, Hucklebridge F, Hunt K, Lambert S (2000) Social class, sex, and age differences in mucosal immunity in a large community sample. *Brain Behav Immun 14*: 41–48.
17. Challacombe SJ, Percival RS, Marsh PD (1995) Age-related changes in immunoglobulin isotypes in whole and parotid saliva and serum in healthy individuals. *Oral Microbiol Immunol 10*: 202–207.
18. Grynpas M (1993) Age and disease-related changes in the mineral of bone. *Calcif Tissue Int 53*(suppl 1): S57–64.
19. Hebling E (2012) Effects of Human Ageing on Periodontal Tissues. In: J Manakil (ed.) *Periodontal Diseases: A Clinician's Guide*. Available at www.intechopen.com/books/periodontal-diseases-a-clinician-s-guide/effects-of-human-ageing-on-periodontal-tissues, accessed 28 September 2019.
20. Evert J, Lawler E, Bogan H, Perls T (2003) Morbidity profiles of centenarians: survivors, delayers, and escapers. *J Gerontol A Biol Sci Med Sci 58*(3): 232–237.
21. Kaufman LB, Setiono TK, Doros G, Andersen S, et al. (2014) An oral health study of centenarians and children of centenarians. *J Am Geriatr Soc 62*(6): 1168–1173.
22. Friedman PK, Lamster IB (2016) Tooth loss as a predictor of shortened longevity: exploring the hypothesis. *Periodontol 2000 72*(1): 142–152.
23. Petersen PE, Kwan S (2004) Evaluation of community-based oral health promotion and oral disease prevention – WHO recommendations for improved evidence in public health practice. *Community Dental Health 21*(suppl.): 319–329.
24. Ueno M, Yanagisawa T, Shinada K, Ohara S, Kawaguchi Y (2008) Masticatory ability and functional tooth units in Japanese adults. *J Oral Rehabil 35*(5): 337–344.
25. Scott J, Valentine JA, St Hill CA, Balasooriya BA (1983) A quantitative histological analysis of the effects of age and sex on human lingual epithelium. *J Biol Buccale 11*(4): 303–315.

CHAPTER 2

1. Marcotte H, Lavoie MC (1998) Oral microbial ecology and the role of salivary immunoglobulin A. *Microbiology and Molecular Biology Reviews 62*(1): 71–109.
2. Jiao S, Chen W, Wang E, Wang J, et al. (2016) Microbial succession in response to pollutants in batch-enrichment culture. *Scientific Reports 6*: 21791.
3. Mandel ID (1989) The role of saliva in maintaining oral homeostasis. *JADA 119*(2): 298–304.
4. Grant DA, Stern IB, Listgarten MA (eds) (1988) Saliva. In: *Periodontics*, 6th edn. St Louis: CV Mosby. pp.135–146. As cited in: Humphrey SP, Williamson RT (2001) A review of saliva: normal composition, flow and function. *The Journal of Prosthetic Dentistry 85*(2): 162–169.
5. Humphrey SP, Williamson RT (2001) A review of saliva: normal composition, flow and function. *The Journal of Prosthetic Dentistry 85*(2): 162–169.
6. Baliga D, Muglikar S, Kale R (2013) Salivary pH: a diagnostic biomarker. *J Indian Soc Periodontol 17*(4): 461–465.
7. Humphrey SP, Williamson RT (2001) A review of saliva: normal composition, flow and function. *The Journal of Prosthetic Dentistry 85*(2): 162–169.
8. Edgar WM (1990) Saliva and dental health. Clinical implications of saliva: report of a consensus meeting. *Br Dent J 169*: 96–98.
9. McDermid AS, McKee AS, Marsh PD (1988) Effect of environmental pH on enzyme activity and growth of Bacteroides gingivalis W50. *Infection and Immunity 56*(5): 1096–1100.
10. Marcotte H, Lavoie MC (1998) Oral microbial ecology and the role of salivary immunoglobulin A. *Microbiology and Molecular Biology Reviews 62*(1): 71–109.
11. Ibid.
12. Ibid.
13. Herbert TB, Cohen S (1993) Stress and immunity in humans: a meta-analytic review. *Psychosomatic Medicine 55*: 364–379.
14. Jemmott JB 3rd, Borysenko JZ, Borysenko M, McClelland DC, et al. (1983) Academic stress, power motivation, and decrease in secretion rate of salivary secretory immunoglobulin A. *Lancet 1*(8339): 1400–1402.
15. Marcotte H, Lavoie MC (1998) Oral microbial ecology and the role of salivary immunoglobulin A. *Microbiology and Molecular Biology Reviews 62*(1): 71–109.
16. Marsh PD, Percival RS, Challacombe SJ (1992) The influence of denture-wearing and age on the oral microflora. *J Dent Res 71*(7): 1374–1381.
17. Zambon JJ, Grossi SG, Machtei EE, Ho AW, Dunford R, Genco RJ (1996) Cigarette smoking increases the risk for subgingival infection with periodontal pathogens. *Journal of Periodontology 67*(suppl. 10S): 1050–1054.
18. Zachariasen RD (1993) The effect of elevated ovarian hormones on periodontal health: oral contraceptives and pregnancy. *Women & Health 20*(2): 21–30.
19. Marsh PD (2009) Dental plaque as a biofilm: the significance of pH in health and caries. *Compend Contin Educ Dent 30*(2): 76–78.

ENDNOTES

20 Costalonga M, Herzberg MC (2014) The oral microbiome and the immunobiology of periodontal disease and caries. *Immunology Letters* 162: 22-38.

21 Simón-Soro A, Tomás I, Cabrera-Rubio R, Catalan MD, Nyvad B, Mira A (2013) Microbial geography of the oral cavity. *J Dent Res* 92(7): 616-621.

22 Wilson M (2001) Bacterial biofilms and human disease. *Science Progress* 84(3): 235-254.

23 Ibid.

24 Moore WEC, Moore LVH (1994) The bacteria of periodontal diseases. *Periodontology 2000* 5: 66-77.

25 Aas JA, Paster BJ, Stokes LN, Olsen I, Dewhirst FE (2005) Defining the normal bacterial flora of the oral cavity. *Journal of Clinical Microbiology* 43(11): 5721-5732.

26 Humphrey SP, Williamson RT (2001) A review of saliva: normal composition, flow and function. *The Journal of Prosthetic Dentistry* 85(2): 162-169.

27 Greabu M, Battino M, Mohora M, Totan A, *et al.* (2009) Saliva – a diagnostic window to the body, both in health and in disease. *Journal of Medicine and Life* 2(2): 124-132.

28 Mager DL, Ximenez-Fyvie LA, Haffajee AD, Socransky SS (2003) Distribution of selected bacterial species on intraoral surfaces. *J Clin Periodontol* 30: 644-654.

29 Carpenter GH (2013) The secretion, components, and properties of saliva. *Annu Rev Food Sci Technol* 4: 267-276.

30 Ibid.

31 Costalonga M, Herzberg MC (2014) The oral microbiome and the immunobiology of periodontal disease and caries. *Immunology Letters* 162: 22-38.

32 Marcotte H, Lavoie MC (1998) Oral microbial ecology and the role of salivary immunoglobulin A. *Microbiology and Molecular Biology Reviews* 62(1): 71-109.

33 Humphrey SP, Williamson RT (2001) A review of saliva: normal composition, flow and function. *The Journal of Prosthetic Dentistry* 85(2): 162-169.

34 Mandel ID (1987) The functions of saliva. *J Dent Res* 66(1 suppl.): 623-627.

35 Nieuw Amerongen AV, Veerman ECI (2002) Saliva – the defender of the oral cavity. *Oral Diseases* 8: 12-22.

36 Tiwari M (2011) Science behind human saliva. *J Nat Sci Biol Med* 2(1): 53-58.

37 Humphrey SP, Williamson RT (2001) A review of saliva: normal composition, flow and function. *The Journal of Prosthetic Dentistry* 85(2): 162-169.

38 Neyraud E, Palicki O, Schwartz C, Nicklaus S, Feron G (2012) Variability of human saliva composition: possible relationships with fat perception and liking. *Archives of Oral Biology* 57: 556-566.

39 Engelen L, van den Keybus PAM, deWijk RA, Veerman ECI, *et al.* (2007) The effect of saliva composition on texture perception of semi-solids. *Archives of Oral Biology* 52: 518-525.

40 Helmerhost EJ (2007) Whole saliva proteolysis: wealth of information for diagnostic exploitation. *Ann N Y Acad Sci* 1098: 454-460.

41 Drago SR, Panouillé M, Saint-Eve A, Neyraud E, Feron G, Souchon I (2011) Relationships between saliva and food bolus properties from model dairy products. *Food Hydrocolloids* 25: 659-667.

42 Stewart JE, Feinle-Bisset C, Golding M, Delahunty C, Clifton PM, Keast RSJ (2010) Oral sensitivity to fatty acids, food consumption and BMI in human subjects. *British Journal of Nutrition* 104: 145-152.

43 Dawes C (2003) Estimates, from salivary analyses, of the turnover time of the oral mucosal epithelium in humans and the number of bacteria in an edentulous mouth. *Archives of Oral Biology* 48: 329-336.

44 Fábián TK, Hermann P, Beck A, Fejérdy P, Fábián G (2012) Salivary defense proteins: their network and role in innate and acquired oral immunity. *Int J Mol Sci* 12: 4295-4320.

45 Humphrey SP, Williamson RT (2001) A review of saliva: normal composition, flow and function. *The Journal of Prosthetic Dentistry* 85(2): 162-169.

46 Mandel ID (1993) Impact of saliva on dental caries. *Compend Suppl* 1989: S476-481. As cited in: Humphrey SP, Williamson RT (2001) A review of saliva: normal composition, flow and function. *The Journal of Prosthetic Dentistry* 85(2): 162-169.

47 Dawes C, Pedersen AML, Villa A, Ekström J, *et al.* (2015) The functions of human saliva: a review sponsored by the World Workshop on Oral Medicine VI. *Archives of Oral Biology* 60: 863-874.

48 Humphrey SP, Williamson RT (2001) A review of saliva: normal composition, flow and function. *The Journal of Prosthetic Dentistry* 85(2): 162-169.

49 Williams RC, Gibbons RJ (1972) Inhibition of bacterial adherence by secretory immunoglobulin A: a mechanism of antigen disposal. *Science* 177: 697-699.

50 Phalipon A, Cardona A, Kraehenbuhl J-P, Edelman L, Sansonetti PJ, Corthésy B (2002) Secretory component: a new role in secretory IgA-mediated immune exclusion in vivo. *Immunity* 17: 107-115.

51 Choi DH, Moon IS, Choi BK, Paik JW, *et al.* (2004) Effects of sub-antimicrobial dose doxycycline therapy on crevicular fluid MMP-8, and gingival tissue MMP-9, TIMP-1 and IL-6 levels in chronic periodontitis. *J Periodontal Res* 39(1): 20-26.

52 Wong JW, Gallant-Behm C, Wiebe C, Mak K, et al. (2009) Wound healing in oral mucosa results in reduced scar formation as compared with skin: evidence from the red Duroc pig model and humans. *Wound Repair and Regeneration* 17(5): 717-729.
53 Dawes C, Pedersen AML, Villa A, Ekström J, et al. (2015) The functions of human saliva: a review sponsored by the World Workshop on Oral Medicine VI. *Archives of Oral Biology 60*: 863-874.
54 Keswani SG, Balaji W, Le LD, Leung A, et al. (2013) Role of salivary vascular endothelial growth factor (VEGF) in palatal mucosal wound healing. *Wound Repair Regen* 21(4): 554-562.
55 Pogrel MA, Low MA, Stern R (2003) Hyaluronan (hyaluronic acid) and its regulation in human saliva by hyaluronidase and its inhibitors. *Journal of Oral Science* 45(2): 85-91.
56 Greabu M, Battino M, Mohora M, Totan A, et al. (2009) Saliva – a diagnostic window to the body, both in health and in disease. *Journal of Medicine and Life* 2(2): 124-132.
57 Holsinger FC, Bui DT (2007) Anatomy, Function and Evaluation of the Salivary Glands. In: EN Myers, RL Ferris (eds) *Salivary Gland Disorders*. Berlin, Heidelberg: Springer. Available at https://link.springer.com/chapter/10.1007%2F978-3-540-47072-4_1, accessed 24 October 2018.
58 Van Nieuw Amerongen A, Bolscher JGM, Veerman ECI (2004) Salivary proteins: protective and diagnostic value in cariology? *Caries Res* 38: 247-253.
59 Crawford JM, Taubman MA, Smith DJ (1975) Minor salivary glands as a major source of secretory immunoglobulin A in the human oral cavity. *Science* 190(4220): 1206-1209.
60 Subrahmanyam MV, Sangeetha M (2003) Gingival crevicular fluid a marker of the periodontal disease activity. *Indian Journal of Clinical Biochemistry* 18(1): 5-7.
61 Buduneli N, Buduneli E, Çetin EÖ, Kırılmaz L, Kütükçüler N (2010) Clinical findings and gingival crevicular fluid prostaglandin E2 and interleukin-1-beta levels following initial periodontal treatment and short-term meloxicam administration. *Expert Opinion on Pharmacotherapy* 11(11): 1805-1812.
62 Rüdiger SG, Carlén A, Meurman JH, Kari K, Olsson J (2002) Dental biofilms at healthy and inflamed gingival margins. *Journal of Clinical Periodontology* 29(6): 524-530.
63 Humphreys I (undated) Immunity in the salivary gland. Bitesized Immunology: British Society for Immunology. Available at www.immunology.org/public-information/bitesized-immunology/organs-and-tissues/immunity-in-the-salivary-gland, accessed 24 October 2018.
64 Pereira LJ, Pereira CV, Murata RM, Pardi V, Pereira-Dourado SM (2020) Biological and social aspects of Coronavirus disease 2019 (COVID-19) related to oral health. *Braz Oral Res* 34: e041.
65 Ren YF, Rasubala L, Malmstrom H, Eliav E (2020) Dental care and oral health under the clouds of COVID-19. *JDR Clinical and Translational Research* 5(3): 202-210.
66 Xu J, Li Y, Gan F, Du Y, Yao Y (2020) Salivary glands: potential reservoirs for COVID-19 asymptomatic infection. *J Dent Res* 99(8): 989.
67 Carreras-Presas C, Sánchez JA, López-Sánchez AF, Jané-Salas E, Pérez MLS (2020) Oral vesiculobullous lesions associated with SARS-CoV-2 infection. *Oral Diseases* 10.1111/odi.13382 [epub ahead of print].
68 Humphrey SP, Williamson RT (2001) A review of saliva: normal composition, flow and function. *The Journal of Prosthetic Dentistry* 85(2): 162-169.
69 Roth G, Calmes R (eds) (1981) Salivary Glands and Saliva. In: *Oral Biology*. St Louis: CV Mosby. pp.196-236. As cited in: Humphrey SP, Williamson RT (2001) A review of saliva: normal composition, flow and function. *The Journal of Prosthetic Dentistry* 85(2): 162-169.
70 Oho T, Yu H, Yamashita Y, Koga T (1998) Binding of salivary glycoprotein-secretory immunoglobulin A complex to the surface protein antigen of Streptococcus mutans. *Infection and Immunity* 66(1): 115-121.
71 Thomsson KA, Prakobphol A, Leffler H, Reddy MS, et al. (2002) The salivary mucin MG1 (MUC5B) carries a repertoire of unique oligosaccharides that is large and diverse. *Glycobiology* 12(1): 1-14.
72 Guillemin GJ, Essa MM, Song B-J, Manivasagam T (2017) Dietary supplements/antioxidants: impact on redox status in brain diseases. *Oxidative Medicine and Cellular Longevity* 2017: 5048432.
73 Fraunberger EA, Scoa G, Laliberté VLM, Duong A, Andreazza AC (2016) Redox modulations, antioxidants, and neuropsychiatric disorders. *Oxidative Medicine and Cellular Longevity* 2016: 4729192.
74 Soory M (2009) Redox status in periodontal and systemic inflammatory conditions including associated neoplasias: antioxidants as adjunctive therapy? *Infectious Disorders Drug Targets* 9: 415-427.
75 Bains VK, Bains R (2015) The antioxidant master glutathione and periodontal health. *Dental Research Journal* 12(5): 389-405.
76 Li T-L, Gleeson M (2004) The effect of single and repeated bouts of prolonged cyclin and circadian variation on saliva flow rate, immunoglobulin A and α-amylase responses. *Journal of Sports Sciences* 22: 1015-1024.

77. Nieman DC (2000) Is infection risk linked to exercise workload? *Med Sci Sports Exerc 32*(7 suppl.): S406–411.

78. Bishop NC, Gleeson M (2009) Acute and chronic effects of exercise on markers of mucosal immunity. *Frontiers in Bioscience 14*: 4444–4456.

CHAPTER 3

1. Snyder DJ, Bartoshuk LM (2016) Oral sensory nerve damage: causes and consequences. *Rev Endocr Metab Disord 17*(2): 149–158.
2. Herness S, Zhao F-L, Kaya N, Sehn T, Lu S-G, Cao Y (2005) Communication routes within the taste bud by neurotransmitters and neuropeptides. *Chem Senses 30*(suppl. 1): i37–i38.
3. Heath TP, Melichar JK, Nutt DJ, Donaldson LF (2006) Human taste thresholds are modulated by serotonin and noradrenaline. *The Journal of Neuroscience 26*(49): 12664–12671.
4. English Oxford Living Dictionaries (2018) Cavity. Available at https://en.oxforddictionaries.com/definition/cavity, accessed 4 June 2018.

CHAPTER 4

1. Association for Psychological Science (2012) *Q & A with Psychological Scientist Linda Bartoshuk*. Available at www.psychologicalscience.org/publications/observer/obsonline/q-a-with-taste-expert-linda-bartoshuk.html, accessed 23 June 2018.
2. deAraujo IE, Simon SA (2009) The gustatory cortex and multisensory integration. *Int J Obes (Lond) 33*(suppl. 2): S34–S43.
3. Møller P (2014) Orosensory Perception. In: D Bar-Shalom and K Rose (eds) *Pediatric Formulations: A Roadmap*. Springer. AAPS Advances in the Pharmaceutical Sciences Series, Vol 11. pp.105–121.
4. Keast RSJ, Costanzo A (2015) Is fat the sixth taste primary? Evidence and implications. *Flavour 4*: 5.
5. deAraujo IE, Simon SA (2009) The gustatory cortex and multisensory integration. *Int J Obes (Lond) 33*(suppl. 2): S34–S43.
6. Mayo Clinic, May Medical Laboratories (1995–2018) Test ID: NACCL Sodium, Serum. Available at www.mayocliniclabs.com/test-catalog/Clinical+and+Interpretive/602353, accessed 29 May 2021.
7. DeSimone JA, Lyall V, Heck FL, Feldman GM (2001) Acid detection by taste receptor cells. *Respiration Physiology 129*: 231–245.
8. Christensen CM, Brand JG, Malamud D (1987) Salivary changes in solution pH: a source of individual differences in sour taste perception. *Physiology & Behavior 40*(2): 221–227.
9. Zhang Y, Hoon MA, Chandrashekar J, Mueller KL, *et al.* (2003) Coding of sweet, bitter, and umami tastes: different receptor cells sharing similar signaling pathways. *Cell 112*: 293–301.
10. He W, Yasumatsu K, Varadarajan V, Yamada A, *et al.* (2004) Umami taste responses are mediated by α-transducin and α-gustducin. *The Journal of Neuroscience 24*(35): 7674–7680.
11. Patel NN, Workman AD, Cohen NA (2018) Role of taste receptors as sentinels of innate immunity in the upper airway. *Journal of Pathogens 2018*: 9541987.
12. Bezençon C, leCoutre J, Damak S (2007) Taste-signaling proteins are coexpressed in solitary intestinal epithelial cells. *Chem Senses 32*: 41–49.
13. Ren X, Zhou L, Terwilliger R, Newton SS, deAraujo IE (2009) Sweet taste signalling functions as a hypothalamic glucose sensor. *Frontiers in Integrative Neuroscience 3*: 12.
14. Singh N, Vrontakis M, Parkinson F, Chelikiani P (2011) Functional bitter taste receptors are expressed in brain cells. *Biochemical and Biophysical Research Communications 406*: 146–151.
15. González JA, Jensen LT, Fugger L, Burdakov D (2008) Metabolism-independent sugar sensing in central orexin neurons. *Diabetes 57*: 2569–2576.
16. O'Connor CM, Adams JU (2010) *Essentials of Cell Biology*. Cambridge, MA: NPG Education. Unit 4.2 G-Protein-Coupled Receptors Play Many Different Roles in Eukaryotic Signaling. Available at www.nature.com/scitable/ebooks/essentials-of-cell-biology-14749010/122997540, accessed 14 June 2021.
17. Schulman H (2013) Intracellular Signaling. In LR Squire, D Berg, FE Bloom, S duLac, A Ghosh, NC Spitzer (eds) *Fundamental Neuroscience* (4th edn). Waltham, MA: Elsevier, Academic Press.
18. Gilchrist A (2007) Modulating G-protein-coupled receptors: from traditional pharmacology to allosterics. *TRENDS in Pharmacological Sciences 28*(8): 431–437.
19. Rask-Andersen M, Almén MS, Schiöth HB (2011) Trends in the exploitation of novel drug targets. *Nature Reviews 10*: 579–590.
20. Smith RG, Burtner AP (1994) Oral side-effects of the most frequently prescribed drugs. *Spec Care Dentist 14*(3): 96–102.

21. National Cancer Institute (2018) Mouth and Throat Problems during Cancer Treatment. NIH. Available at www.cancer.gov/about-cancer/treatment/side-effects/mouth-throat, accessed 25 July 2018.
22. Hovan AL, Williams PM, Stevenson-Moore P, Wahlin YB, *et al.* (2010) A systematic review of dysgeusia induced by cancer therapies. *Support Care Cancer* 18: 1081–1087.
23. Japan Patent Office (2002) Kikunae Ikeda Sodium Glutamate. Available at www.jpo.go.jp/e/introduction/rekishi/10hatsumeika/kikunae_ikeda.html, accessed 19 August 2018.
24. Yamaguchi S (1991) Basic properties of umami and effects on humans. *Physiology & Behaviour* 49(5): 833–841.
25. Kurihara K (2009) Glutamate: from discovery as a food flavour to role as a basic taste (umami). *Am J Clin Nutr* 90(suppl.): 719S–722S.
26. Kurihara K (2015) Umami the fifth basic taste: history of studies on receptor mechanisms and role as a food flavor. *BioMed Research International 2015*: 189402.
27. Jenness R (1979) The composition of human milk. *Semin Pernatol* 3(3): 225–239.
28. Carratù B, Boniglia C, Scalise F, Ambruzzi AM, Sanzini E (2003) Nitrogenous components of human milk: non-protein nitrogen, true protein and free amino acids. *Food Chemistry* 81: 357–362.
29. Beauchamp GK, Mennella JA (2011) Flavor perception in human infants: development and functional significance. *Digestion* 83(suppl. 1): 1–6.
30. Roper SD, Chaudhari N (2017) Taste buds: cells, signals and synapses. *Nat Rev Neurosci* 18(8): 485–497.
31. Kurihara K (2015) Umami the fifth basic taste: history of studies on receptor mechanisms and role as a food flavor. *BioMed Research International 2015*: 189402.
32. Behrens M, Meyerhof W (2013) Bitter taste receptor research comes of age: from characterization to modulation of TAS2Rs. *Seminars in Cell & Developmental Biology* 24: 215–221.
33. Reichling C, Meyerhof W, Behrens M (2008) Functions of human bitter taste receptors depend on N-glycosylation. *Journal of Neurochemistry* 106: 1138–1148.
34. Meyerhof W, Batram C, Kuhn C, Brockhoff A, *et al.* (2010) The molecular receptive ranges of human TAS2R bitter taste receptors. *Chem Senses* 35: 157–170.
35. Wu SV, Rozengurt N, Yang M, Young SH, Sinnett-Smith J, Rozengurt E (2002) Expression of bitter taste receptors of the T2R family in the gastrointestinal tract and enteroendocrine STC-1 cells. *Proc Natl Acad Sci USA* 99(4): 2392–2397.
36. Finger TE, Böttger B, Hansen A, Anderson KT, Alimohammadi H, Silver WL (2003) Solitary chemoreceptor cells in the nasal cavity serve as sentinels of respiration. *Proceedings of the National Academy of Sciences of the United States of America* 100: 8981–8986.
37. Singh N, Vrontakis M, Parkinson F, Chelikiani P (2011) Functional bitter taste receptors are expressed in brain cells. *Biochemical and Biophysical Research Communications* 406: 146–151.
38. Prandi S, Bromke M, Hübner S, Voigt A, *et al.* (2013) A subset of mouse colonic goblet cells expresses the bitter taste receptor Ras2r131. *PLOS ONE* 8(12): e82820.
39. Höfer D, Püschel B, Drenckhahn D (1996) Taste receptor-like cells in the rat gut identified by expression of alpha-gustducin. *Proc Natl Acad Sci USA* 93: 6631–6634.
40. Wu SV, Rozengurt N, Yang M, Young SH, Sinnett-Smith J, Rozengurt E (2002) Expression of bitter taste receptors of the T2R family in the gastrointestinal tract and enteroendocrine STC-1 cells. *Proc Natl Acad Sci USA* 99: 2392–2397.
41. Höfer D, Drenckhahn D (1998) Identification of the taste cell G-protein, α-gustducin, in brush cells of the rat pancreatic duct system. *Histochem Cell Biol* 110: 303–309.
42. Rozengurt E (2006) Taste receptors in the gastrointestinal tract. 1. Bitter taste receptors and α-gustducin in the mammalian gut. *Am J Physiol Gastroint Liver Physiol* 291: G171–G177.
43. Janssen S, Laermans J, Verhulst P-J, Thijs T, Tack J, Depoortere I (2011) Bitter taste receptors and α-gustducin regulate the secretion of ghrelin with functional effects on food intake and gastric emptying. *PNAS* 108(5): 2094–2099.
44. Ibid.
45. Janssen S, Depoortere I (2013) Nutrient sensing in the gut: new roads to therapeutics? *Trends in Endocrinology and Metabolism* 24(2): 92–100.
46. Ibid.
47. Yamamoto K, Ishimaru Y (2013) Oral and extra-oral taste perception. *Seminars in Cell & Developmental Biology* 24: 240–246.
48. Lu P, Zhang C-H, Lifshitz LM, ZhuGe R (2017) Extraoral bitter taste receptors in health and disease. *J Gen Physiol* 149(2): 181–197.
49. Patel NN, Workman AD, Cohen NA (2018) Role of taste receptors as sentinels of innate immunity in the upper airway. *Journal of Pathogens* 2018: 9541987.
50. Low JYQ, McBride RL, Lacy KE, Keast RSJ (2017) Psychophysical evaluation of sweetness functions across multiple sweeteners. *Chemical Senses* 42: 111–120.
51. Mainland JD, Matsunami H (2009) Taste perception: how sweet it is (to be transcribed by you). *Curr Biol* 19(15): R655–R656.

ENDNOTES

52 Margolskee RF, Dyer J, Kokrashvili Z, Salmon DSH, et al. (2007) T1R3 and gustducin in gut sense sugars to regulate expression of Na+-glucose cotransporter 1. *PNAS 104*(38): 15075–15080.

53 Shah K, DeSilva S, Abbruscato T (2012) The role of glucose transporters in brain disease: diabetes and Alzheimer's disease. *Int J Mol Sci 13*: 12629–12655.

54 Wooding S, Kim U-k, Bamshad MK, Larsen J, Jorde LB, Drayna D (2004) Natural selection and molecular evolution in PTC, a bitter-taste receptor gene. *Am J Hum Genet 74*(4): 637–646.

55 Kaminski LC, Henderson SA, Drewnowski A (2000) Young women's food preferences and taste responsiveness to 6-n-propylthiouracil (PROP). *Physiology & Behavior 68*: 691–697.

56 Bartoshuk LM, Duffy VB, Miller IJ (1994) PTC/PROP tasting: anatomy, psychophysics, and sex effects. *Physiology & Behavior 56*(6): 1165–1171.

57 Bradbury J (2004) Taste perception: cracking the code. *PLoS Biology 2*(3): e64.

58 Bartoshuk LM, Duffy VB, Miller IJ (1994) PTC/PROP tasting: anatomy, psychophysics, and sex effects. *Physiology & Behavior 56*(6): 1165–1171.

59 Prutkin J, Duffy VB, Etter L, Fast K, et al. (2000) Genetic variation and inferences about perceived taste intensity in mice and men. *Physiology & Behavior 69*: 161–173.

60 Gorovic N, Afzal S, Tjønneland A, Overvad K, et al. (2011) Genetic variation in the hTAS2R38 taste receptor and brassica vegetable intake. *Scandinavian Journal of Clinical & Laboratory Investigation 71*: 274–279.

61 Hayes JE, Feeney EL, Allen AL (2013) Do polymorphisms in chemosensory genes matter for human ingestive behaviour? *Food Quality and Preference 30*: 202–216.

62 Martin LE, Nikonova LV, Kay K, Paedae AB, Contreras RJ, Torregrossa A-M (2018) Salivary proteins alter taste-guided behaviors and taste nerve signalling in rat. *Physiology & Behavior 184*: 150–161.

63 Vriens J, Nilius B, Vennekens R (2008) Herbal compounds and toxins modulating TRP channels. *Current Neuropharmacology 6*: 79–96.

64 McNamara FN, Randal A, Gunthorpe MJ (2005) Effects of piperine, the pungent component of black pepper, at the human vanilloid receptor (TRPV1). *British Journal of Pharmacology 144*: 781–790.

65 Koizumi K, Iwasaki Y, Narukawa M, Iitsuka Y, et al. (2009) Diallyl sulphides in garlic activate both TRPA1 and TRPV1. *Biochemical and Biophysical Research Communications 382*: 545–548.

66 Bautista DM, Movahed P, Hinman A, Axelsson HE, et al. (2005) Pungent products from garlic activate the sensory ion channel TRPA1. *PNAS 102*(34): 12248–12252.

67 Bandell M, Story GM, Hwang SW, Viswanath V, et al. (2004) Noxious cold ion channel TRPA1 is activated by pungent compounds and bradykinin. *Neuron 41*: 849–857.

68 Jordt S-E, Bautista DM, Chuang H-H, McKemy DD, et al. (2004) Mustard oils and cannabinoids excite sensory nerve fibres through the TRP channel ANKTM1. *Nature 427*: 260–265.

69 Holzer P (2004) TRPV1 and the gut: from a tasty receptor for a painful vanilloid to a key player in hyperalgesia. *Eur J Pharmac 500*: 231–241.

70 Tirado-Lee L (2014) This is Your Brain on Capsaicin. Available at https://helix.northwestern.edu/blog/2014/07/your-brain-capsaicin, accessed 25 May 2019.

71 Tang H-B, Li Y-S, Miyano K, Nakata Y (2008) Phosphorylation of TRPV1 by neurokinin-1 receptor agonist exaggerates the capsaicin-mediated substance P release from cultured rat dorsal root ganglion neurons. *Neuropharmacology 55*: 1405–1411.

72 Sprouse-Blum AS, Smith G, Sugai D, Parsa FD (2010) Understanding endorphins and their importance in pain management. *Hawaii Medical Journal 69*: 70–71.

73 Tirado-Lee L (2014) This is Your Brain on Capsaicin. Available at https://helix.northwestern.edu/blog/2014/07/your-brain-capsaicin, accessed 25 May 2019.

74 Carstens E, Carstens MI, Dessirier J-M, O'Mahony M, et al. (2002) It hurts so good: oral irritation by spices and carbonated drinks and the underlying neural mechanisms. *Food Quality and Preference 13*: 431–443.

75 Riera CE, Vogel H, Simon SA, leCoutre J (2007) Artificial sweeteners and salts producing a metallic taste sensation activate TRPV1 receptors. *Am J Physiol Regul Integr Comp Physiol 293*(2): R626–R634.

76 Ibid.

77 Schiffman SS (2018) Influence of medications on taste and smell. *World Journal of Otorhinolaryngology – Head and Neck Surgery 4*: 84–91.

78 Ibid.

79 Xu H, Tian W, Fu Y, Oyama TT, Anderson S, Cohen DM (2007) Functional effects of nonsynonymous polymorphisms in the human TRPV1 gene. *Am J Physiol Renal Physiol 293*: F1865–F1876.

80 Riera CE, Vogel H, Simon SA, leCoutre J (2007) Artificial sweeteners and salts producing a metallic taste sensation activate TRPV1 receptors. *Am J Physiol Regul Integr Comp Physiol 293*(2): R626–R634.

81 Talavera K, Yasumatsu K, Voets T, Droogmans G, et al. (2005) Heat activation of TRPM5 underlies thermal sensitivity of sweet taste. *Nature 438*: 1022–1025.

82. Engelen L, deWijk RA, Prinz JF, Janssen AM, Weenen H, Bosman F (2003) The effect of oral and product temperature on the perception of flavor and texture attributes of semi-solids. *Appetite 41*: 273–281.
83. Masic U, Yeomans MR (2014) Umami flavor enhances appetite but also increases satiety. *Am J Clin Nutr 100*: 532–538.
84. Gerhold KA, Bautista DM (2009) Molecular and cellular mechanisms of trigeminal chemosensation. *Ann NY Acad Sci 1170*: 184–189.
85. Chambers ES, Bridge MW, Jones DA (2009) Carbohydrate sensing in the human mouth: effects on exercise performance and brain activity. *J Physiol 587*(8): 1779–1794.
86. Rowltt G, Bottoms L, Edmonds CJ, Buscombe R (2017) The effect of carbohydrate mouth rinsing on fencing performance and cognitive function following fatigue-inducing fencing. *Eur J Sport Sci 17*(4): 433–440.

CHAPTER 5

1. Arizona State University (2017) Sugar-coated world: probing the mysteries of glycan structure and function. *ScienceDaily*, 18 December. Available at www.sciencedaily.com/releases/2017/12/171218120356.htm, accessed 8 January 2019.
2. Touger-Decker R, van Loveren C (2003) Sugars and dental caries. *Am J Clin Nutr 78*(suppl.): 881S–892S.
3. Note that *this is fucose, not fructose*. Fructose is not considered to be an 'essential saccharide'.
4. Mondoa EI, Kitei M (2001) *Sugars That Heal: The New Healing Science of Glyconutrients*. New York: Ballantine Books.
5. Arizona State University (2017) Sugar-coated world: probing the mysteries of glycan structure and function. *ScienceDaily*, 18 December. Available at www.sciencedaily.com/releases/2017/12/171218120356.htm, accessed 8 January 2019.
6. Ibid.
7. Dutchen S, MacLachlan A (2011) Why Sugars May Be the Body's Superstars. Available at www.livescience.com/17349-sugars-glycans-nigms.html, accessed 23 December 2018.
8. Glenville M (2016) *Natural Alternatives to Sugar*. Tunbridge Wells, Kent: Lifestyle Press.
9. McCooey A (undated) various webpages. Available at www.sugar-and-sweetener-guide.com/glycemic-index-for-sweeteners.html, accessed 19 December 2018.
10. Diabetes Canada (2018) Sugars and Sweeteners. Available at https://guidelines.diabetes.ca/docs/patient-resources/sugars-and-sweeteners.pdf, accessed 14 January 2019.
11. Rafiqul ISM, Mimi Sakinah AM (2012) A perspective: bioproduction of xylitol by enzyme technology and future prospects. *International Food Research Journal 19*(2): 405–408.
12. Nayak PA, Nayak UA, Khandelwal V (2014) The effect of xylitol on dental caries and oral flora. *Clinical, Cosmetic and Investigational Dentistry 6*: 89–94.
13. Dawes C (2012) Factors Influencing Salivary Flow Rate and Composition. In: M Edgar, C Dawes, D O'Mullane (eds) *Saliva and Oral Health*, 4th edition (Wrigley Oral Healthcare Programme). Duns Tew, Oxfordshire: Stephen Hancocks.
14. Aguirre-Zero O, Zero DT, Proskin HM (1993) Effect of chewing xylitol chewing gum on salivary flow rate and the acidogenic potential of dental plaque. *Caries Res 27*(1): 55–59.
15. Nordblad A, Suominen-Taipale L, Murtomaa H, Vartiainen E, Koskela K (1995) Smart Habit xylitol campaign, a new approach in oral health promotion. *Community Dent Health 12*: 230–234. As cited in: Nyak PA, Nyak UA, Khandelwal V (2014) The effect of xylitol on dental caries and oral flora. *Clinical, Cosmetic and Investigational Dentistry 6*: 89–94.
16. Scheinin A, Mäkinen KK, Ylitalo K (1976) Turku sugar studies. V. Final report on the effect of sucrose, fructose and xylitol diets on the caries incidence in man. *Acta Odontol Scand. 34*(4): 179–216.
17. Castro MR (undated) Artificial Sweeteners: Any Effect on Blood Sugar? Available at www.mayoclinic.org/diseases-conditions/diabetes/expert-answers/artificial-sweeteners/faq-20058038, accessed 13 January 2019.
18. Van Loveren C (2004) Sugar alcohols: what is the evidence for caries-preventive and caries-therapeutic effects? *Caries Res 38*: 286–293.
19. Riley P, Moore D, Ahmed F, Sharif MO, Worthington HV (2015) Xylitol-containing products for preventing dental caries in children and adults. *Cochrane Database Syst Rev 3*: CD010743.
20. Ly KA, Milgrom P, Rothen M (2006) Xylitol, sweeteners, and dental caries. *Pediatr Dent 28*(2): 154–163.
21. Söderling E (2009) Controversies around xylitol. *European Journal of Dentistry 3*: 81–82.
22. Castro MR (undated) Artificial Sweeteners: Any Effect on Blood Sugar? Available at www.mayoclinic.org/diseases-conditions/diabetes/expert-answers/artificial-sweeteners/faq-20058038, accessed 13 January 2019.

ENDNOTES

23. Diabetes UK (undated) Sugar, Sweeteners and Diabetes. Available at www.diabetes.org.uk/guide-to-diabetes/enjoy-food/carbohydrates-and-diabetes/sugar-sweeteners-and-diabetes, accessed 14 January 2019.
24. Grembecka M (2015) Sugar alcohols – their role in the modern world of sweeteners: a review. *Eur Food Res Technol 241*: 1–14.
25. Burt BA (2006) The use of sorbitol- and xylitol-sweetened chewing gum in caries control. *JADA 137*: 190–196.
26. Grembecka M (2015) Sugar alcohols – their role in the modern world of sweeteners: a review. *Eur Food Res Technol 241*: 1–14.
27. Yale New Haven Health Hospital (undated) Eat Any Sugar Alcohol Lately? Available at www.ynhh.org/services/nutrition/sugar-alcohol.aspx, accessed 14 January 2019.
28. Hiele M, Ghoos Y, Rutgeerts P, Vantrappen G (1993) Metabolism of erythritol in humans: comparison with glucose and lactitol. *British Journal of Nutrition 69*(1): 169–176.
29. Grembecka M (2015) Sugar alcohols – their role in the modern world of sweeteners: a review. *Eur Food Res Technol 241*: 1–14.
30. De Cock P (1999) Erythritol: a novel noncaloric sweetener ingredient. In: Low-Calorie Sweeteners: Present and Future. Corti A (ed.) *World Rev Nutr Diet 85*: 110–116.
31. Axe J (2018) Erythritol: Is This Common Sweetener Safe? Available at https://draxe.com/nutrition/erythritol, accessed 13 January 2019.
32. De Cock P (1999) Erythritol: a novel noncaloric sweetener ingredient. In: Low-Calorie Sweeteners: Present and Future. Corti A (ed.) *World Rev Nutr Diet 85*: 110–116.
33. Grembecka M (2015) Sugar alcohols – their role in the modern world of sweeteners: a review. *Eur Food Res Technol 241*: 1–14.
34. denHartog GJ, Boots AW, Adam-Perrot A, Brouns F, et al. (2010) Erythritol is a sweet antioxidant. *Nutrition 26*(4): 449–458.
35. Hino H, Kasai S, Hattori N, Kenjo K (2000) A case of allergic urticarial caused by erythritol. *J Dermatol 27*(3): 163–165.
36. Wölnerhanssen BK, Cajacob L, Keller N, Doody A, et al. (2016) Gut hormone secretion, gastric emptying, and glycemic responses to erythritol and xylitol in lean and obese subjects. *Am J Physiol Endocrinol Metab 310*: E1053–E1061.
37. Honkala S, Runnel R, Saag M, Olak J, et al. (2014) Effect of erythritol and xylitol on dental caries prevention in children. *Caries Res 48*(5): 482–490.
38. Mäkinen KK, Saag M, Isotupa KP, Olak J, et al. (2005) Similarity of the effects of erythritol and xylitol on some risk factors of dental caries. *Caries Res 39*(3): 207–215.
39. Grembecka M (2015) Sugar alcohols – their role in the modern world of sweeteners: a review. *Eur Food Res Technol 241*: 1–14.
40. Cury JA, Rebelo MAB, Del Bel Cury AA, Derbyshire MTVC, Tabchoury CPM (2000) Biochemical composition and cariogenicity of dental plaque formed in the presence of sucrose or glucose and fructose. *Caries Res 34*: 491–497.
41. Ahmadi-Motamayel F, Rezaei-Soufi L, Kiani L, Alikhani MY, Poorolajal J, Moghadam M (2013) Effects of honey, glucose and fructose on the enamel demineralization depth. *Journal of Dental Sciences 8*: 147–150.
42. Molan PC (1992) The antibacterial activity of honey: 1 The nature of the antibacterial activity. *Bee World 73*: 5–28.
43. Ikeda T, Hirasawa M, Kurita T (1982) Cariogenesis of nystose as a substrate in vitro. In Proceedings of Neo Sugar Meeting. Vol.1, pp.77–86. Meiji Seika Ltd, Tokyo (in Japanese). As cited in: Ohyama T, Ito O, Yasuyoshi S, Ikarashi T, et al. (1990) Composition of storage carbohydrate in tubers of yacon (Polymnia sonchifolia). *Soil Science and Plant Nutrition 36*(1): 167–171.
44. Madison Avenue Dentists (undated) Popular Sugar Alternatives – Paleo Dentist's Perspective. Available at www.mavedds.com/blog/popular-sugar-alternatives-paleo-dentists-perspective, accessed 22 March 2020.
45. Food and Drug Adminstration, HHS (2006) Food labelling: health claims; dietary noncariogenic carbohydrate sweeteners and dental caries. Final rule. *Fed Regist 71*(60): 15559–15564.
46. Qin XF (2002) Impaired inactivation of digestive proteases by deconjugated bilirubin: the possible mechanisms for inflammatory bowel disease. *Medical Hypotheses 59*(2): 159–163.
47. Fowler SPG, Williams K, Hazuda HP (2015) Diet soda intake is associated with long-term increases in waist circumference in a bi-ethnic cohort of older adults: The San Antonio Longitudinal Study of Aging. *J Am Geriatr Soc 63*(4): 708–715.
48. Suez J, Korem T, Zeevi D, Zilberman-Schapira G, et al. (2014) Artificial sweeteners induce glucose intolerance by altering the gut microbiota. *Nature 514*(7521): 181–186.
49. Swithers SE (2013) Artificial sweeteners produce the counterintuitive effect of inducing metabolic derangements. *Trends in Endocrinology and Metabolism 24*(9): 431–441.
50. Glenville M (2016) *Natural Alternatives to Sugar*. Tunbridge Wells, Kent: Lifestyle Press.
51. Gardana C, Simonetti P, Canzi E, Zanchi R, Pietta P (2003) Metabolism of stevioside and rebaudioside A from Stevia rebaudiana extracts by human microflora. *J Agric Food Chem 51*: 6618–6622.

52. Pure Circle Stevia Institute (undated) Stevia in Metabolism. Available at www.purecirclesteviainstitute.com, accessed 20 April 2019.
53. Brambilla E, Cgetti MG, Ionecu A, Campus G, Lingström P (2013) An in vitro and in vivo comparison of the effect of Stevia rebaudiana extracts on different caries-related variables: a randomized controlled trial pilot study. *Caries Research* 48(1): 19–23.
54. Mohammadi Sichani M, Karbasizadeh V, Aghai F, Mofid MR (2012) Effect of different extracts of Stevia rebaudiana leaves on Streptococcus mutans growth. *Journal of Medicinal Plants Research* 6(32): 4731–4734.
55. Zheng Y, Liu Z, Ebersole J, Huang CB (2009) A new antibacterial compound from Luo Han Kuo fruit extract (Siraitia grosvenori). *J Asian Nat Prod Res* 11(8): 761–765.
56. Lipatova O, Campolattaro MM (2016) The miracle fruit: an undergraduate laboratory exercise in taste sensation and perception. *The Journal of Undergraduate Neuroscience Education* 15(1): A56–A60.
57. Edmonds M (undated) How Flavor Tripping Works. Available at https://people.howstuffworks.com/flavor-tripping.htm accessed 29 May 2019.
58. Goodson A (2018) 6 Impressive Health Benefits of Gymnema Sylvestre. Available at www.healthline.com/nutrition/gymnema-sylvestre-benefits, accessed 29 May 2019.
59. Shih M (2019) Gymnema Sylvestre: The Plant That Helps Control Your Sugar Cravings. Available at www.sweetdefeat.com/blogs/science-of-sd/gymnema-sylvestre, accessed 29 May 2019.
60. Kanetkar P, Singhal R, Kamat M (2007) Gymnema sylvestre: a memoir. *J Clin Biochem Nutr* 41: 77–81.
61. Brala PM, Hagen RL (1983) Effects of sweetness perception and caloric value of a preload on short term intake. *Physiol Behav* 30(1): 1–9.
62. Joffe DJ, Freed SH (2001) Effect of extended release Gymnema sylvestre leaf extract (beta fast GXR). *Diabetes in Control Newsletter* 76(1): 30 October.
63. Pothuraju R, Sharma RK, Chagalamarri J, Jangra S, Kumar Kavadi P (2014) A systematic review of Gymnema sylvestre in obesity and diabetes management. *J Sci Food Agric* 94(5): 834–840.
64. Shimizu K, Iino A, Nakajima J, Tanaka K, et al. (1997) Suppression of glucose absorption by some fractions extracted from Gymnema sylvestre leaves. *J Vet Med Sci* 59(4): 245–251.
65. Al-Romaiyan A, Liu B, Docherty R, Huang GC, et al. (2012) Investigation of intracellular signalling cascades mediating stimulatory effect of a Gymnema sylvestre extract on insulin secretion from isolated mouse and human islets of Langerhans. *Diabetes Obes Metab* 14(12): 1104–1113.
66. Meiselman HL, Halpern BP (1970) Human judgments of Gymnema sylvestre and sucrose mixtures. *Physiology & Behavior* 5(8): 945–948.
67. Shih M (2019) Gymnema Sylvestre: The Plant That Helps Control Your Sugar Cravings. Available at www.sweetdefeat.com/blogs/science-of-sd/gymnema-sylvestre, accessed 29 May 2019.
68. Johnson JM, Conforti FD (2003) Fructose. In: *Encyclopedia of Food Sciences and Nutrition*, 2nd edn. Amsterdam: Academic Press. pp.2748–2752.
69. Campbell E, Schlappal A, Geller E, Castonguay TW (2014) Fructose-Induced Hypertriglyeridemia: A Review. In: RR Watson (ed.) *Nutrition in the Prevention and Treatment of Abdominal Obesity*. London: Academic Press.
70. Thomsson KA, Prakobphol A, Leffler H, Reddy MS, et al. (2002) The salivary mucin MG1 (MUC5B) carries a repertoire of unique oligosaccharides that is large and diverse. *Glycobiology* 12(1): 1–14.
71. Mondoa EI, Kitei M (2001) *Sugars That Heal: The New Healing Science of Glyconutrients*. New York: Ballantine Books.
72. Arizona State University (2017) Sugar-coated world: probing the mysteries of glycan structure and function. *ScienceDaily*, 18 December. Available at www.sciencedaily.com/releases/2017/12/171218120356.htm, accessed 8 January 2019.
73. Royle L, Roos A, Harvey DJ, Wormald MR, et al. (2003) Secretory IgA N- and O-Glycans provide a link between the innate and adaptive immune systems. *The Journal of Biological Chemistry* 278(22): 20140–20153.

CHAPTER 6

1. Socransky SS, Haffajee AD (1992) The bacterial etiology of destructive periodontal disease: current concepts. *J Periodontol* 63: 322–331.
2. Socransky SS, Haffajee AD, Dzink JL, Hillman JD (1988) Association between microbial species in subgingival plaque samples. *Oral Microbiol Immunol* 3: 1–7.

ENDNOTES

3. Holt SC, Kesavalu L, Walker S, Genco CA (1999) Virulence factors of Porphyromonas gingivalis. *Periodontol 2000 20*: 168-238.
4. Bartold PM, VanDyke TE (2013) Periodontitis: a host-mediated disruption of microbial homeostasis. Unlearning learned concepts. *Periodontol 2000 62*(1): 203-217.
5. Marsh PD (2011) How is the development of dental biofilms influenced by the host? *J Clin Periodontol 38*(suppl. 11): 28-35.
6. Bartold PM, VanDyke TE (2013) Periodontitis: a host-mediated disruption of microbial homeostasis. Unlearning learned concepts. *Periodontol 2000 62*(1): 203-217.
7. Ibid.
8. Marsh PD (2009) Dental plaque as a biofilm: the significance of pH in health and caries. *Compend Contin Educ Dent 30*(2): 76-78.
9. Flemming H-C, Wingender J (2010) The biofilm matrix. *Nature Reviews Microbiology 8*: 623-633.
10. Byun R, Nadkarni MA, Chhour K-L, Martin FE, Jacques NA, Hunter N (2004) Quantitative analysis of diverse Lactobacillus species present in advanced dental caries. *Journal of Clinical Microbiology 42*(7): 3128-3136.
11. Selwitz RH, Ismail A, Pitts NB (2007) Dental caries. *Lancet 369*: 51-59.
12. Caglar E, Cildir SK, Ergeneli S, Sandalli N, Twetman S (2006) Salivary mutans streptococci and lactobacilli levels after ingestion of the probiotic bacterium Lactobacillus reuteri ATCC 55730 by straws or tablets. *Acta Odontol Scand 64*(5): 314-318.
13. Caglar E, Kuscu OO, Cildir SK, Kuvvetli SS, Sandalli N (2008) A probiotic lozenge administered medical device and its effect on salivary mutans streptococci and lactobacilli. *Int J Paediatr Dent 18*(1): 35-39.
14. Caufield PW, Li Y, Dasanayake A, Saxena D (2007) Diversity of lactobacilli in the oral cavities of young women with dental caries. *Caries Res 41*: 2-8.
15. Koo H, Xiao J, Klein MI, Jeon JG (2010) Exopolysaccharides produced by Streptococcus mutans glucosyltransferases modulate the establishment of microcolonies within multispecies biofilms. *Journal of Bacteriology 192*(12): 3024-3032.
16. Humphrey SP, Williamson RT (2001) A review of saliva: normal composition, flow and function. *The Journal of Prosthetic Dentistry 85*(2): 162-169.
17. Edgar WM (1990) Saliva and dental health. Clinical implications of saliva: report of a consensus meeting. *Br Dent J 169*: 96-98.
18. Humphrey SP, Williamson RT (2001) A review of saliva: normal composition, flow and function. *The Journal of Prosthetic Dentistry 85*(2): 162-169.
19. Marsh PD (2009) Dental plaque as a biofilm: the significance of pH in health and caries. *Compend Contin Educ Dent 30*(2): 76-78.
20. Ibid.
21. Marsh PD (2003) Are dental diseases examples of ecological catastrophes? *Microbiology 149*: 279-294.
22. Marsh PD (1994) Microbial ecology of dental plaque and its significance in health and disease. *Adv Dent Res 8*: 263-271.
23. Kumar PS, Griffen AL, Barton JA, Paster BJ, Moeschberger ML, Leys EJ (2003) New bacterial species associated with chronic periodontitis. *J Dent Res 82*(5): 338-344.
24. Marcotte H, Lavoie MC (1998) Oral microbial ecology and the role of salivary immunoglobulin A. *Microbiology and Molecular Biology Reviews 62*(1): 71-109.
25. Darby I (2006) Drugs and gingival bleeding. *Australian Prescriber 29*(6): 154-155.
26. Jacob RA, Sotoudeh G (2002) Vitamin C function and status in chronic disease. *Nutr Clin Care 5*: 66-74.
27. Calkins CC, Platt K, Potempa J, Travis J (1998) Inactivation of tumor necrosis factor-alpha by proteinases (gingipains) from the periodontal pathogen, Porphyromonas gingivalis. Implications of immune evasion. *The Journal of Biological Chemistry 273*(12): 6611-6614.
28. Sroka A, Sztukowska M, Potempa J, Travis J, Genco CA (2001) Degradation of host heme proteins by lysine- and arginine-specific cysteine proteinases (gingipains) of porphyromonas gingivalis. *Journal of Bacteriology 183*(19): 5609-5616.
29. How KY, Song KP, Chan KG (2016) Porphyromonas gingivalis: an overview of periodontopathic pathogen below the gum line. *Frontiers in Microbiology 7*: 53.
30. Soukos NS, Som S, Abernethy AD, Ruggiero K, et al. (2005) Phototargeting oral black-pigmented bacteria. *Antimicrobial Agents and Chemotherapy 49*(4): 1391-1396.
31. Touger-Decker R, van Loveren C (2003) Sugars and dental caries. *Am J Clin Nutr 78*(suppl.): 881S-892S.
32. Marcotte H, Lavoie MC (1998) Oral microbial ecology and the role of salivary immunoglobulin A. *Microbiology and Molecular Biology Reviews 62*(1): 71-109.
33. Alwan AH (2015) Determination of interleukin-1β (IL-1β) and interleukin-6 (IL 6) in gingival crevicular fluid in patient with chronic periodontitis. *IOSR-JDMS 14*(11, Ver.IV): 81-90.
34. Toker H, Poyraz O, Eren K (2008) Effect of periodontal treatment on IL-1beta, IL-1ra, and IL-10 levels in gingival crevicular fluid in patients with aggressive periodontitis. *J Clin Periodontol 35*(6): 507-513.

35 Kleinberg I (2002) A mixed-bacteria ecological approach to understanding the role of the oral bacteria in dental caries causation: an alternative to Streptococcus mutans and the specific-plaque hypothesis. *Crit Rev Oral Biol Med* 13(2): 108–125.

36 Hajishengallis G, Lamont RJ (2012) Beyond the red complex and into more complexity: the polymicrobial synergy and dysbiosis (PSD) model of periodontal disease etiology. *Mol Oral Microbiol* 27(6): 409–419.

37 Costalonga M, Herzberg MC (2014) The oral microbiome and the immunobiology of periodontal disease and caries. *Immunology Letters* 162: 22–38.

38 Lovegrove JM (2004) Dental plaque revisited: bacteria associated with periodontal disease. *JNZ Soc Periodontol* 2004(87): 7–21.

39 Costalonga M, Herzberg MC (2014) The oral microbiome and the immunobiology of periodontal disease and caries. *Immunology Letters* 162: 22–38.

40 Marsh PD (2003) Are dental diseases examples of ecological catastrophes? *Microbiology* 149: 279–294.

41 Manikandan GR, Ajithkumar KC (2016) Diabetes mellitus and periodontal disease: unravelling the two way relationship. *Kerala Medical Journal* 9(3): 111–119.

42 Golub LM, Lee HM, Greenwald RA, Ryan ME, et al. (1997) A matrix metalloproteinase inhibitor reduces bone-type collagen degradation fragments and specific collagenases in gingival crevicular fluid during adult periodontitis. *Inflammation Research* 26(8): 310–319.

43 Smith QT, Harriman L, Au GS, Stoltenberg JL, et al. (1995) Neutrophil elastase in crevicular fluid: comparison of a middle-aged general population with healthy and periodontitis groups. *J Clin Periodontol* 22(12): 935–941.

44 Hernández M, Gamornal J, Tervahartiala T, Mäntylä P, et al. (2010) Associations between matrix metalloproteinase-8 and -14 and myeloperoxidase in gingival crevicular fluid from subjects with progressive chronic periodontitis: a longitudinal study. *Journal of Periodontology* 81(11): 1644–1652.

45 Slots J (2010) Human viruses in periodontitis. *Periodontology 2000* 53: 89–110.

46 Marcotte H, Lavoie MC (1998) Oral microbial ecology and the role of salivary immunoglobulin A. *Microbiology and Molecular Biology Reviews* 62(1): 71–109.

47 Albander JM (2002) Global risk facts and risk indicators for periodontal diseases. *Periodontal 2000* 29: 177–206. As cited in: Slots J (2010) Human viruses in periodontitis. *Periodontology 2000* 53: 89–110.

48 Holt SC, Kesavalu L, Walker S, Genco CA (1999) Virulence factors of Porphyromonas gingivalis. *Periodontology 2000* 20: 168–238.

49 Bhattacharjee MK, Childs CB, Ali E (2011) Sensitivity of the periodontal pathogen Aggregativacter actinomycetemcomitans at mildly acidic pH. *J Periodontol* 82(6): 917–925.

50 Park S-R, Kim D-J, Han S-Y, Kang M-J, et al. (2014) Diverse toll-like receptors mediate cytokine production by Fusobacterium nucleatum and Aggregatibacter actinomycetemcomitans in macrophages. *Infection and Immunity* 82(5): 1914–1920.

51 Han YW (2015) Fusobacterium nucleatum: a commensal-turned pathogen. *Curr Opin Microbiol* 23: 141–147.

52 Kesic L, Milasin J, Igic M, Obradovic R (2008) Microbial etiology of periodontal disease – mini review. Facta Universitatis Series: *Medicine and Biology* 15(1): 1–6.

53 Haffajee AD, Teles RP, Socransky SS (2006) Association of Eubacterium nodatum and Treponema denticola with human periodontitis lesions. *Oral Microbiol Immunol* 21(5): 269–282.

54 Zheng P, Zhou W (2015) Relation between periodontitis and helicobacter pylori infection. *Int J Clin Exp Med* 8(9): 16741–16744.

55 Adler I, Muiño, Aguas S, Harada L, et al. (2014) Helicobacter pylori and oral pathology: relationship with the gastric infection. *World J Gastroenterol* 20(29): 9922–9935.

56 Griffen AL, Becker MR, Lyons SR, Moeschberger ML, Leys EJ (1998) Prevalence of Porphyromonas gingivalis and periodontal health status. *Journal of Clinical Microbiology* 36(11): 3239–3242.

57 vanWinkelhoff AJ, Loos BG, van der Reijden WA, van der Velden U (2002) Porphyromonas gingivalis, Bacteroides forsythus and other putative periodontal pathogens in subjects with and without periodontal destruction. *J Clin Periodontol* 29: 1023–1028.

58 Ibid.

59 Darveau RP, Hajishengallis G, Curtsi MA (2012) Porphyromonas gingivalis as a potential community activist for disease. *J Dent Res* 91(9): 816–820.

60 Bostanci N, Belibasakis GN (2012) Porphyromonas gingivalis: an invasive and evasive opportunistic oral pathogen. *FEMS Microbiol Lett* 333: 1–9.

61 Darveau RP, Hajishengallis G, Curtsi MA (2012) Porphyromonas gingivalis as a potential community activist for disease. *J Dent Res* 91(9): 816–820.

62 Mysak J, Podzimek S, Sommerova P, Lyuya-Mi Y, et al. (2014) Porphyromonas gingivalis: major periodontopathic pathogen overview. *Journal of Immunology Research* 2014: 476068.

ENDNOTES

63. Gibson FC III, Genco CA (2001) Prevention of Porphyromonas gingivalis-induced oral bone loss following immunization with gingipain. *Infection and Immunity 69*: 7959-7963.
64. Bostanci N, Belibasakis GN (2012) Porphyromonas gingivalis: an invasive and evasive opportunistic oral pathogen. *FEMS Microbiol Lett 333*: 1-9.
65. Smalley JW, Birss AJ, Szmigielski B, Potempa J (2006) The HA2 haemagglutinin domain of the lysine-specific gingipain (Kgp) of Porphyromonas gingivalis promotes micro-oxo bishaem formation from monomeric iron(III) protoporphyrin IX. *Microbiology 152*: 1839-1845.
66. McKee AS, McDermid AS, Baskerville A, Dowsett AB, Ellwood DC, Marsh PD (1986) Effect of hemin on the physiology and virulence of bacteroides gingivalis W50. *Infection and Immunity 52*(2): 349-355.
67. Liang S, Krauss JL, Domon H, McIntosh ML, et al. (2011) The C5a receptor impairs IL-12-dependent clearance of Porphyromonas gingivalis and is required for induction of periodontal bone loss. *The Journal of Immunology 186*: 869-877.
68. Bostanci N, Belibasakis GN (2012) Porphyromonas gingivalis: an invasive and evasive opportunistic oral pathogen. *FEMS Microbiol Lett 333*: 1-9.
69. Mysak J, Podzimek S, Sommerova P, Lyuya-Mi Y, et al. (2014) Porphyromonas gingivalis: major periodontopathic pathogen overview. *Journal of Immunology Research 2014*: 476068.
70. Holt SC, Kesavalu L, Walker S, Genco CA (1999) Virulence factors of Porphyromonas gingivalis. *Periodontology 2000 20*: 168-238.
71. Lee J, Sojar H, Bedi G, Genco R (1992) Synthetic peptides analogous to the fimbrillin sequence inhibit adherence of Porphyromonas gingivalis. *Infect Immun 60*: 1662-1670.
72. Calkins CC, Platt K, Potempa J, Travis J (1998) Inactivation of tumor necrosis factor-α by proteinases (gingipains) from the periodontal pathogen, Porphyromonas gingivalis. Implications of immune evasion. *The Journal of Biological Chemistry 273*(12): 6611-6614.
73. Wang P-L, Azuma Y, Shinohara M, Ohura K (2000) Toll-like receptor 4-mediated signal pathway induced by Porphyromonas gingivalis lipopolysaccharide in human gingival fibroblasts. *Biochemical and Biophysical Research Communications 273*: 1161-1167.
74. Mysak J, Podzimek S, Sommerova P, Lyuya-Mi Y, et al. (2014) Porphyromonas gingivalis: major periodontopathic pathogen overview. *Journal of Immunology Research 2014*: 476068.
75. Tobias PS, Gegner J, Tapping R, Orr S, et al. (1997) Lipopolysaccharide dependent cellular activation. *J Periodont Res 32*: 99-103.
76. Mayrand D, Holt SC (1988) Biology of asaccharolytic black-pigmented Bacteroides species. *Microbiological Reviews 52*(1): 134-152.
77. Pandit N, Changela R, Bali D, Tikoo P, Gugnani S (2015) Porphyromonas gingivalis: its virulence and vaccine. *Journal of the International Clinical Dental Research Organization 7*(1): 51-58.
78. Holt SC, Ebersole JF (2005) Porphyromonas gingivalis, Treponema denticola, and Tannerella forsythia: the 'red complex', a prototype polybacterial pathogenic consortium in periodontitis. *Periodontology 2000 38*: 72-122.
79. Sakamoto M, Suzuki M, Umeda M, Ishikawa I, Benno Y (2002) Reclassification of Bacteroides forsythus (Tanner et al. 1986) as Tannerella forsythensis corrig., gen. nov., comb. nov. *International Journal of Systematic and Evolutionary Microbiology 52*: 841-849.
80. Holt SC, Ebersole JF (2005) Porphyromonas gingivalis, Treponema denticola, and Tannerella forsythia: the 'red complex', a prototype polybacterial pathogenic consortium in periodontitis. *Periodontology 2000 38*: 72-122.
81. Tanner ACR, Strzempko MN, Belsky CA, McKinley GA (1985) API ZYM and API An-Ident reactions of fastidious oral gram-negative species. *Journal of Clinical Microbiology 22*(3): 333-335.
82. Posch G, Andrukhov O, Vinogradov E, Lindner B, et al. (2013) Structure and immunogenicity of the rough-type lipopolysaccharide from the periodontal pathogen Tannerella forsythia. *Clinical and Vaccine Immunology 20*(6): 945-953.
83. Dashper SG, Seers CA, Tan KH, Reynolds EC (2011) Virulence factors of the oral spirochete Treponema denticola. *J Dent Res 90*(6): 691-703.
84. Miyamoto M, Ishihara K, Okuda K (2006) The Treponema denticola surface protease dentilisin degrades interleukin-1β (IL-β), IL-6, and tumor necrosis factor alpha. *Infection and Immunity 74*(4): 2462-2467.
85. Dashper SG, Seers CA, Tan KH, Reynolds EC (2011) Virulence factors of the oral spirochete Treponema denticola. *J Dent Res 90*(6): 691-703.
86. Tan KH, Seers CA, Dashper SG, Mitchell HL, et al. (2014) Porphyromonas gingivalis and Treponema denticola exhibit metabolic symbioses. *PLoS Pathog 10*(3): e1003955.
87. Bonner M, Amard V, Bar-Pinatel C, Charpentier F, et al. (2014) Detection of the amoeba Entamoeba gingivalis in periodontal pockets. *Parasite 21*: 30.
88. CDC (2019) Entamoeba Gingivalis. Available at www.cdc.gov/dpdx/entamoebagingivalis, accessed 29 May 2021.
89. Trim RD, Skinner MA, Farone MB, DuBois JD, Newsome AL (2011) Use of PCR to detect Entamoeba gingivalis in diseased gingival pockets and demonstrate its absence in healthy gingival sites. *Parasitol Res 109*: 857-864.

90 Bonner M, Amard V, Bar-Pinatel C, Charpentier F, *et al.* (2014) Detection of the amoeba Entamoeba gingivalis in periodontal pockets. *Parasite* 21: 30.
91 Slots J (2009) Herpesviral-bacterial interactions in periodontal diseases. *Periodontology 2000* 51: 1-24.
92 Crough T, Khanna R (2009) Immunobiology of human cytomegalovirus: from bench to bedside. *Clinical Microbiology Reviews* 22(1): 76-98.
93 Slots J (2009) Herpesviral-bacterial interactions in periodontal diseases. *Periodontology 2000* 51: 1-24.
94 Ibid.
95 Asai D, Hakashima H (2018) Pathogenic viruses commonly present in the oral cavity and relevant antiviral compounds derived from natural products. *Medicines* 5: 120.
96 Slots J (2005) Herpes viruses in periodontal diseases. *Periodontology 2000* 38: 33-62.
97 Slots J (2010) Human viruses in periodontitis. *Periodontology 2000* 53: 89-110.
98 Slots J (2009) Herpesviral-bacterial interactions in periodontal diseases. *Periodontology 2000* 51: 1-24.

CHAPTER 7

1 DellaCorte KW, Perrar I, Pencyzynski KJ, Schwingshackl L, Herder C, Buyken AE (2018) Effect of dietary sugar intake on biomarkers of subclinical inflammation: a systematic review and meta-analysis of intervention studies. *Nutrients* 10: 606.
2 Hert KA, Fisk II PS, Rhee YS, Brunt AR (2014) Decreased consumption of sugar-sweetened beverages improved selected biomarkers of chronic disease risk among US adults: 1999 to 2010. *Nutrition Research* 34(1): 58-65.
3 Gurav AN (2013) Advanced glycation end products: a link between periodontitis and diabetes mellitus? *Curr Diabetes Rev* 9(5): 355-361.
4 Takeda M, Ojima M, Yoshioka H, Inaba H, *et al.* (2006) Relationship of serum advanced glycation end products with deterioration of periodontitis in type 2 diabetes patients. *J Periodontol* 77: 15-20.
5 Vlassara H, Uribarri J (2014) Advanced glycation end products (AGE) and diabetes: cause, effect, or both? *Curr Diab Rep* 141: 453.
6 Jabr F (2013) Is Sugar Really Toxic? Sifting through the Evidence. Available at https://blogs.scientificamerican.com/brainwaves/is-sugar-really-toxic-sifting-through-the-evidence, accessed 14 November 2020.
7 Ahmed N (2005) Advanced glycation endproducts - role in pathology of diabetic complications. *Diabetes Research and Clinical Practice* 67: 3-21.
8 Paul RG, Bailey AJ (1996) Glycation of collagen: the basis of its central role in the late complications of ageing and diabetes. *Int J Biochem Cell Biol* 28(12): 1297-1310.
9 Ahmed N (2005) Advanced glycation endproducts - role in pathology of diabetic complications. *Diabetes Research and Clinical Practice* 67: 3-21.
10 Gkogkolou P, Böhm M (2012) Advanced glycation end products: key players in skin aging? *Dermato-Endocrinology* 4(3): 259-270.
11 Paul RG, Bailey AJ (1996) Glycation of collagen: the basis of its central role in the late complications of ageing and diabetes. *Int J Biochem Cell Biol* 28(12): 1297-1310.
12 Pietropaoli D, Monaco A, DelPinto R, Cifone MG, Marzo G, Giannoni M (2012) Advanced glycation end products: possible link between metabolic syndrome and periodontal diseases. *Int J Immunopath Pharmac* 25(1): 9-17.
13 Gkogkolou P, Böhm M (2012) Advanced glycation end products: key players in skin aging? *Dermato-Endocrinology* 4(3): 259-270.
14 Schmidt AM, Weidman E, Lalla E, Yan SD, *et al.* (1996) Advanced glycation endproducts (AGEs) induce oxidant stress in the gingiva: a potential mechanism underlying accelerated periodontal disease associated with diabetes. *Journal of Periodontal Research* 31(7): 508-515.
15 Lalla E, Lamster IB, Stern DM, Schmidt AM (2001) Receptor for advanced glycation end products, inflammation, and accelerated periodontal disease in diabetes: mechanisms and insights into therapeutic modalities. *Ann Periodontol* 6(1): 113-118.
16 Katz J, Bhattacharyya I, Farkhondeh-Kish F, Perez FM, Caudle RM, Heft MW (2005) Expression of the receptor of advanced glycation end products in gingival tissues of type 2 diabetes patients with chronic periodontal disease: a study utilizing immunohistochemistry and RT-PCR. *Journal of Clinical Periodontology* 32(1): 40-44.
17 Elenkova M, Tipton DA, Karydis A, Stein SH (2019) Vitamin D attenuates human gingival fibroblast inflammatory cytokine production following advanced glycation end product interaction with receptors for AGE. *J Periodontal Res* 54(2): 154-163.
18 Chang PC, Chien LY, Chong LY, Kuo YP, Hsiao JK (2013) Glycated matrix up-regulates inflammatory signalling similarly to Porphyromonas gingivalis lipopolysaccharide. *J Periodontal Res* 48(2): 184-193.

19. Sánchez-Domínguez B, López-López J, Jané-Salas E, Castellanos-Cosano L, Velasco-Ortega E, Segura-Egea JJ (2015) Glycated hemoglobin levels and prevalence of apical periodontitis in type 2 diabetic patients. *J Endod 41*(5): 601-606.
20. Grossi SG, Skrepcinski FB, DeCaro T, Robertson DC, *et al*. (1997) Treatment of periodontal disease in diabeteics reduces glycated haemoglobin. *J Periodontol 68*(8): 713-719.
21. Cerami C, Founds H, Nicholl I, Mitsuhashi T, *et al*. (1997) Tobacco smoke is a source of toxic reactive glycation products. *PNAS, USA 94*: 13915-13920.
22. Fleming TH, Humpert PM, Nawroth PP, Bierhaus A (2011) Reactive metabolites and AGE/RAGE-mediated cellular dysfunction affect the aging process: a mini-review. *Gerontology 57*: 435-443.
23. Van der Lugt T, Weseler AR, Gebbink WA, Vrolijk MF, Opperhuizen A, Bast A (2018) Dietary advanced glycation endproducts induce an inflammatory response in human macrophages in vitro. *Nutrients 10*(12): 1868.
24. Uribarri J, delCastillo MD, de la Maza MP, Filip R, *et al*. (2015) Dietary advanced glycation end products and their role in health and disease. *Adv Nutr 6*: 461-473.
25. Bengmark S (2007) Advanced glycation and lipoxidation end products – amplifiers of inflammation: the role of food. *JPEN 31*(5): 430-440.
26. Fleming TH, Humpert PM, Nawroth PP, Bierhaus A (2011) Reactive metabolites and AGE/RAGE-mediated cellular dysfunction affect the aging process: a mini-review. *Gerontology 57*: 435-443.
27. Majtan J, Klaudiny J, Bohova J, Kohutova L, *et al*. (2012) Methylglyoxal-induced modifications of significant honeybee proteinous components in manuka honey: possible therapeutic implications. *Fitoterapia 83*(4): 671-677.
28. Thornalley PJ (2003) Glyoxalase I – structure, function and acritical role in the enzymatic defence against glycation. *Biochem Soc Trans 31*(Pt 6): 1343-1348.
29. Rabbani N, Godfrey L, Xue M, Shaheen F, *et al*. (2011) Glycation of LDL by methylglyoxal increases arterial atherogenicity: a possible contributor to increased risk of cardiovascular disease in diabetes. *Diabetes 60*: 1973-1980.
30. Uribarri J, delCastillo MD, de la Maza MP, Filip R, *et al*. (2015) Dietary advanced glycation end products and their role in health and disease. *Adv Nutr 6*: 461-473.
31. Franco C, Patricia H-R, Timo S, Claudia B, Marcela H (2017) Matrix metalloproteinases as regulators of periodontal inflammation. *Int J Mol Sci 18*: 440.
32. Guo Y, Nguyen K-A, Potempa J (2010) Dichotomy of gingipains action as virulence factors: from cleaving substrates with a precision of a surgeon's knife to a meat chopper-like brutal degradation of proteins. *Periodontol 2000 54*(1): 15-44.
33. Potempa J, Banbula A, Travis J (2000) Role of bacterial proteinases in matrix destruction and modulation of host responses. *Periodontology 2000 24*(1): 153-192.
34. Smalley JW (1994) Pathogenic mechanisms in periodontal disease. *Adv Dent Res 8*(2): 320-328.
35. Li N, Collyer CA (2011) Gingipains from Porphyromonas gingivalis – complex domain structures confer diverse functions. *European Journal of Microbiology and Immunology (Bp) 1*(1): 41-58.
36. Nema NK, Maity N, Sarkar BK, Mukherjee PK (2013) Matrix metalloproteinase, hyaluronidase and elastase inhibitory potential of standardized extract of Centella asiatica. *Pharm Biol 51*(9): 1182-1187.
37. Sastravaha G, Gassmann G, Sangtherapitikul P, Grim W-D (2005) Adjunctive periodontal treatment with Centella asiatica and Punica granatum extracts in supportive periodontal therapy. *J Int Acad Periodontol 7*(3): 70-79.
38. Tanaka M, Masuko-Hongo K, Kato T, Nishioka K, Nakamura H (2006) Suppressive effects of hyaluronan on MMP-1 and RANTES production from chondrocytes. *Rheumatol Int 26*(3): 185-190.
39. Politis C, Schoenaers J, Jacobs R, Agbaje JO (2016) Wound healing problems in the mouth. *Frontiers in Physiology 7*: 507.
40. Oudhoff MJ, Bolscher JGM, Nazmi K, Kalay H, *et al*. (2008) Histatins are the major wound-closure stimulating factors in human saliva as identified in a cell culture assay. *FASEB J 22*: 3805-3812.
41. Pogrel MA, Low MA, Stern R (2003) Hyaluronan (hyaluronic acid) and its regulation in human saliva by hyaluronidase and its inhibitors. *Journal of Oral Science 45*(2): 85-91.
42. Politis C, Schoenaers J, Jacobs R, Agbaje JO (2016) Wound healing problems in the mouth. *Frontiers in Physiology 7*: 507.
43. Ibid.
44. Ibid.
45. Discepoli N, Vignoletti F, Laino L, DeSanctis M, Muñoz F, Sanz M (2013) Early healing of the alveolar process after tooth extraction: an experimental study in the beagle dog. *J Clin Periodontol 40*: 638-644.
46. Larjava H (2012) *Oral Wound Healing: Cell Biology and Clinical Management*. West Sussex: John Wiley & Sons.
47. Politis C, Schoenaers J, Jacobs R, Agbaje JO (2016) Wound healing problems in the mouth. *Frontiers in Physiology 7*: 507.

48 Windham B (ed.) (undated) Incidence Levels and Chronic Health Effects Related to Cavitations. Available at www.biodentistalabama.com/research/windham-cavitations.pdf, accessed 27 January 2019.

49 Eni Juliana A, Shahrul Hisham ZA, Rohaya MAW, Nik Marzuki S (2009) Molecular existence of mature odontoblast and osteoblast cells in adult human pulp tissues. *Asian Journal of Biochemistry* 4: 36–44.

50 Windham B (ed.) (undated) Incidence Levels and Chronic Health Effects Related to Cavitations. Available at www.biodentistalabama.com/research/windham-cavitations.pdf, accessed 27 January 2019.

51 Marincola M (2014) Jawbone cavitation and its implications in implant dentistry. *Implants* 1: 20–24.

52 Bouquot JE, Christian J (1995) Long-term effects of jawbone curettage on the pain of facial neuralgia. *Journal of Oral and Maxillofacial Surgery* 53(4): 387–397.

53 Williams L (2012) Dental Cavitation Surgery. Available at www.westonaprice.org/health-topics/dentistry/dental-cavitation-surgery, accessed 2 February 2019.

54 IAOMT (The International Academy of Oral Medicine and Toxicology) (2014) IAOMT Position Paper on Human Jawbone Osteonecrosis. Available at https://iaomt.org, accessed 2 February 2019.

55 Levy JA (2009) The unexpected pleiotropic activities of RANTES. *Journal of Immunology* 182(7): 3945–3946.

56 Soria G, Ben-Baruch A (2008) The inflammatory chemokines CCL2 and CCL5 in breast cancer. *Cancer Lett* 267: 271–285.

57 Eissa SAL, Zaki SA, El-Maghraby SM, Kadry DY (2005) Importance of serum IL-18 and RANTES as markers for breast carcinoma progression. *Journal of the Egyptian Nat Cancer Inst* 17(1): 51–55.

58 Lechner J, von Baehr V (2014) Hyperactivated signaling pathways of chemokine RANTES/CCL5 in osteopathies of jawbone in breast cancer patients – case report and research. *Breast Cancer: Basic and Clinical Research* 8: 89–96.

59 Lechner J, von Baehr V (2013) RANTES and fibroblast growth factor 2 in jawbone cavitations: triggers for systemic disease? *International Journal of General Medicine* 6: 277–290.

60 Appay V, Rowland-Jones SL (2001) RANTES: a versatile and controversial chemokine. *TRENDS in Immunology* 22(2): 83–87.

61 Agere SA, Akhtar N, Watson JM, Ahmed S (2017) RANTES/CCL5 induces collagen degradation by activating MMP-1 and MMP-13 expression in human rheumatoid arthritis synovial fibroblasts. *Front Immunol* 8: 1341.

62 Holmström SB, Clark R, Zwicker S, Bureik D, et al. (2017) Gingival tissue inflammation promotes increased matrix metalloproteinase-12 production by CD200Rlow monocyte-derived cells in periodontitis. *J Immunol* 199: 4023–4035.

63 Al-Majid A, Alassiri S, Rathnayake N, Tervahartiala T, Gieselmann D-R, Sorsa T (2018) Matrix metalloproteinase-8 as an inflammatory and prevention biomarker in periodontal and peri-implant diseases. *Int J Dent 2018*: 7891323.

64 Lechner J, Schuett S, von Baehr V (2017) Aseptic-avascular osteonecrosis: local 'silent inflammation' in the jawbone and RANTES/CCL5 overexpression. *Clinical, Cosmetic and Investigational Dentistry* 9: 99–109.

65 Lechner J, Mayer W (2010) Immune messengers in neuralgia inducing cavitational osteonecrosis (NICO) in jaw bone and systemic interference. *European Journal of Integrative Medicine* 2: 71–77.

66 Lechner J, von Baehr V (2013) RANTES and fibroblast growth factor 2 in jawbone cavitations: triggers for systemic disease? *International Journal of General Medicine* 6: 277–290.

67 Lechner J, von Baehr V (2014) Hyperactivated signaling pathways of chemokine RANTES/CCL5 in osteopathies of jawbone in breast cancer patients – case report and research. *Breast Cancer: Basic and Clinical Research* 8: 89–96.

68 Liao WC, Lin Y-H, Chang T-M, Huang W-Y (2012) Identification of two licorice species, Glycyrrhiza uranlensis and Glycyrrhiza glabra, based on separation and identification of their bioactive components. *Food Chemistry* 132(4): 2188–2193.

69 Ko HC, Wei BL, Chiou WF (2006) The effect of medicinal plants used in Chinese folk medicine on RANTES secretion by virus-infected human epithelial cells. *J Ethnopharmacol* 107(2): 205–210.

70 Mak NK, Leung CY, Wei XY, Shen XL, et al. (2004) Inhibition of RANTES expression by indirubin in influenza virus-infected human bronchial epithelial cells. *Biochem Pharmacol* 67(1): 167–174.

CHAPTER 8

1 DaSilva Dantas A, Lee KK, Raziunaite I, Schaefer K, et al. (2016) Cell biology of Candida albicans – host interactions. *Current Opinion in Microbiology* 34: 111–118.

2 Falsetta M, Klein MI, Colonne PM, Scott-Anne K, et al. (2014) Symbiotic relationship between Streptococcus mutans and Candida albicans synergizes virulence of plaque biofilms in vivo. *Infection and Immunity* 82(5): 1968–1981.

ENDNOTES

3. Scully C, Porter S (2000) ABC of oral health: swellings and red, white and pigmented lesions. *BMJ 321*: 225–228.
4. Redding SW, Zellars RC, Kirkpatrick WR, McAtee RK, et al. (1999) Epidemiology of oropharyngeal Candida colonization and infection in patients receiving radiation for head and neck cancer. *Journal of Clinical Microbiology 27*(12): 3896–3900.
5. Stanford Medicine (undated) Examination of the Tongue. Available at https://stanfordmedicine25.stanford.edu/the25/tongue.html, accessed 6 May 2019.
6. Cirino E (2019) How to Stop Biting Your Tongue in Your Sleep. Available at www.healthline.com/health/biting-tongue-in-sleep, accessed 3 August 2019.
7. Stanley M (2010) HPV – immune response to infection and vaccination. *Infectious Agents and Cancer 5*: 19.
8. Centers for Disease Control and Prevention (2017) Human Papillomavirus (HPV) Statistics. Available at www.cdc.gov/std/hpv/stats.htm, accessed 15 May 2019.
9. Alzahrani AA (2017) Association between human herpes virus and aggressive periodontitis: a systematic review. *The Saudi Journal for Dental Research 8*: 97–104.
10. Becker Y, Olshevsky U, Levitt J (1967) The role of arginine in the replication of herpes simplex virus. *J Gen Virol 1*: 471–478.
11. Singh BB, Udani J, Vinjamury SP, Der-Martirosian C, et al. (2005) Safety and effectiveness of an L-lysine, zinc and herbal-based product on the treatment of facial and circumoral herpes. *Altern Med Rev 10*(2): 123–127.
12. Griffith RS, Walsh DE, Myrmel KH, Thompson RW, Behforooz A (1987) Success of L-lysine therapy in frequently recurrent herpes simplex infection. Treatment and prophylaxis. *Dermatologica 175*(4): 183–190.
13. Schuhmacher A, Reichling J, Schnitzler P (2003) Virucidal effect of peppermint oil on the enveloped viruses herpes simplex virus type 1 and type 2 in vitro. *Phytomedicine 10*: 504–510.
14. Carson CF, Ashton L, Dry L, Smith DW, Riley TV (2001) Melaleuca alternifolia (tea tree) oil gel (6%) for the treatment of recurrent herpes labialis. *Journal of Antimicrobial Chemotherapy 48*: 445–458.
15. Koytchev R, Alken RG, Dundarov S (1999) Balm mint extract (Lo-701) for topical treatment of recurring Herpes labialis. *Phytomedicine 6*(4): 225–230.
16. Wölbling RH, Leonhardt K (1994) Local therapy of herpes simplex with dried extract from Melissa offinalis. *Phytomedicine 1*(1): 25–31.
17. Shahid Z, Kalayanamitra R, McClafferty B, Kepko D, et al. (2020) COVID-19 and older adults: what we know. *JAGS 68*: 926–929.
18. Dziedzic A, Wojtyczka R (2020) The impact of coronavirus infectious disease 19 (COVID-19) on oral health. *Oral Diseases 27*(suppl. 3): 703–706.
19. Telles-Araujo GdeT, Caminha RD'AG, Kallás MS, Santos PSdaS (2020) Teledentistry support in COVID-19 oral care. *Clinics 75*: e2030.
20. Azarpazhooh A, Leake JL (2006) Systematic review of the association between respiratory diseases and oral health. *Periodontol 77*: 1465–1482.
21. Scully C, Shotts R (2000) ABC of oral health: mouth ulcers and other causes of orofacial soreness and pain. *BMJ 321*(7254): 162–165.
22. Ibid.
23. Ibid.
24. Adler I, Muiño, Aguas S, Harada L, et al. (2014) Helicobacter pylori and oral pathology: relationship with the gastric infection. *World J Gastroenterol 20*(29): 9922–9935.
25. Avcu N, Avcu F, Beyan C, Ural AU, et al. (2001) The relationship between gastric-oral Helicobacter pylori and oral hygiene in patients with vitamin B12-deficiency anemia. *Oral Surgery, Oral Medicine, Oral Pathology, Oral Radiology, and Endodontology 92*(2): 166–169.
26. Zou QH, Li RQ (2011) Helicobacter pylori in the oral cavity and gastric mucosa: a meta-analysis. *J Oral Pathol Med 40*(4): 317–324.
27. Sarari AS, Farraj MA, Hamoudi W, Essawi TA (2008) Helicobacter pylori, a causative agent of vitamin B12 deficiency. *J Infect Dev Ctries 2*(5): 346–349.
28. Adler I, Muiño, Aguas S, Harada L, et al. (2014) Helicobacter pylori and oral pathology: relationship with the gastric infection. *World J Gastroenterol 20*(29): 9922–9935.
29. Mayo Clinic (undated) Pemphigus. Available at www.mayoclinic.org/diseases-conditions/pemphigus/symptoms-causes/syc-20350404, accessed 24 February 2019.
30. Ellis ME (2017) Pemphigoid. Available at www.healthline.com/health/bullous-pemphigoid, accessed 24 February 2019.
31. Oakley A (2015) Erythema Multiforme. Available at https://dermnetnz.org/topics/erythema-multiforme, accessed 24 February 2019.
32. NHS (2018) Overview: Epidermolysis Bullosa. Available at www.nhs.uk/conditions/epidermolysis-bullosa, accessed 24 February 2019.
33. Duffill M (2008) Angina Bullosa Haemorrhagica. Available at https://dermnetnz.org/topics/angina-bullosa-haemorrhagica, accessed 24 February 2019.
34. Scully C, Shotts R (2000) ABC of oral health: mouth ulcers and other causes of orofacial soreness and pain. *BMJ 321*(7254): 162–165.
35. Lisi O, D'Urso V, Vaccalluzzo V, Bongiorno G, et al. (2014) Persistence of phlebotomine *Leishmania* vectors in urban sites of Catania (Sicily, Italy). *Parasites & Vectors 7*: 560.

36 Herlofson BB, Barkvoll P (1996) The effect of two toothpaste detergents on the frequency of recurrent aphthous ulcers. *Acta Odontol Scand* 54(3): 150–153.
37 Wu IB, Schwartz RA (2008) Reiter's syndrome: the classic triad and more. *J Am Acad Dermatol* 59(1): 113–121.
38 Scully C, Shotts R (2000) ABC of oral health: mouth ulcers and other causes of orofacial soreness and pain. *BMJ 321*(7254): 162–165.
39 Coventry J, Griffiths G, Scully C, Tonetti M (2000) ABC of oral health: periodontal disease. *BMJ 321*: 36–39.
40 Scully C, Shotts R (2000) ABC of oral health: mouth ulcers and other causes of orofacial soreness and pain. *BMJ 321*(7254): 162–165.
41 Ibid.
42 Lamey J, Lamb AB, Hughes A, Milligan KA, Forsyth A (1994) Type 3 burning mouth syndrome: psychological and allergic aspects. *J Oral Pathol Med 23*: 216–219. As cited in: Cerchiari DP, de Morica RD, Sanjar FA, Rapoport PB, Moretti G, Guerra MM (2006) Burning mouth syndrome: etiology. *Rev Bras Otorrinolaringol 72*(3): 419–424.
43 Bartoshuk LM, Snyder DJ, Grushka M, Berger AM, Duffy VB, Kveton JF (2005) Taste damage: previously unsuspected consequences. *Chem Senses 30*(suppl.1): i218–i219.
44 Alramadhn E, Hanna MS, Hanna MS, Goldstein TA, Avila SM, Weeks BS (2012) Dietary and botanical anxiolytics. *Med Sci Monit 18*(4): RA42–RA48.
45 Scully C, Porter S (2000) ABC of oral health: swellings and red, white and pigmented lesions. *BMJ 321*: 225–228.
46 Stanford Medicine (undated) Examination of the Tongue. Available at https://stanfordmedicine25.stanford.edu/the25/tongue.html, accessed 6 May 2019.
47 Scully C, Porter S (2000) ABC of oral health: swellings and red, white and pigmented lesions. *BMJ 321*: 225–228.
48 Kurapati KRV, Stluri VS, Samikkannu T, Garcia G, Nair MPN (2016) Natural products as anti-HIV agents and role in HIV-associated neurocognitive disorders (HAND): a brief overview. *Frontiers in Microbiology 6*: 1444.
49 Scully C, Porter S (2000) ABC of oral health: swellings and red, white and pigmented lesions. *BMJ 321*: 225–228.
50 Guan X-b, Bain J-p, Fu J, Zhang H-n, Wang L-h, Li P (2011) Clinical evaluation on treatment of oral lichen planus with Yiqiyangyin Mixture and its mechanism. *Electronic Journal of Biology 7*(2): 20–25.
51 Scully C, Porter S (2000) ABC of oral health: swellings and red, white and pigmented lesions. *BMJ 321*: 225–228.
52 Ibid.
53 Ibid.
54 Ozbayrak S, Dumlu A, Ercalik-Yalcinkaya S (2000) Treatment of melanin-pigmented gingiva and oral mucosa by CO2 laser. *Oral Surg Oral Med Oral Pathol Oral Radiol Endod 90*: 14–15.
55 Amir E, Gorsky M, Buhner A, Sarnat H, Gat H (1991) Physiologic pigmentation of the oral mucosa in Israeli children. *Oral Surg Oral Med Oral Pathol 71*: 396–398.
56 Çiçek Y (2003) The normal and pathological pigmentation of oral mucous membrane: a review. *J Contemp Dent Pract 4*(3): 76–86.
57 Ibid.
58 AlShoubaki RE, AlZahrani AS (2018) Outcomes of gingival depigmentation among smokers and non-smokers: a comparative study. *International Journal of Pharmaceutical Research & Allied Sciences 7*(1): 148–155.
59 Anand R, Chingra C, Menon I, Prasad S (2014) Betel nut chewing and its deleterious effects on oral cavity. *Journal of Cancer Research and Therapeutics 10*(3): 499–505.
60 Pol A, Renkema GH, Tangerman A, Winkel EG, et al. (2018) Mutations in SELENBP1, encoding a novel human methanethiol oxidase, cause extra-oral halitosis. *Nat Genet 50*(1): 120–129.
61 Scully C, Porter S (2000) ABC of oral health: swellings and red, white and pigmented lesions. *BMJ 321*: 225–228.
62 Bouquot JE (undated) The Little Book of Lists (Version 19,05). From seminar slides – personal communication.
63 Scully C, Porter S (2000) ABC of oral health: swellings and red, white and pigmented lesions. *BMJ 321*: 225–228.
64 Mohamad I, Yaroko AA (2013) Peritonsillar swelling is not always quinsy. *Malays Fam Physician 8*(2): 53–55.
65 Dawes C, Pedersen AML, Villa A, Ekström J, et al. (2015) The functions of human saliva: a review sponsored by the World Workshop on Oral Medicine VI. *Archives of Oral Biology 60*: 863–874.
66 Sideras K, Hallemeier CL, Loprinzi CL (2013) Oral Complications. In: JE Niederhuber, JO Armitage, JH Doroshow, MB Kastan, JE Tepper (eds) *Abeloff's Clinical Oncology*, 5th edition, revised. Philadelphia, PA: Elsevier Health Sciences.
67 Aps JKM, Martens LC (2005) Review: the physiology of saliva and transfer of drugs into saliva. *Forensic Science International 150*: 119–131.
68 Divya VC, Sathasivasubramanian S (2015) Submandibular sialolithiasis – a report of two cases. *J Med Res 1*: 5–7.
69 Hammett JT, Walker C (updated 2019, Oct 24) Sialolithiasis. Available at www.ncbi.nlm.nih.gov/books/NBK549845, accessed 27 August 2021.

ENDNOTES

70 Divya VC, Sathasivasubramanian S (2015) Submandibular sialolithiasis – a report of two cases. *J Med Res 1*: 5–7.
71 Arifa SS, Christopher PJ, Kumar S, Kengasubbiah S, Shenoy V (2019) Sialolithiasis of the submandibular gland: report of cases. *Cureus 11*(3): e4180.
72 Hammett JT, Walker C (updated 2019, Oct 24) Sialolithiasis. Available at www.ncbi.nlm.nih.gov/books/NBK549845, accessed 27 August 2021.
73 Martínez-Pérez EF, Juárez ZN, Hernández LR, Bach H (2018) Natural antispasmodics: source, stereochemical configuration, and biological activity. *BioMed Research International 2018*: 2819714.
74 Dulguerov P, Marchal F, Lehmann W (1999) Postparotidectomy facial nerve paralysis: possible etiologic factors and results with routine facial nerve monitoring. *Laryngoscope 109*(5): 754–762. As cited in: Torres-Lagares D, Barranco-Piedra S, Serrera-Figallo MA, Hita-Iglesias P, Martínez-Sahuquillo-Márquez A, Gutiérrez-Pérez JL (2006) Parotid sialolithiasis in Stensen's duct. *Med Oral Patol Oral Cir Bucal 11*: E80–84.
75 Hammett JT, Walker C (updated 2019, Oct 24) Sialolithiasis. Available at www.ncbi.nlm.nih.gov/books/NBK549845, accessed 27 August 2021.
76 Divya VC, Sathasivasubramanian S (2015) Submandibular sialolithiasis – a report of two cases. *J Med Res 1*: 5–7.
77 Oteri G, Procopio RM, Cicciù M (2011) Giant salivary gland calculi (GSGC): report of two cases. *The Open Dentistry Journal 5*: 90–95.
78 Eylgor H, Osma U, Yilmaz MD, Selcuk OT (2012) Multiple sialolithiasis in sublingual gland causing dysphagia. *Am J Case Rep 13*: 44–46.
79 Torres-Lagares D, Barranco-Piedra S, Serrera-Figallo MA, Hita-Iglesias P, Martínez-Sahuquillo-Márquez A, Gutiérrez-Pérez JL (2006) Parotid sialolithiasis in Stensen's duct. *Med Oral Patol Oral Cir Bucal 11*: E80–84.
80 Eylgor H, Osma U, Yilmaz MD, Selcuk OT (2012) Multiple sialolithiasis in sublingual gland causing dysphagia. *Am J Case Rep 13*: 44–46.
81 Divya VC, Sathasivasubramanian S (2015) Submandibular sialolithiasis – a report of two cases. *J Med Res 1*: 5–7.
82 Harrison JD (2009) Causes, natural history, and incidence of salivary stones and obstructions. *Otolarygnol Clin North Am 42*(6): 927–947.
83 Oteri G, Procopio RM, Cicciù M (2011) Giant salivary gland calculi (GSGC): report of two cases. *The Open Dentistry Journal 5*: 90–95.
84 Marchal F, Kurt A-M, Dulguerov P, Lehmann W (2001) Retrograde theory of sialolithiasis formation. *Arch Otolaryngol Head Neck Surg 127*: 66–68.
85 Oteri G, Procopio RM, Cicciù M (2011) Giant salivary gland calculi (GSGC): report of two cases. *The Open Dentistry Journal 5*: 90–95.
86 Eylgor H, Osma U, Yilmaz MD, Selcuk OT (2012) Multiple sialolithiasis in sublingual gland causing dysphagia. *Am J Case Rep 13*: 44–46.
87 Oteri G, Procopio RM, Cicciù M (2011) Giant salivary gland calculi (GSGC): report of two cases. *The Open Dentistry Journal 5*: 90–95.
88 Redding SW, Zellars RC, Kirkpatrick WR, McAtee RK, et al. (1999) Epidemiology of oropharyngeal candida colonization and infection in patients receiving radiation for head and neck cancer. *Journal of Clinical Microbiology 27*(12): 3896–3900.
89 Mayo Clinic (2017) Sjogren's Syndrome. Available at www.mayoclinic.org/diseases-conditions/sjogrens-syndrome/symptoms-causes/syc-20353216, accessed 24 February 2019.
90 Ibid.
91 Bond A, Alavi A, Axford SJ, Bourke BE, et al. (1997) A detailed lectin analysis of IgG glycosylation, demonstrating disease specific changes in terminal galactose and N-acetylglucosamine. *Journal of Autoimmunity 10*: 77–85.
92 Mondoa EI, Kitei M (2001) *Sugars That Heal: The New Healing Science of Glyconutrients*. New York: Ballantine Books.
93 Basset C, Durand V, Jamin C, Clément J, et al. (2000) Increased N-linked glycosylation leading to oversialylation of monomeric immunoglobulin A1 from patients with Sjögren's syndrome. *Scand J Immunol 51*(3): 300–306.
94 Bluestone R, Gumpel JM, Goldberg LS, Holborow EJ (1972) Salivary immunoglobulins in Sjögren's syndrome. *Int Arch Allergy 42*: 686–692.
95 Hsu P-Y, Yang S-H, Tsang N-M, Fan K-H, et al. (2016) Efficacy of Traditional Chinese medicine in xerostomia and quality of life during radiotherapy for head and neck cancer: a prospective pilot study. *Evidence-Based Complementary and Alternative Medicine 2016*: 8359251.
96 Seo WH, Cho ER, Thomas RJ, An S-Y, et al. (2013) The association between periodontitis and obstructive sleep apnea: a preliminary study. *J Periodon Res 48*: 500–506.
97 Oksenberg A, Froom P, Melamed S (2006) Dry mouth upon awakening in obstructive sleep apnea. *J Sleep Res 15*: 317–320.
98 Bergeron C, Kimoff J, Hamid Q (2005) Obstructive sleep apnea syndrome and inflammation. *J Allergy Clin Immunol 116*(6): 1393–1396.
99 Brownfield E (2004) Hypersalivation. Available at www.medscape.com/viewarticle/477613, accessed 11 December 2018.
100 Ibid.

101 Mignogna MD, Fedele S, Russo LL, Muzio LL (2003) Sialorrhea as early oral clinical manifestation of primary Sjögren's syndrome. *Rheumatology 42*: 1113–1114.
102 Scully C, Porter S (2000) ABC of oral health: oral cancer. *BMJ 321*: 97–100.
103 Ibid.
104 Ibid.
105 Riboli E, Norat T (2003) Epidemiologic evidence of the protective effect of fruit and vegetables on cancer risk. *Am J Clin Nutr 78*(suppl.): 559S–569S.
106 Luther F, Layton S, McDonald F (2010) Orthodontics for treating temporomandibular joint (TMJ) disorders. *Cochrane Database Syst Rev 7*(7): CD006541.
107 Cairns BE (2010) Pathophysiology of TMD pain – basic mechanisms and their implications for pharmacotherapy. *J Oral Rehabil 37*(6): 391–410.
108 Scully C, Shotts R (2000) ABC of oral health: mouth ulcers and other causes of orofacial soreness and pain. *BMJ 321*(7254): 162–165.
109 Ibid.
110 Dinis-Oliveira RJ, Caldas I, Carvalho F, Magalhães T (2010) Bruxism after 3,4-methylenedioxymethamphetamine (ecstasy) abuse. *Clinical Toxicology 48*(8): 863–864.
111 Scully C, Shotts R (2000) ABC of oral health: mouth ulcers and other causes of orofacial soreness and pain. *BMJ 321*(7254): 162–165.
112 Bradford A (2015) *Oil Pulling: Benefits & Side Effects*. Available online at www.livescience.com/50896-oil-pulling-facts.html, accessed 5 June 2019.
113 Dryden M, Gaff H, McCombs G, Medlock J, Pietzsch M (2015) The dangers of tick-borne diseases: considerations for dental professionals. *DH&T October*: 26–29.
114 College of Dental Hygienists of Ontario (2014) Lyme Disease. Available at www.cdho.org/Advisories/CDHO_Factsheet_Lyme_Disease.pdf, accessed 2 March 2019.
115 Alqahtani MQ (2014) Tooth-bleaching procedures and their controversial effects: a literature review. *The Saudi Dental Journal 26*: 33–46.
116 Sulieman M (2004) An overview of bleaching techniques: 1. History, chemistry, safety and legal aspects. *Dent Update 31*: 608–616.
117 Alqahtani MQ (2014) Tooth-bleaching procedures and their controversial effects: a literature review. *The Saudi Dental Journal 26*: 33–46.
118 Leonard RH Jr, Van Haywood B, Caplan DJ, Tart ND (2003) Nightguard vital bleaching of tetracycline-stained teeth: 90 months post treatment. *J Esthet Restor Dent 15*(3): 142–152. Discussion 153.
119 Alqahtani MQ (2014) Tooth-bleaching procedures and their controversial effects: a literature review. *The Saudi Dental Journal 26*: 33–46.
120 Wallman IS, Hilton HB (1962) Teeth pigmented by tetracycline. *Lancet 1*: 827–829. As cited in: Watts A, Addy M (2001) Tooth discolouration and staining: a review of the literature. *British Dental Journal 190*(6): 309–316.
121 Watts A, Addy M (2001) Tooth discolouration and staining: a review of the literature. *British Dental Journal 190*(6): 309–316.
122 *British National Formulary* (March 1999) 37: 254–256. London, UK: BMJ Books. As cited in: Watts A, Addy M (2001) Tooth discolouration and staining: a review of the literature. *British Dental Journal 190*(6): 309–316.
123 Moffitt JM, Cooley RO, Olsen NH, Hefferen JJ (1974) Prediction of tetracycline induced tooth discolouration. *J Am Dent Assoc 88*: 547–552.
124 van der Bijl P, Pitigoi-Aron G (1995) Tetracyclines and calcified tissues. *Ann Dent 54*: 69–72. As cited in: Watts A, Addy M (2001) Tooth discolouration and staining: a review of the literature. *British Dental Journal 190*(6): 309–316.
125 Watts A, Addy M (2001) Tooth discolouration and staining: a review of the literature. *British Dental Journal 190*(6): 309–316.
126 Ibid.
127 Wei SHY, Ingram MJ (1969) Analyses of the amalgam–tooth interface using the electron microprobe. *J Dent Res 48*(2): 317–320.
128 Alqahtani MQ (2014) Tooth-bleaching procedures and their controversial effects: a literature review. *The Saudi Dental Journal 26*: 33–46.
129 Flötra L, Gjermo P, Rölla G, Waergaug J (1971) Side effects of chlorhexidine mouth washes. *European Journal of Oral Sciences 79*(2): 119–125.
130 Watts A, Addy M (2001) Tooth discolouration and staining: a review of the literature. *British Dental Journal 190*(6): 309–316.
131 Alqahtani MQ (2014) Tooth-bleaching procedures and their controversial effects: a literature review. *The Saudi Dental Journal 26*: 33–46.
132 Watts A, Addy M (2001) Tooth discolouration and staining: a review of the literature. *British Dental Journal 190*(6): 309–316.
133 Ahmad R, Ariffin EHZM, Vengrasalam I, Kasim NHA (2005) Patients' perceptions and knowledge on tooth bleaching. *Annal Dent Univ Malaya 12*: 24–30.
134 Sulieman M (2004) An overview of bleaching techniques: 1. History, chemistry, safety and legal aspects. *Dent Update 31*: 608–616.
135 Plessas A, Pepelassi E (2012) Dental and periodontal complications of lip and tongue piercing: prevalence and influencing factors. *Australian Dental Journal 57*: 71–78.
136 DeMoor RJG, DeWitte AMJC, Delmé KIM, DeBruyne MAA, Hommez GMG, Goyvaerts D (2005) Dental and oral complications of lip and tongue piercings. *British Dental Journal 1998*: 506–509.

137 Go Ask Alice! Columbia University Health Q&A (undated) Pondering the Pros and Cons of Tongue Piercing. Available at https://goaskalice.columbia.edu/answered-questions/pondering-pros-and-cons-tongue-piercing, accessed 3 August 2019.

138 Zadik Y, Burnstein S, Derazne E, Sandler V, Ianculovici C, Halperin T (2010) Colonization of Candida: prevalence among tongue-pierced and non-pierced immunocompetent adults. *Oral Dis* 16(2): 172–175.

139 Go Ask Alice! Columbia University Health Q&A (undated) Pondering the Pros and Cons of Tongue Piercing. Available at https://goaskalice.columbia.edu/answered-questions/pondering-pros-and-cons-tongue-piercing, accessed 3 August 2019.

140 WebMD (2019) Oral Piercings: What You Should Know. Available at www.webmd.com/oral-health/guide/oral-piercing, accessed 3 August 2019.

141 Scully C, Shotts R (2000) ABC of oral health: mouth ulcers and other causes of orofacial soreness and pain. *BMJ* 321(7254): 162–165.

142 Gedikli O, Doğru H, Aydin G, Tüz M, Uygur K, Sari A (2001) Histopathological changes of chorda tympani in chronic otitis media. *Laryngoscope* 111(4): 724–727.

143 Snyder DJ, Bartoshuk LM (2016) Oral sensory nerve damage: causes and consequences. *Rev Endocr Metab Disord* 17(2): 149–158.

144 Association for Psychological Science (2012) Q & A with Psychological Scientist Linda Bartoshuk. Available at www.psychologicalscience.org/publications/observer/obsonline/q-a-with-taste-expert-linda-bartoshuk.html, accessed 23 June 2018.

145 Schiffman SS, Graham BG (2000) Taste and smell perception affect appetite and immunity in the elderly. *European Journal of Clinical Nutrition* 54(suppl. 3): S54–S63.

146 Nelson GM (1998) Biology of taste buds and the clinical problem of taste loss. *Anat Rec* 253: 70–78.

147 Getchell TV, Doty RL, Bartoshuk LM, Snow JB Jr (1991) *Smell and Taste in Health and Disease.* New York: Raven. As cited in: Nelson GM (1998) Biology of taste buds and the clinical problem of taste loss. *Anat Rec* 253: 70–78.

148 National Institutes of Health (2017) Taste Disorders. NIH Pub. No. 14-3231A. Available at www.nidcd.nih.gov/health/taste-disorders, accessed 8 May 2019.

149 Nelson GM (1998) Biology of taste buds and the clinical problem of taste loss. *Anat Rec* 253: 70–78.

150 Schatzman AR, Henkin RI (1981) Gustin concentration changes relative to salivary zinc and taste in humans. *Proc Natl Acad Sci USA* 78(6): 3867–3871.

151 Thatcher BJ, Doherty AE, Orvisky E, Martin BM, Henkin RI (1998) Gustin from human parotid saliva is carbonic anhydrase VI. *Biochemical and Biophysical Research Communications* 250: 635–641.

152 Caló C, Padiglia A, Zonza A, Corrias L, *et al.* (2011) Polymorphisms in TAS2R38 and the taste bud trophic factor, gustin gene co-operate in modulating PROP taste phenotype. *Physiology & Behavior* 104: 1065–1071.

CHAPTER 9

1 Azarpazhooh A, Tenenbaum HC (2012) Separating fact from fiction: use of high-level evidence from research syntheses to identify diseases and disorders associated with periodontal disease. *J Can Dent Assoc* 78: c25.

2 Han YW, Wang X (2013) Mobile microbiome: oral bacteria in extra-oral infections and inflammation. *J Dent Res* 92(6): 485–491.

3 Scannapieco FA (1999) Role of oral bacteria in respiratory infection. *J Periodontol* 70: 793–802.

4 Carinci F, Martinelli M, Contaldo M, Santoro R, *et al.* (2018) Focus on periodontal disease and development of endocarditis. *J Biol Regul Homeost Agents* 32(suppl. 1): 143–147.

5 Douglas CWI, Heath J, Hampton KK, Preston FE (1993) Identity of viridans streptococci isolated from cases of infective endocarditis. *J Med Microbiol* 39: 179–182.

6 Buduneli N, Baylas H, Buduneli E, Turkoglu O, Kose T, Dahlen G (2005) Periodontal infections and pre-term low birth weight: a case-control study. *J Clin Periodontol* 32: 174–181.

7 Dodman T, Robson J, Pincus D (2000) Kingella kingae infections in children. *J Pediatr Child Health* 36(1): 87–90.

8 Hajishengallis G (2014) Aging and its impact on innate immunity and inflammation: implications for periodontitis. *J Oral Biosci* 56(1): 30–37.

9 Steele J, O'Sullivan I (2011) NHS: Executive Summary: Adult Dental Health Survey 2009. Available at https://files.digital.nhs.uk/publicationimport/pub01xxx/pub01086/adul-dent-heal-surv-summ-them-exec-2009-rep2.pdf accessed 30 May 2021.

10. Knowler WC, Bennett PH, Hamman RF, Miller M (1978) Diabetes incidence and prevalence in Pima Indians: a 19-fold greater incidence than in Rochester, Minnesota. *American Journal of Epidemiology* 108(6): 497–505.
11. Bennett PH, Burch TA, Miller M (1971) Diabetes mellitus in American (Pima) Indians. *The Lancet* 298(7716): 125–128.
12. Löe H (1993) Periodontal disease. The sixth complication of diabetes mellitus. *Diabetes Care* 16(1): 329–334.
13. Saremi A, Nelson RG, Tuloch-Reid M, Hanson RL, et al. (2005) Periodontal disease and mortality in type 2 diabetes. *Diabetes Care* 28(1): 27–32.
14. Löe H (1993) Periodontal disease. The sixth complication of diabetes mellitus. *Diabetes Care* 16(1): 329–334.
15. Darling-Fisher CS, Kanjirath PP, Peters MC, Borgnakke WS (2015) Oral health: an untapped resource in managing glycemic control in diabetes and promoting overall health. *The Journal for Nurse Practitioners* 11(9): 889–896.
16. Genco RJ, Borgnakke WS (2013) Risk factors for periodontal disease. *Periodontology 2000* 62(1): 59–94. As cited in: Genco RJ, Genco FD (2014) Common risk factors in the management of periodontal and associated systemic diseases: the dental setting and interprofessional collaboration. *J Evid Base Dent Pract* 14S1: 4–16.
17. Dunning T (2009) Periodontal disease – the overlooked diabetes complication. *Nephrology Nursing Journal* 36(5): 489–496.
18. Li DX, Deng TZ, Lv J, Ke J (2014) Advanced glycation end products (AGEs) and their receptor (RAGE) induce apoptosis of periodontal ligament fibroblasts. *Braz J Med Biol Res* 47(12): 1036–1043.
19. Dandona P, Aljada A, Mohanty P, Ghanim H, et al. (2001) Insulin inhibits intranuclear nuclear factor κB and stimulates IκB in mononuclear cells in obese subjects: evidence for an anti-inflammatory effect? *J Clin Endocrinol Metab* 86(7): 3257–3265.
20. Gurav AN (2012) Periodontal therapy – an adjuvant for glycemic control. *Diabetes & Metabolic Syndrome: Clinical Research & Reviews* 6: 218–223.
21. Acharya AB, Thakur S, Muddapur MV, Kulkarni RD (2017) Cytokine ratios in chronic periodontitis and type 2 diabetes mellitus. *Diabetes & Metabolic Syndrome: Clinical Research & Reviews* 11: 277–278.
22. Manikandan GR, Ajithkumar KC (2016) Diabetes mellitus and periodontal disease: unravelling the two way relationship. *Kerala Medical Journal* 9(3): 111–119.
23. Jawed M, Shahid SM, Qader SA, Azhar A (2011) Dental caries in diabetes mellitus: role of salivary flow rate and minerals. *Journal of Diabetes and Its Complications* 25: 183–186.
24. Saruta J, Tsukinoki K, Sasaguri K, Ishii H, et al. (2005) Expression and localization of chromogranin A gene and protein in human submandibular gland. *Cells Tissue Organs* 180: 237–244.
25. O'Connor DT & Bernstein KN (1984) Radio-immunoassay of chromogranin A in plasma as a measure of exocytotoxic sympathoadrenal activity in normal subjects and patients with pheochromocytoma. *N Engl J Med* 311: 764–770.
26. Zheng A & Moritani T (2008) Effect of the combination of ginseng, oriental bezoar and glycyrrhiza on autonomic nervous activity and immune system under mental arithmetic stress. *J-STAGE* 54(3): 244–249.
27. Haririan H, Bertl K, Laky M, Rausch W-D, et al. (2012) Salivary and serum chromogranin A and α-amylase in periodontal health and disease. *Journal of Periodontology* 83(10): 1314–1321.
28. Tatemoto K, Efendić S, Mutt V, Makk G, Feistner GJ, Barchas JD (1986) Pancreastatin, a novel pancreatic peptide that inhibits insulin secretion. *Nature* 324: 476–478.
29. Kogawa EM, Grisi DC, Falcão DP, Amorim IA, et al. (2016) Impact of glycemic control on oral health status in type 2 diabetes individuals and its association with salivary and plasma levels of chromogranin A. *Archives of Oral Biology* 62: 10–19.
30. Chaffee BW, Weston SJ (2010) Association between chronic periodontal disease and obesity: a systematic review and meta-analysis. *J Periodontol* 81(12): 1708–1724.
31. Saito T, Shimazaki Y, Sakamoto M (1998) Obesity and periodontitis. *N Engl J Med* 339(7): 482–483.
32. Hotamisligil GS, Arner P, Caro JF, Atkinson RL, Spiegelman BM (1995) Increased adipose tissue expression of tumor necrosis factor-α in human obesity and insulin resistance. *J Clin Invest* 95: 2409–2415.
33. Kumar M, Mishra L, Mohanty R, Nayak R (2014) Diabetes and gum disease: the diabolic duo. *Diabetes & Metabolic Syndrome: Clinical Research & Reviews* 8: 255–258.
34. Hotamisligil GS, Peraldi P, Budavari A, Ellis R, White MF, Speigelman BM (1996) IRS-1-mediated inhibition of insulin receptor tyrosine kinase activity in TNF-α-and obesity-induced insulin resistance. *Science* 271(5249): 665–668.
35. Stephens JM, Lee J, Pilch PF (1997) Tumor necrosis factor-alpha-induced insulin resistance in 3T3-L1 adipocytes is accompanied by a loss of insulin receptor substrate-1 and GLUT-4 expression without a loss of insulin receptor-mediated signal transduction. *J Biol Chem* 272: 971–976.
36. Long SD, Pekala PH (1996) Regulation of GLUT-4 mRNA stability by tumor necrosis factor alpha: alterations in both protein binding to the 30 untranslated region and initiation of translation. *Biochem Biophys Res Commun* 220: 949–953.

37. Hansen LL, Ikeda Y, Olsen GS, Busch AK, Mosthaaf L (1999) Insulin signaling is inhibited by micromolar concentration of H2O2. Evidence for a role of H2O2 in tumor necrosis factor-alpha-mediated insulin resistance. *J Biol Chem 274*: 25078-25084.
38. Feingold KR, Doerrler W, Dinarello CA, Fiers W, Grunfeld C (1992) Stimulation of lipolysis in cultured fat cells by tumor necrosis factor, interleukin-1, and the interferons is blocked by inhibition of prostaglandin synthesis. *Endocrinology 130*: 10-16.
39. Su Y, Wang D, Xuan D, Ni J, et al. (2013) Periodontitis as a novel contributor of adipose tissue inflammation promotes insulin resistance in a rat model. *J Periodontol 84*(11): 1617-1626.
40. Khosravi R, Ka K, Huang T, Khalili S, et al. (2013) Tumor necrosis factor-α and interleukin-6: potential interorgan inflammatory mediators contributing to destructive periodontal disease in obesity or metabolic syndrome. *Mediators of Inflammation 2013*: 728987.
41. Chauhan A, Yadav SS, Dwivedi P, Lai N, Usman K, Khattri S (2016) Correlation of serum and salivary cytokines level with clinical parameters in metabolic syndrome with periodontitis. *J Clin Lab Anal 30*(5): 649-655.
42. Bullon P, Morillo JM, Ramirez-Tortosa MC, Quiles JL, Newman HN, Battino M (2009) Metabolic syndrome and periodontitis: is oxidative stress a common link? *J Dent Res 88*(6): 503-518.
43. Umeki H, Tokuyama R, Ide S, Okubo M, et al. (2014) Leptin promotes wound healing in the oral mucosa. *PLOS ONE 9*(7): e101984.
44. Nokhbehsaim M, Kesser S, Nogueira AVB, Jäger A, et al. (2014) Leptin effects on the regenerative capacity of human periodontal cells. *International Journal of Endocrinology 2014*: 180304.
45. Umeki H, Tokuyama R, Ide S, Okubo M, et al. (2014) Leptin promotes wound healing in the oral mucosa. *PLOS ONE 9*(7): e101984.
46. Keswani SG, Balaji W, Le LD, Leung A, et al. (2013) Role of salivary vascular endothelial growth factor (VEGF) in palatal mucosal wound healing. *Wound Repair Regen 21*(4): 554-562.
47. Kettner NM, Mayo SA, Hua J, Lee C, Moore DD, Fu L (2015) Circadian dysfunction induces leptin resistance in mice. *Cell Metabolism 22*: 448-459.
48. Cutando A, Gómez-Moreno G, Arana C, Acuña-Castroviejo D, Reiter RJ (2007) Melatonin: potential functions in the oral cavity. *J Periodontol 78*: 1094-1102.
49. Dawes C, Pedersen AML, Villa A, Ekström J, Proctor GB, et al. (2015) The functions of human saliva: a review sponsored by the World Workshop on Oral Medicine VI. *Archives of Oral Biology 60*: 863-874.
50. Cutando A, Aneiros-Fernánez J, López-Valverde A, Arias-Santiago S, Aneiros-Cachaza J, Reiter RJ (2011) A new perspective in oral health: potential importance and actions of melatonin receptors MT1, MT2, MT3 and RZR/ROR in the oral cavity. *Archives of Oral Biology 56*: 944-950.
51. Ibid.
52. Karesek M (2004) Melatonin, human aging, and age-related diseases. *Experimental Gerontology 39*: 1723-1729.
53. Carpentieri AR, Lopez MEP, Aguilar J, Solá VM (2017) Melatonin and periodontal tissues: molecular and clinical perspectives. *Pharmacological Research 125*: 224-231.
54. Cutando A, Gómez-Moreno G, Arana C, Acuña-Castroviejo D, Reiter RJ (2007) Melatonin: potential functions in the oral cavity. *J Periodontol 78*: 1094-1102.
55. Cutando A, Aneiros-Fernánez J, López-Valverde A, Arias-Santiago S, Aneiros-Cachaza J, Reiter RJ (2011) A new perspective in oral health: potential importance and actions of melatonin receptors MT1, MT2, MT3 and RZR/ROR in the oral cavity. *Archives of Oral Biology 56*: 944-950.
56. Rangé H, Poitou C, Boillot A, Ciangura C, et al. (2013) Orosomucoid, a new biomarker in the association between obesity and periodontitis. *PLOS ONE 8*(3): e57645.
57. Dede FO, Gokmenoglu C, Sahin IO (2018) Induces of periodontitis increases salivary orosomucoid levels. *Annals of Medical Research 25*(3): 466-471.
58. Levine RS (2013) Obesity, diabetes and periodontitis – a triangular relationship? *British Dental Journal 215*(1): 35-39.
59. D'Aiuto F, Sabbah W, Netuveli G, Donos N, et al. (2008) Association of the metabolic syndrome with severe periodontitis in a large U.S. population-based survey. *The Journal of Clinical Endocrinology & Metabolism 93*(10): 3989-3994.
60. Furuta M, Liu A, Shinagawa T, Takeuci K, et al. (2016) Tooth loss and metabolic syndrome in middle-aged Japanese adults. *J Clin Periodontol 43*(6): 482-491.
61. Zhou X, Zhang W, Liu X, Zhang W, Li Y (2015) Interrelationship between diabetes and periodontitis: role of hyperlipidemia. *Archives of Oral Biology 60*: 667-674.
62. Fentoglu O, Bozkurt FY (2008) The bi-directional relationship between periodontal disease and hyperlipidemia. *European Journal of Dentistry 2*: 142-149.
63. Campbell LA, Rosenfeld ME (2015) Infection and atherosclerosis development. *Arch Med Res 46*(5): 339-350.

64. Bozoglan A, Ertugrul AS, Taspinar M, Yuzbasioglu B (2017) Determining the relationship between atherosclerosis and periodontopathogenic microorganisms in chronic periodontitis patients. *Acta Odontol Scand* 75(4): 233–242.
65. Bains A, Rashid MA (2013) Junk food and heart disease: the missing tooth. *J R Soc Med* 106(12): 472–473.
66. Janket SJ, Baird AE, Chuang SK, Jones JA (2003) Meta-analysis of periodontal disease and risk of coronary heart disease and stroke. *Oral Surg Oral Med Oral Pathol Oral Radiol Endod* 95(5): 559–569.
67. Mustapha IZ, Debrey S, Oladubu M, Ugarte R (2007) Markers of systemic bacterial exposure in periodontal disease and cardiovascular disease risk: a systematic review and meta-analysis. *J Periodontol* 78: 2289–2302.
68. Noack B, Genco RJ, Trevisan M, Grossi S, Zambon JJ, DeNardin E (2001) Periodontal infections contribute to elevated systemic C-reactive protein level. *Journal of Periodontology* 72(9): 1221–1227.
69. Teixeira FB, Saito MT, Matheus FC, Prediger RD, et al. (2017) Periodontitis and Alzheimer's disease: a possible comorbidity between oral chronic inflammatory condition and neuroinflammation. *Front Aging Neurosci* 9: 327.
70. Gomes-Filho IS, Coelho JMF, daCruz SS, Passos JS, et al. (2011) Chronic periodontitis and C-reactive protein levels. *J Periodontol* 82: 868–978.
71. Mustapha IZ, Debrey S, Oladubu M, Ugarte R (2007) Markers of systemic bacterial exposure in periodontal disease and cardiovascular disease risk: a systematic review and meta-analysis. *J Periodontol* 78: 2289–2302.
72. Casey R, Newcombe J, McFadden JJ, Bodman-Smith KB (2008) The acute-phase reactant C-reactive protein binds to phosphorylcholine-expressing neisseria meningitides and increases uptake by human phagocytes. *Infection and Immunity* 76(3): 1298–1304.
73. Pepys MB, Hirschfield GM (2003) C-reactive protein: a critical update. *The Journal of Clinical Investigation* 111(12): 1805–1812.
74. Ma X, Shang-Rong JI, Wu Y (2013) Regulated conformation changes in C-reactive protein orchestrate its role in atherogenesis. *Chinese Science Bulletin* 58(14): 1642–1649.
75. Pepys MB, Baltz ML (1983) Acute phase proteins with special reference to C-reactive protein and related proteins (pentaxins) and serum amyloid A protein. *Adv Immunol* 34: 141–212.
76. Gomes-Filho IS, Coelho JMF, daCruz SS, Passos JS, et al. (2011) Chronic periodontitis and C-reactive protein levels. *J Periodontol* 82: 868–978.
77. Wu T, Trevisan M, Genco RJ, Dorn JP, Falkner KL, Sempos CT (2000) Periodontal disease and risk of cerebrovascular disease: the first national health and nutrition examination survey and its follow-up study. *Arch Intern Med* 160: 2749–2755.
78. Ibid.
79. Öztekin G, Baser U, Kucukcoskun M, Tanrikulu-Kucuk S, et al. (2014) The association between periodontal disease and chronic obstructive pulmonary disease: a case control study. *COPD* 11(4): 424–430.
80. Leukfeld I, Obregon-Whittle MV, Lund MB, Geiran O, Bjørtuft O, Olsen I (2008) Severe chronic obstructive pulmonary disease: association with marginal bone loss in periodontitis. *Respiratory Medicine* 102: 488–494.
81. Yaghobee S, Paknejad M, Khorsand A (2008) Association between asthma and periodontal disease. *Journal of Dentistry, Tehran University of Medical Science, Tehran, Iran* 5(2): 47–51.
82. Manikandan GR, Ajithkumar KC (2016) Diabetes mellitus and periodontal disease: unravelling the two way relationship. *Kerala Medical Journal* 9(3): 111–119.
83. Yilmaz M, Kendirli SG, Altintas D, Bingöl G, Antmen B (2001) Cytokine levels in serum of patients with juvenile rheumatoid arthritis. *Clin Rheumatol* 20(1): 30–35.
84. Lotz M (1995) Interleukin-6: A Comprehensive Review. In: R. Kurzrock, M. Talpaz (eds) *Cytokines: Interleukins and Their Receptors*. Cancer Treatment and Research, vol. 80. Boston, MA: Springer.
85. deSmit M, Westra J, Vissink A, Doornbos-van der Meer B, Brouwer E, vanWinkelhoff AJ (2012) Periodontitis in established rheumatoid arthritis patients: a cross-sectional clinical, microbiological and serological study. *Arthritis Research & Therapy* 14: R222.
86. Susanto H, Nesse W, Kertia N, Soeroso J, et al. (2013) Prevalence and severity of periodontitis in Indonesian rheumatoid arthritis patients. *J Periodontol* 84(8): 1067–1074.
87. Krall EA, Garcia RI, Dawson-Hughes B (1996) Increased risk of tooth loss is related to bone loss at the whole body, hip and spine. *Calcif Tissue Int* 59(6): 433–437.
88. Golub LM, Ramamurthy NS, Llavaneras A, Ryan ME, et al. (1999) A chemically modified nonantimicrobial tetracycline (CMT-8) inhibits gingival matrix metalloproteinases, periodontal breakdown, and extra-oral bone loss in ovariectomized rats. *Ann N Y Acad Sci* 878: 290–310.
89. Craig RG, Yip JK, So MK, Boylan RJ, Socransky SS, Haffajee AD (2003) Relationship of destructive periodontal disease to the acute-phase response. *J Periodontol* 74(7): 1007–1016.

ENDNOTES

90. Beklen A, Ainola M, Hukkanen M, Gürgan C, Sors T, Konttinen YT (2007) MMPs, IL-1, and TNF are regulated by IL-17 in periodontitis. *J Dent Res* 86(4): 347–351.
91. Graves DT, Oskoui M, Volejnikova S, Naguib G, et al. (2001) Tumor necrosis factor modulates fibroblast apoptosis, PMN recruitment, and osteoclast formation in response to P. gingivalis infection. *J Dent Res* 80(10): 1875–1879.
92. Wang C-W, McCauley LK (2016) Osteoporosis and periodontitis. *Curr Osteoporos Rep* 14(6): 284–291.
93. Huang Y-F, Chang C-T, Liu S-P, Muo C-H, et al. (2016) The impact of oral hygiene maintenance on the association between periodontitis and osteoporosis: a nationwide population-based cross sectional study. *Medicine (Baltimore)* 95(6): e2348.
94. Lee J-H, Lee J-S, Park J-Y, Choi J-K, et al. (2015) Association of lifestyle-related comorbidities with periodontitis: a nationwide cohort study in Korea. *Medicine* 94(37): e1567.
95. Schulze-Späte U, Turner R, Wang Y, Chao R, et al. (2015) Relationship of bone metabolism biomarkers and periodontal disease: the osteoporotic fractures in men (MrOS) study. *J Clin Endocrinol Metab* 100(6): 2425–2433.
96. Assos-Soares JS, Vianna IP, Gomes-Filho IS, Cruz SS, et al. (2017) Association between osteoporosis treatment and severe periodontitis in postmenopausal women. *Menopause* 24(7): 789–795.
97. Wang J, Massoudi D, Ren Y, Muir AM, et al. (2017) BMP1 and TLL1 are required for maintaining periodontal homeostasis. *J Dent Res* 96(5): 578–585.
98. Hartigan N, Garrigue-Antar L, Kadler KE (2003) Bone morphogenetic protein-1 (BMP-1). *The Journal of Biological Chemistry* 278(20): 18045–18049.
99. Sun Y, Weng Y, Zhang C, Liu Y, et al. (2015) Glycosylation of dentin matrix protein 1 is critical for osteogenesis. *Sci Rep* 5: 17518.
100. Lee J-H, Lee J-S, Park J-Y, Choi J-K, et al. (2015) Association of lifestyle-related comorbidities with periodontitis: a nationwide cohort study in Korea. *Medicine* 94(37): e1567.
101. Shariff JA, Ingleshwar A, Lee KC, Zavras AI (2016) Relationship between chronic periodontitis and erectile dysfunction: a narrative review. *Journal of Oral Diseases 2016*: 7824321.
102. Práger N, Pásztor N, Vángy Á, Kozinszky Z, et al. (2017) Idiopathic male infertility related to periodontal and caries status. *J Clin Periodontol* 44(9): 872–880.
103. Luddi A, Governini L, Wilmskötter D, Gudermann T, Boekhoff I, Piomboni P (2019) Taste receptors: new players in sperm biology. *Int J Mol Sci* 20(4): 967.
104. Ide M, Papapanou PN (2013) Epidemiology of association between maternal periodontal disease and adverse pregnancy outcomes – systematic review. *J Clin Periodontol* 40(suppl. 14): S181–194.
105. Bobetsis VA, Barros SP, Offebacher S (2006) Exploring the relationship between periodontal disease and pregnancy complications. *JADA* 137(10 suppl.): 7S–13S.
106. Polyzos NP, Polyzos IP, Mauri D, Tzioras S, et al. (2009) Effect of periodontal disease treatment during pregnancy on preterm birth incidence: a metaanalysis of randomized trials. *American Journal of Obstetrics and Gynecology* 200(3): 225–232.
107. Meraz-Ríos MA, Toral-Rios D, Franco-Bocanegra D, Villeda-Hernández J, Campos-Peña V (2013) Inflammatory process in Alzheimer's disease. *Frontiers in Integrative Neuroscience* 7: 59.
108. Barnum CJ, Tansey MG (2012) Neuroinflammation and non-motor symptoms: the dark passenger of Parkinson's disease? *Curr Neurol Neurosci Rep* 12(4): 350–358.
109. Hanaoka A, Kashihara K (2009) Increased frequencies of caries, periodontal disease and tooth loss in patients with Parkinson's disease. *Journal of Clinical Neuroscience* 16: 1279–1282.
110. Li J, Xu H, Pan W, Wu B (2017) Association between tooth loss and cognitive decline: a 13-year longitudinal study of Chinese older adults. *PLOS ONE* 12(2): e171404.
111. Ono Y, Yamamoto T, Kubo KY, Onozuka M (2010) Occlusion and brain function: mastication as a prevention of cognitive dysfunction. *J Oral Rehabil* 37(8): 624–640.
112. Ide M, Harris M, Stevens A, Sussams R, et al. (2016) Periodontitis and cognitive decline in Alzheimer's disease. *PLOS ONE* 11(3): e015081.
113. Harding A, Gonder U, Robinson SJ, Crean SJ, Singhrao SK (2017) Exploring the association between Alzheimer's disease, oral health, microbial endocrinology and nutrition. *Front Aging Neurosci* 9: 398.
114. Teixeira FB, Saito MT, Matheus FC, Prediger RD, et al. (2017) Periodontitis and Alzheimer's disease: a possible comorbidity between oral chronic inflammatory condition and neuroinflammation. *Front Aging Neurosci* 9: 327.
115. Gomes-Filho IS, Coelho JMF, daCruz SS, Passos JS, et al. (2011) Chronic periodontitis and C-reactive protein levels. *J Periodontol* 82: 868–978.
116. Ilievski V, Zuchowska PK, Green SJ, Toth PT, et al. (2018) Chronic oral application of a periodontal pathogen results in brain inflammation, neurodegeneration and amyloid beta production in wild type mice. *PLOS ONE* 13(10): e0204941.

117 Castellani RJ, Lee H-g, Siedlak SL, Nunomura A, et al. (2009) Reexamining Alzheimer's disease: evidence for a protective role for amyloid-β protein precursor and amyloid-β. *J Alzheimers Dis* 18(2): 447–452.

118 Haley BE (2007) The relationship of the toxic effects of mercury to exacerbation of the medical condition classified as Alzheimer's disease. *Medical Veritas* 4: 1484–1498.

119 Said HS, Sua W, Nakagome S, Chinen H, et al. (2014) Dysbiosis of salivary microbiota in inflammatory bowel disease and its association with oral immunological biomarkers. *DNA Research* 21: 15–25.

120 Atarashi K, Sua W, Luo C, Kawaguchi T, et al. (2017) Ectopic colonization of oral bacteria in the intestine drives TH1 cell induction and inflammation. *Science* 358(6361): 359–365.

121 Qin N, Yang F, Li A, Prifti E, et al. (2014) Alterations of the human gut microbiome in liver cirrhosis. *Nature* 513(7516): 59–64.

122 Zou QH, Li RQ (2011) Helicobacter pylori in the oral cavity and gastric mucosa: a meta-analysis. *J Oral Pathol Med* 40(4): 317–324.

123 Olsen I, Yamazaki K (2019) Can oral bacteria affect the microbiome of the gut? *Journal of Oral Microbiology* 11: 1586422.

124 Alzahrani AA (2017) Association between human herpes virus and aggressive periodontitis: a systematic review. *Saudi Journal for Dental Research* 8: 97–104.

125 Heron SE, Elahi S (2017) HIV infection and compromised mucosal immunity: oral manifestations and systemic inflammation. *Frontiers in Immunology* 8: 241.

126 Jacob JA (2016) Study links periodontal disease bacteria to pancreatic cancer risk. *JAMA* 315(24): 2653–2654.

127 Gao S, Li S, Ma Z, Liang S, et al. (2016) Presence of Porphyromonas gingivalis in esophagus and its association with the clinicopathological characteristics and survival in patients with esophageal cancer. *Infectious Agents and Cancer* 11: 3.

128 Farquar DR, Divaris K, Mazul AL, Weissler MC, Zevallos JP (2017) Poor oral health affects survival in head and neck cancer. *Oral Oncology* 73: 111–117.

129 Söder B, Yakob M, Klinge B, Söder P-Ö (2011) Periodontal disease may associate with breast cancer. *Breast Cancer Res Treat* 127(2): 497–502.

130 Freudenheim JL, Genco RJ, LaMonte MJ, Millen AE, et al. (2015) Periodontal disease and breast cancer: prospective cohort study of postmenopausal women. *Cancer Epidemiol Biomarkers Prev* 25(1): 43–50.

131 Willershausen I, Schmidtmann I, Azaripour A, Kledtke J, Willershausen B, Hasenburg A (2019) Association between breast cancer chemotherapy, oral health and chronic dental infections: a pilot study. *Odontology* 107(3): 401–408.

132 Grube BD (2018) Oral Pathogens and Brain Degeneration. Is There a Link? Presentation on 8 November 2018 at ACIM Brain Regeneration Congress, Orlando, FLA, USA.

133 Levy T (2017) The Cause of All Disease: A Unified Theory. Presentation on 22 April 2017 at IHCAN Conferences, London, UK.

134 Allin KH, Nordestgaard BG (2011) Elevated C-reactive protein in the diagnosis, prognosis and cause of cancer. *Crit Rev Clin Lab Sci* 48(4): 155–170.

135 Johansen JS, Jensen BV, Rosilind A, Nielsen D, Price PA (2006) Serum YKL-40, a new prognostic biomarker in cancer patients? *Cancer Epidemiol Biomarkers Prev* 15(2): 194–202.

136 Keles ZP, Keles GC, Avci B, Cetinkaya BO, Emingil G (2014) Analysis of YKL-40 acute-phase protein and interleukin-6 levels in periodontal disease. *J Periodontol* 85: 1240–1246.

137 Hiraki A, Matsuo K, Suzuki T, Kawase T, Tajima K (2008) Teeth loss and risk of cancer at 14 common sites in Japanese. *Cancer Epidemiol Biomarkers Prev* 17(5): 1222–1227.

138 Cle MF, Arnold RR, Rhodes MJ, McGhee JR (1977) Immune dysfunction and dental caries: a preliminary report. *J Dent Res* 56(3): 198–204.

139 Jockers D (2016) Are Root Canals Really a Cause of Cancer? Available at https://thetruthaboutcancer.com/root-canals-cause-cancer, accessed 2 February 2019.

140 Windham B (ed.) (undated) Incidence Levels and Chronic Health Effects Related to Cavitations. Available at www.biodentistalabama.com/research/windham-cavitations.pdf, accessed 27 January 2019.

141 Crowther G (undated) Kryptopyrroluria – The Elephant in the Room. Available at https://aonm.org/kryptopyrroluria-the-elephant-in-the-room, accessed 19 September 2019.

142 Strienz J (2011) Leben mit KPU Kryptopyrrolurie, Ein Ratgeber für Patienten. Germering: München (Living with KPU Kryptopyrroluria, only available in German). As cited in: Crowther G (undated) Kryptopyrroluria – The Elephant in the Room. Available at https://aonm.org/kryptopyrroluria-the-elephant-in-the-room, accessed 19 September 2019.

143 Steele J, O'Sullivan I (2011) NHS: Executive Summary: Adult Dental Health Survey 2009. Available at https://files.digital.nhs.uk/publicationimport/pub01xxx/pub01086/adul-dent-heal-surv-summ-them-exec-2009-rep2.pdf, accessed 30 May 2021.

CHAPTER 10

1. Evans JJ, Wilkinson AR, Aickin DR (1984) Salivary estriol concentration during normal pregnancy, and a comparison with plasma estriol. *Clin Chem 30*: 120–121.
2. Morishita M, Aoyama H, Tokumoto K, Iwamoto Y (1988) The concentration of salivary steroid hormones and the prevalence of gingivitis at puberty. *Adv Dent Res 2*(2): 397–400.
3. Markou E, Eleana B, Lazaros T, Antonios K (2009) The influence of sex steroid hormones of gingiva of women. *The Open Dentistry Journal 3*: 114–119.
4. Hileman B (2006) Fluoride risks are still a challenge. *Chemical & Engineering News 84*(36): 34–37.
5. Long H, Jin Y, Lin M, Sun Y, Zhang L, Clinch C (2009) Fluoride toxicity in the male reproductive system. *Fluoride 42*(4): 260–276.
6. Connett P, Beck J, Micklem HS (2010) *The Case Against Fluoride*. White River Junction, VT: Chelsea Green Publishing. p.150.
7. Bertoldo BB, daSilva CB, Rodrigues DBR, Geraldo-Martins VR, Ferriani VPL, Nogueira RD (2017) Comparisons of IgA response in saliva and colostrum against oral streptococci species. *Braz Oral Res 31*: e39.
8. Li Y, Wang W, Caufield PW (2000) The fidelity of mutans streptococci transmission and caries status correlate with breast-feeding experience among Chinese families. *Caries Res 34*: 123–132.
9. Avila WM, Pordeus IA, Paiva SM, Martins CC (2015) Breast and bottle feeding as risk factors for dental caries: a systematic review and meta-analysis. *PLOS ONE 10*(11): e0142922.
10. Gussy MG, Waters EG, Walsh O, Kilpatrick NM (2006) Early childhood caries: current evidence for aetiology and prevention. *Journal of Paediatrics and Child Health 42*: 37–43.
11. Cole MF, Bryan S, Evans MK, Pearce CL et al. (1998) Humoral immunity to commensal oral bacteria in human infants: salivary antibodies reactive with actinomyces naeslundii genospecies 1 and 2 during colonization. *Infection and Immunity 66*(9): 4283–4289.
12. Cole MF, Bryan S, Evans MK, Pearce CL, et al. (1999) Humoral immunity to commensal oral bacteria in human infants: salivary secretory immunoglobulin A antibodies reactive with streptococcus mitis biovar 1, Streptococcus oralis, Streptococcus mutans, and Enterococcus faecalis during the first two years of life. *Infection and Immunity 67*(4): 1878–1886.
13. Miletic ID, Schiffman SS, Miletic VD, Sattely-Miller EA (1996) Salivary IgA secretion rate in young and elderly persons. *Physiology & Behavior 60*(1): 243–248.
14. Vissink A, Spijkervet FK, Van Nieuw Amerongen A (1996) Aging and saliva: a review of the literature. *Spec Care Dentist 16*(3): 95–103.
15. Scott J, Valentine JA, St.Hill CA, Balasooriya BA (1983) A quantitative histological analysis of the effects of age and sex on human lingual epithelium. *J Biol Buccale 11*(4): 303–315.
16. Aps JKM, Martens LC (2005) Review: the physiology of saliva and transfer of drugs into saliva. *Forensic Science International 150*: 119–131.
17. Hebling E (2012) Effects of Human Ageing on Periodontal Tissues. In: J Manakil (ed.) *Periodontal Diseases: A Clinician's Guide*. Available at www.intechopen.com/books/periodontal-diseases-a-clinician-s-guide/effects-of-human-ageing-on-periodontal-tissues, accessed 28 September 2019.
18. Percival RS, Challacombe SJ, Marsh PD (1991) Age-related microbiological changes in the salivary and plaque microflora of healthy adults. *J Med Microbiol 35*: 5–11.
19. Franceschi C, Campisi J (2014) Chronic inflammation (inflammaging) and its potential contribution to age-associated diseases. *J Gerontol A Biol Sci Med Sci 69*(S1): S4–S9.
20. Percival RS, Challacombe SJ, Marsh PD (1991) Age-related microbiological changes in the salivary and plaque microflora of healthy adults. *J Med Microbiol 35*: 5–11.
21. Lerner UH (2005) Inflammation-induced bone remodelling in periodontal disease and the influence of post-menopausal osteoporosis. *J Dent Res 85*(7): 596–607.
22. Dutt P, Chaudhary SR, Kumar P (2013) Oral health and menopause: a comprehensive review on current knowledge and associated dental management. *Annals of Medical and Health Sciences Research 3*(3): 320–323.
23. Mascarenhas P, Gapski R, Al-Shammari K, Wang HL (2003) Influence of sex hormones on the periodontium. *J Clin Periodontol 30*: 671–681.
24. Välimaa H, Savolainen S, Soukka T, Silvoniemi P, et al. (2004) Estrogen receptor-beta is the predominant estrogen receptor subtype in human oral epithelium and salivary glands. *J Endocrinol 180*: 55–62.
25. Leimola-Virtanen R, Salo T, Toikkanen S, Pulkkinen J, Syrjänen S (2000) Expression of estrogen receptor (ER) in oral mucosa and salivary glands. *Maturitas 36*: 131–137.
26. Scardina GA, Messina P (2012) Oral microcirculation in post-menopause: a possible correlation with periodontitis. *Gerodontology 29*: e1045–1051.

27. Yalçin F, Gurgan S, Gurgan T (2005) The effect of menopause, hormone replacement therapy (HRT), alendronate (ALN), and calcium supplements on saliva. *J Contemp Dent Pract* 6: 10–17.
28. Reinhardt RA, Payne JB, Maze C, Babbitt M, Nummikoski PV, Dunning D (1998) Gingival fluid IL-1beta in postmenopausal females on supportive periodontal therapy. A longitudinal 2-year study. *J Clin Periodontol* 25: 1029–1035.
29. Yalçin F, Gurgan S, Gurgan T (2005) The effect of menopause, hormone replacement therapy (HRT), alendronate (ALN), and calcium supplements on saliva. *J Contemp Dent Pract* 6: 10–17.
30. Allen IE, Monroe M, Connelly J, Cintron R, Ross SD (2000) Effect of postmenopausal hormone replacement therapy on dental outcomes: systematic review of the literature and pharmacoeconomic analysis. *Manag Care Interface* 13: 93–99.
31. Suri V, Suri V (2014) Menopause and oral health. *J Midlife Health* 5(3): 115–120.
32. Foutsizoglou S (2017) Anatomy of the ageing lip. *PMFA Journal* 4(2).
33. Scheid RC, Woelfel JB (2007) *Woelfel's Dental Anatomy: Its Relevance to Dentistry*. Lippincott Williams & Wilkins. p.81.
34. Law Smith MJ, Deady DK, Moore FR, Jones BC, et al. (2012) Maternal tendencies in women are associated with estrogen levels and facial femininity. *Hormones and Behaviour* 61: 12–16.
35. Casale M, Moffa A, Vella P, Sabatino L et al. (2016) Hyaluronic acid: perspectives in dentistry. A systematic review. *International Journal of Immunopathology and Pharmacology* 29(4): 572–582.
36. Tamer TM (2013) Hyaluronan and synovial joint: function, distribution and healing. *Interdiscip Toxicol* 6(3): 111–125.
37. Stern R (2004) Hyaluronan catabolism: a new metabolic pathway. *Eur J Cell Biol* 83: 317–325.
38. Culty M, Nguyen HA, Underhill CB (1992) The hyaluronan receptor (CD44) participates in the uptake and degradation of hyaluronan. *The Journal of Cell Biology* 116(4): 1055–1062.
39. Dahiya P, Kamal R (2013) Hyaluronic acid: a boon in periodontal therapy. *N Am J Med Sci* 5(5): 309–315.
40. Sukumar S, Dřízhal I (2007) Hyaluronic acid and periodontitis. *Acta Medica (Hradec Králové)* 51(4): 225–228.
41. Pagnacco A, Vangelisti R, Erra C, Poma A (1997) Double-blind clinical trial versus placebo of a new sodium-hyaluronate-based gingival gel. *Attual Ter In* 15: 1–7.
42. Sukumar S, Dřízhal I (2007) Hyaluronic acid and periodontitis. *Acta Medica (Hradec Králové)* 51(4): 225–228.
43. Klinger MM, Rahemtulla F, Prince CW, Lucas LC, Lemons JE (1998) Proteoglycans at the bone–implant interface. *Crit Rev Oral Biol Med* 9(4): 449–463.
44. Nolan A, Baillie C, Badminton J, Rudralingham M, Seymour RA (2006) The efficacy of topical hyaluronic acid in the management of recurrent aphthous ulceration. *J Oral Pathol & Med* 35(8): 461–465.
45. Hanifl PH, Davis G, Balbinot J, Pokorsky-Loy L (2010) US Patent Application: Oral Moisturizer for Alleviating Dry Mouth. Appl. No. 12/178,212. Filed 2008. Pub. No.:2010/0022471 A1.
46. Longas MO, Russell CS, He X-Y (1987) Evidence for structural changes in dermatan sulfate and hyaluronic acid with aging. *Carbohydrate Research* 159(1): 127–136.
47. Meletis C, Rousett D (2010) *The Hyaluronic Acid Miracle: Instant Facelift, and Anti-Aging, Rejuvenation*. Topanga, CA: Freedom Press.
48. Leung CW, Laraia BA, Needham BL, Rehkopf DH, et al. (2014) Soda and cell aging: associations between sugar-sweetened beverage consumption and leukocyte telomere length in healthy adults from the National Health and Nutrition Examination Surveys. *Am J Public Health* 104(12): 2425–2431.
49. Fitzpatrick AL, Kronmal RA, Gardner JP, Psaty BM, et al. (2007) Leukocyte telomere length and cardiovascular disease in the Cardiovascular Health Study. *American Journal of Epidemiology* 165(1): 14–21.
50. Masi S, Salpea KD, Lii KW, Parkar M, et al. (2011) Oxidative stress, chronic inflammation, and telomere length in patients with periodontitis. *Free Radical Biology and Medicine* 50(6): 730–735.
51. Schiffman SS, Zervakis J (2002) Taste and smell perception in the elderly: effect of medications and disease. *Advances in Food and Nutrition Research* 44: 247–346.
52. Schiffman SS (1983) Taste and smell in disease (second of two parts). *N Engl J Med* 308(22): 1337–1343.
53. Schiffman SS, Zervakis J (2002) Taste and smell perception in the elderly: effect of medications and disease. *Advances in Food and Nutrition Research* 44: 247–346.
54. Handelman SL, Baric JM, Espeland MA, Berglund KL (1986) Prevalence of drugs causing hyposalivation in an institutionalized geriatric population. *Oral Surgery, Oral Medicine, Oral Pathology* 62(1): 26–31.
55. Schiffman SS, Lockhead E, Maes FW (1983) Amiloride deduces the taste intensity of Na+ and Li+ salts and sweeteners. *Proc Natl Acad Sci USA* 80: 6136e6140.

56 Ohkoshi N, Shoji S (2002) Reversible ageusia induced by losartan: a case report. *European Journal of Neurology 9*: 315–322.
57 Prutkin J, Duffy VB, Etter L, Fast K, et al. (2000) Genetic variation and inferences about perceived taste intensity in mice and men. *Physiology & Behavior 69*: 161–173.
58 Schiffman SS (1997) Taste and smell losses in normal aging and disease. *JAMA 278*: 1357–1362.
59 Schiffman SS, Zervakis J (2002) Taste and smell perception in the elderly: effect of medications and disease. *Advances in Food and Nutrition Research 44*: 247–346.
60 Schiffman SS, Graham BG (2000) Taste and smell perception affect appetite and immunity in the elderly. *European Journal of Clinical Nutrition 54*(S3): S54–S63.
61 Joshi A, Rao G (2020, 21 March) Coronavirus: Expert Says New Symptom Could Be Loss of Taste or Smell. Available at https://news.sky.com/story/coronavirus-experts-say-new-symptoms-could-be-loss-taste-or-smell-11961439, accessed 21 March 2020.
62 Boyce JM, Shone GR (2006) Effects of ageing on smell and taste. *Postgrad Med J 82*: 239–241.
63 Jackson JA (1967) Heavy smoking and sodium chloride hypogeusia. *J Dent Res 46*: 742–744.
64 Perrin MJ, Krut LH, Bronte-Stewart B (1961) Smoking and food preferences. *Br Med J 1*(5223): 387–388.
65 Mashhadi NS, Ghiasvand R, Askari G, Hariri M, Darvishi L, Mofid MR (2013) Anti-oxidative and anti-inflammatory effects of ginger in health and physical activity: review of current evidence. *Int J Prev Med 4*(suppl. 1): S36–S42.
66 Arreola R, Quintero-Fabián S, López-Roa RI, Flores-Gutiérrez EO, et al. (2015) Immunomodulation and anti-inflammatory effects of garlic compounds. *Journal of Immunology Research 2015*: 401630.
67 Rao PV, Gan SH (2014) Cinnamon: a multifaceted medicinal plant. *Evid Based Complement Alternat Med 2014*: 642942.
68 McKay DL, Blumberg JB (2006) A review of the bioactivity and potential health benefits of peppermint tea (Mentha piperita L.). *Phytotherapy Research 20*(8): 619–633.
69 Parthasarathy VA, Chempakam B, Zachariah TJ (2008) *Chemistry of Spices*. Wallingford, Oxfordshire: CAB International, p.420.
70 Gevorgyan A, Segboer C, Gorissen R, van Drunen CM, Fokkens W (2015) Capsaicin for non-allergic rhinitis (Review). *Cochrane Database of Systematic Reviews 7*: CD010591.
71 Shin Y-H, Kim JM, Park K (2016) The effect of capsaicin on salivary gland dysfunction. *Molecules 21*: 835.
72 Moallem SA, Barahoyee A (2010) Evaluation of acute and chronic anti-nociceptive and anti-inflammatory effects of apple cider vinegar. *Iranian Journal of Pharmaceutical Research 3*(suppl. 2): 57 (article 166).
73 Vieira C, Evangelista S, Cirillo R, Lippi A, Maggi CA, Manzini S (2000) Effect of ricinoleic acid in acute and subchronic experimental models of inflammation. *Mediators Inflamm 9*(5): 223–228.
74 Umar S, Asif M, Sajad M, Ansari M, et al. (2012) Anti-inflammatory and antioxidant activity of Trachyspermum ammi seeds in collagen induced arthritis in rats. *International Journal of Drug Development and Research 4*(1): 210–219.
75 Malaty J, Malaty IAC (2013) Smell and taste disorders in primary care. *Am Fam Physician 88*(12): 852–859.
76 Derin S, Koseoglu S, Sahin C, Sahan M (2016) Effect of vitamin B12 deficiency on olfactory function. *Int Forum Allergy Rhinol 6*(10): 1051–1055.
77 Malaty J, Malaty IAC (2013) Smell and taste disorders in primary care. *Am Fam Physician 88*(12): 852–859.
78 Hardikar S, Höchenberger R, Villringer A, Ohla K (2017) Higher sensitivity to sweet and salty taste in obese compared to lean individuals. *Appetite 111*: 158–165.
79 Stice E, Spoor S, Bohon C, Veldhuizen M, Small D (2008) Relation of reward from food intake and anticipated food intake to obesity: a functional magnetic resonance imaging study. *J Abnorm Psychol 117*(4): 924–935.
80 Chatterjee S, Chatterjee A, Bandyopahyay SK (2016) L-theanine: a prospective natural medicine. *Int J Pharm Sci Rev Res 41*(2): 95–103.
81 Redmer J (2018) Adrenal Fatigue. In: D Rakel (ed.) *Integrative Medicine* (4th edn). Philadelphia, PA: Elsevier, pp.404–409.
82 Heath TP, Melichar JK, Nutt DJ, Donaldson LF (2006) Human taste thresholds are modulated by serotonin and noradrenaline. *The Journal of Neuroscience 26*(49): 12664–12671.
83 Umamaheswari G, Vezhavendhan N, Sivaramakrishnan M, Suganya R, Devy AS, Vidyalakshmi S (2017) Sialochemical profile in depressive individuals: a cross-sectional ex vivo study. *SRM J Res Dent Sci 8*: 116–120.
84 Lasschuijt MP, Mars M, deGraaf C, Smeets PAM (2018) Exacting responses: lack of endocrine cephalic phase responses upon oro-sensory exposure. *Frontiers in Endocrinology 9*: 332.
85 Smeets PA, Erkner A, deGraaf C (2010) Cephalic phase responses and appetite. *Nutr Rev 68*(11): 643–655.
86 Anguah KO-B, Lovejoy JC, Craig BA, Gehrke MM, et al. (2017) Can the palatability of healthy, satiety-promoting foods increase with repeated exposure during weight loss? *Foods 6*(2): 16.

87 Arguin H, Tremblay A, Blundell JE, Després J-P, et al. (2017) Impact of a non-restrictive satiating diet on anthropometrics, satiety responsiveness and eating behaviour traits in obese men displaying a high or a low satiety phenotype. *British Journal of Nutrition* 118: 750-760.

88 Jamshidi N, Taylor DA (2001) Anandamide administration into the ventromedial hypothalamus stimulates appetite in rats. *Br J Pharmacol* 134, 1151-1154.

89 Niki M, Jyotaki M, Yoshida R, Yasumatsu K, et al. (2015) Modulation of sweet taste sensitivities by endogenous leptin and endocannabinoids in mice. *J Physiol* 593: 2527-2545.

90 Beauchamp GK (2016) Why do we like sweet taste: a bitter tale? *Physiology & Behavior* 164: 432-437.

91 Drewnowski A, Mennella JA, Johnson SL, Bellisle F (2012) Sweetness and food preference. *Journal of Nutrition* 142(6): 1142S-1148S.

92 Egan JM, Margolskee RF (2008) Taste cells of the gut and gastrointestinal chemosensation. *Mol Interv* 8(2): 78-81.

93 Damak S, Rong M, Yasumatsu K, Kokrashvili Z, et al. (2003) Detection of sweet and umami taste in the absence of taste receptor Tr3. *Science* 301: 850-853.

94 Treesukosol Y, Smith KR, Spector AC (2011) The functional role of the T1R family of receptors in sweet taste and feeding. *Physiol Behav* 105(1): 14-26.

95 Cui M, Jiang P, Maillet E, Max M, Margolskee RF, Osman R (2006) The heterodimeric sweet taste receptor has multiple potential ligand binding sites. *Curr Pharm Des* 12: 4591-4600.

96 Frank GKW, Oberndorfer TA, Simmons AN, Paulus MP, et al. (2008) Sucrose activates human taste pathways differently from artificial sweetener. *NeuroImage* 39: 1559-1569.

97 Drewnowski A, Mennella JA, Johnson SL, Bellisle F (2012) Sweetness and food preference. *Journal of Nutrition* 142(6): 1142S-1148S.

98 Drewnowski A, Krahn DD, Demitrack MA, Nairn K, Gosnell BA (1995) Naloxone, an opiate blocker, reduces the consumption of sweet high-fat foods in obese and lean female binge eaters. *Am J Clin Nutr* 61: 1206-1212.

99 Drewnowski A, Mennella JA, Johnson SL, Bellisle F (2012) Sweetness and food preference. *Journal of Nutrition* 142(6): 1142S-1148S.

100 Reece AS (2007) Dentition of addiction in Queensland: poor dental status and major contributing drugs. *Australian Dental Journal* 52(2): 144-149.

101 Titsas A, Ferguson MM (2002) Impact of opioid use on dentistry. *Australian Dental Journal* 47(2): 94-98.

102 Mysels DJ, Sullivan MA (2010) The relationship between opioid and sugar intake: review of evidence and clinical applications. *J Opioid Manag* 6(6): 445-452.

103 Brownley KA, Boettiger CA, Young L, Cefalu WT (2015) Dietary chromium supplementation for targeted treatment of diabetes patients with comorbid depression and binge eating. *Med Hypotheses* 85(1): 45-48.

104 DiNicolantonio JD, O'Keefe JH, Wilson WL (2018) Sugar addiction: is it real? A narrative review. *Br J Sports Med* 52(14): 910-913.

105 Yagi T, Ueda H, Amitani H, Asakawa A, Miyawaki S, Inui A (2012) The role of ghrelin, salivary secretions, and dental care in eating disorders. *Nutrients* 4: 967-989.

106 DiNicolantonio JD, O'Keefe JH, Wilson WL (2018) Sugar addiction: is it real? A narrative review. *Br J Sports Med* 52(14): 910-913.

107 Glenville M (2016) *Natural Alternatives to Sugar*. Tunbridge Wells, Kent: Lifestyle Press.

108 Tsoukalas D, Fragkiakaki P, Docea AO, Alegakis AK, et al. (2019) Association of nutraceutical supplements with longer telomere length. *Int J Mol Med* 44(1): 218-226.

109 Shin C, Baik I (2016) Leukocyte telomere length is associated with serum vitamin B12 and homocysteine levels in older adults with the presence of systemic inflammation. *Clin Nutr Res* 5: 7-14.

110 Masic U, Yeomans MR (2014) Umami flavor enhances appetite but also increases satiety. *Am J Clin Nutr* 100: 532-538.

111 Glenville M (2016) *Natural Alternatives to Sugar*. Tunbridge Wells, Kent: Lifestyle Press.

CHAPTER 11

1 Pandor S (2019) Insight, Intuition and Mapping the Territory. Presentation at IAOMT Annual Scientific Conference 2019, London, 22-23 June 2019.

2 Saini R (2011) Ozone therapy in dentistry: a strategic review. *J Nat Sci Biol Med* 2(2): 151-153.

3 Nogales CG, Ferrari PH, Kantorovich EO, Lage-Marques JL (2008) Ozone therapy in medicine and dentistry. *Journal of Contemporary Dental Practice* 9(4): 75-84.

4 Srinivasan K, Chitra S (2015) The application of ozone in dentistry: a systematic review of literature. *SJDS* 2(6): 373-377.

5 Saini R (2011) Ozone therapy in dentistry: a strategic review. *J Nat Sci Biol Med* 2(2): 151-153.

6. Tiwari S, Avinash A, Katiyar S, Iyer AA, Jain S (2017) Dental applications of ozone therapy: a review of literature. *The Saudi Journal for Dental Research 8*: 105–111.
7. Gupta S, Deepa D (2016) Applications of ozone therapy in dentistry. *J Oral Res Rev 8*: 86–91.
8. Srinivasan K, Chitra S (2015) The application of ozone in dentistry: a systematic review of literature. *SJDS 2*(6): 373–377.
9. Gupta S, Deepa D (2016) Applications of ozone therapy in dentistry. *J Oral Res Rev 8*: 86–91.
10. Hoseinishad M, Nosratipour A, Moghaddam SM, Khajavi A (2015) Homeopathy in dentistry: a review. *International Journal of Contemporary Dental and Medical Reviews 2015*: 030815.
11. Ibid.
12. Lobbezoo F, van der Zaag J, Visscher CM, Naeije M. (2004) Oral kinesiology. A new postgraduate programme in the Netherlands. *J Oral Rehabil 31*(3): 192–198.
13. World Dental Federation (2008) Use of Acupuncture in Dentistry. Available at www.fdiworlddental.org/use-acupuncture-dentistry, accessed 26 June 2019.
14. Galland L (1991) Magnesium, stress and neuropsychiatric disorders. *Magnes Trace Elem 10*(2–4): 287–301.
15. Córdova A, Navas FJ (1998) Effect of training on zinc metabolism: changes in serum and sweat zinc concentrations in sportsmen. *Ann Nutr Metab 42*(5): 274–282.

CHAPTER 12

1. Bradford A (2015) *Oil Pulling: Benefits & Side Effects*. Available online at www.livescience.com/50896-oil-pulling-facts.html, accessed 5 June 2019.
2. Asokan S, Emmadi P, Chamundeswari R (2009) Effect of oil pulling on plaque induced gingivitis: a randomized, controlled, triple-blind study. *Indian J Dent Res 20*(1): 47–51.
3. Asokan S, Kumar RS, Emmadi P, Raghuraman R, Sivakumar N (2011) Effect of oil pulling on halitosis and microorganisms causing halitosis: a randomized controlled pilot trial. *J Indian Soc Pedod Prev Dent 29*(2): 90–94.
4. Sood P, Devi MA, Narang R, V S, Makkar DK (2014) Comparative efficacy of oil pulling and chlorhexidine on oral malodour: a randomized controlled trial. *J Clin Dian Res 8*(11): ZC18–21.
5. Selvam P, Nandan N, Raj S (2016) Oil pulling – a blessing in disguise. *Journal of Ayurveda and Integrated Medical Sciences 1*(4): 8–13.
6. Bekeleski GM, McCombs G, Melvin WL (2012) Oil pulling: an ancient practice for a modern time. *JIOH 4*(3): 1–10.
7. Peedikayi FC, Sreenivasan P, Narayanan A (2015) Effect of coconut oil in plaque related gingivitis – a preliminary report. *Nigerian Medical Journal 56*(2): 143–147.
8. Asokan S, Rathan J, Muthu MS, Prabhu V, *et al.* (2008) Effect of oil pulling on Streptococcus mutans count in plaque and saliva using Dentocult SM Strip mutans test: a randomized, controlled, triple-blind study. *J Indian Soc Pedod Prevent Dent 26*(1): 12–17.
9. Selvam P, Nandan N, Raj S (2016) Oil pulling – a blessing in disguise. *Journal of Ayurveda and Integrated Medical Sciences 1*(4): 8–13.
10. Ibid.
11. Mouth Healthy/American Dental Association (undated) Oil Pulling. Available at www.mouthhealthy.org/en/az-topics/o/oil-pulling, accessed 5 June 2019.
12. Selvam P, Nandan N, Raj S (2016) Oil pulling – a blessing in disguise. *Journal of Ayurveda and Integrated Medical Sciences 1*(4): 8–13.
13. Shanbhag VKL (2017) Oil pulling for maintaining oral hygiene – a review. *Journal of Traditional and Complementary Medicine 7*(1): 106–109.
14. Schmid U (undated) Healing Teeth Naturally: My Personal Best Toothache Cure. Available at www.healingteethnaturally.com/salt-water-brine-toothache-cure.html, accessed 4 May 2019.
15. Sircus M (2013) Real Salt, Celtic Salt and Himalayan Salt. Available at https://drsircus.com/general/real-salt-celtic-salt-and-himalayan-salt, accessed 11 June 2019.
16. Wormer EJ (1999) A Taste for Salt in the History of Medicine. Available at www.tribunes.com/tribune/sel/worm.htm, accessed 11 June 2019.
17. Hurtig S (2010) Tooth Cleaning Formulation: United States Patent Application Publication. US 2010/0303737 A1. Appl No: 12/792,278.
18. World Health Organization (2013) Poisons Centre Training Manual. Available at https://apps.who.int/iris/handle/10665/329503, accessed 14 June 2019.
19. Kärkkäinen S, Neuvonen PJ (1986) Pharmacokinetics of amitriptyline influenced by oral charcoal and urine pH. *International Journal of Clinical Pharmacology, Therapy and Toxicology 24*(6): 326–332.
20. Burhenne M (2019, updated August 2020) Activated Charcoal Toothpaste: Benefits and Precautions, Plus a Recipe. Available at https://askthedentist.com/charcoal-toothpaste, accessed 13 May 2020.
21. Brooks JK, Bashirelahi N, Reynolds MA (2017) Charcoal and charcoal-based dentifrices. *JADA 148*(9): 661–670.

22. Greenwall L (2017) Charcoal Toothpastes: What We Know So Far. *The Pharmaceutical Journal*. Available at https://pharmaceutical-journal.com/article/letters/charcoal-toothpastes-what-we-know-so-far, accessed 14 June 2019.
23. Williams LB, Haydel SE (2010) Evaluation of the medicinal use of clay minerals as antibacterial agents. *Int Geol Rev 52*(7/8): 745–770.
24. Schemehorn BR (2011) Abrasion, polishing, and stain removal characteristics of various commercial dentifrices in vitro. *J Clin Dent 22*: 11–18.
25. Kennedy BA (1990) *Surface Mining*, 2nd edn. Society for Mining, Metallurgy & Exploration (U.S.). SME. As cited in: Arledge, PA~ (undated) Is Montmorillonite Clay the Same as Bentonite Clay? (by Perry A~, author of *Living Clay, Nature's Own Miracle Cure*). Available at http://www.bentoniteclayinfo.com/clay_info/articles/montmorillonite_bentonite.htm, accessed 31 August 2021.
26. A~, P (undated) Is Montmorillonite Clay the Same as Bentonite Clay? (by Perry A~, author of *Living Clay, Nature's Own Miracle Cure*). Available at https://livingclayco.com/is-montmorillonite-same-as-bentonite-clay, accessed 15 June 2019.
27. Holder BL (2014) Sodium Bentonite vs Calcium Bentonite: Which is Better? Sodium or Calcium? Available at https://purewhitemontmorillonite.wordpress.com/2014/10/31/sodium-bentonite-vs-calcium-bentonite, accessed 15 June 2019.
28. This Green (undated) Hair Bleach with White Clay. Available at https://thisgreen.be/en/decoloration, accessed 15 June 2019.
29. A~, P (undated) Is Montmorillonite Clay the same as Bentonite Clay? Available at https://livingclayco.com/is-montmorillonite-same-as-bentonite-clay, accessed 15 June 2019.
30. Milanovich N, Cameron RB, Curtis JP, Subramanyam R, Prencipe M (2004) US Patent: Dental whitening method. US7601002B2, Application No: US10/811.724.
31. Moosavi M (2017) Bentonite clay as a natural remedy: a brief review. *Iran J Public Health 26*(9): 1176–1183.
32. Williams LB, Haydel SE, Ferrell RE Jr (2009) Bentonite, bandaids, and borborygmi. *Elements (Que) 5*(2): 99–104.
33. Abdullahi SL, Audu AA (2017) Comparative analysis on chemical composition of bentonite clays obtained from ashaka and tango deposits in Gombe State, Nigeria. *CSJ 8*(2): 35–40.
34. Ibid.
35. Nutting PG (1933) *The Bleaching Clays*. United States Department of the Interior. Available at https://pubs.usgs.gov/circ/1933/0003/report.pdf, accessed 15 June 2019.
36. Menzies A (1958) US Patent: Dentifrice Comprising Diatomaceous Silica. Patent no:2,820,000. Ser no:346,791.
37. Orgill C (2015) Bentonite Clay, Diatomaceous Earth, & Activated Charcoal: Information, Strengths and Uses. Available at http://beyondwheatandweeds.com/wp-content/uploads/2015/08/clay_vs_de_vs_charcoal3.pdf, accessed 19 June 2019.
38. The Clay Cure (undated) Zeo Nutri. Available at www.theclaycure.co.uk/zeolite, accessed 19 June 2019.
39. Jurkić LM, Cepanec I, Pavelić SK, Pavelić K (2013) Biological and therapeutic effects of ortho-silicic acid and some ortho-silicic acid-releasing compounds: new perspectives for therapy. *Nutrition & Metabolism 10*: 2.
40. The Clay Cure (undated) Zeo Nutri. Available at www.theclaycure.co.uk/zeolite, accessed 19 June 2019.
41. IAOMT (2016) *Clinical Use of Calcium Bentonite Clay (CBC) in Dentistry and Natural Medicine*. Available at https://iaomt.org/wp-content/uploads/Clinical-Use-of-Calcium-Bentonite-Clay-Scientific-Review-5.10.16.pdf, accessed 14 June 2019.
42. Kadir AKMS, Rabbi AA, Rahman MM (2017) Coenzyme Q10: a new horizon in the treatment of periodontal diseases. *International Dental Journal of Students Research 5*(1): 1–6.
43. Ibid.
44. Soni S, Pk A, Sharma N, Chander S (2012) Co-enzyme Q10 and periodontal health: a review. *International Journal of Oral & Maxillofacial Pathology 3*(2): 21–26.
45. Hanioka T, McRee JT, Folkers K (2002) United States Patent: Therapy with coenzyme Q10 to reduce subgingival microorganisms in patients with periodontal disease. US Patent no: 6,461,593 B1. Appl no:07/838,604.
46. Sharma V, Gupta R, Dahiya P, Kumar M (2016) Comparative evaluation of coenzyme Q10-based gel and 0.8% hyaluronic acid gel in treatment of chronic periodontitis. *J Indian Soc Periodontol 20*(4): 374–380.
47. Raut CP, Sethi KS (2016) Comparative evaluation of co-enzyme Q10 and Melaleuca alternifolia as antioxidant gels in treatment of chronic periodontitis: a clinical study. *Contemp Clin Dent 7*(3): 377–381.
48. Littarru GP, Nakamura R, Ho L, Folkers K, Kuzell WC (1971) Deficiency of coenzyme Q10 in gingival tissue from patients with periodontal disease. *Proc Nat Acad Sci USA 68*(10): 2332–2335.
49. Hanioka T, Tanaka M, Ojima M, Shizukuishi S, Folkers K (1994) Effect of topical application of coenzyme Q10 on adult periodontitis. *Mol Aspects Med 15* suppl.: s241–248.

CHAPTER 13

1. Miller DW Jn (2006) Extrathyroidal benefits of iodine. *Journal of American Physicians and Surgeons* 11(4): 106–110.
2. Susheela AK, Jethanandani P (1996) Circulating testosterone levels in skeletal fluorosis patients. *Journal of Toxicology: Clinical Toxicology* 24(2): 183–189.
3. Long H, Jin Y, Lin M, Sun Y, Zhang L, Clinch C (2009) Fluoride toxicity in the male reproductive system. *Fluoride* 42(4): 260–276.
4. Hileman B (2006) Fluoride risks are still a challenge. *Chemical & Engineering News* 84(36): 34–37.
5. Freni SC (1994) Exposure to high fluoride concentrations in drinking water is associated with decreased birth rates. *J Toxicol Environ Health* 42(1): 109–121.
6. Du L, Wan C, Cao X, Liu J (2008) The effect of fluorine on the developing human brain. *Fluoride* 41(4): 327–330.
7. Hileman B (2006) Fluoride risks are still a challenge. *Chemical & Engineering News* 84(36): 34–37.
8. Valdez-Jiménez L, Fregozo CS, Beltrán MLM, Coronado OG, Vega MIP (2011) Effects of the fluoride on the central nervous system. *Neurología* 26(5): 297–300.
9. Luke J (2001) Fluoride deposition in the aged human pineal gland. *Caries Res* 35(2): 125–128.
10. Xiang Q, Liang Y, Chen L, Wang C, et al. (2003) Effect of fluoride in drinking water on children's intelligence. *Fluoride* 36(2): 84–94.
11. Strunecka A, Patocka J, Blaylock RL, Chinoy NJ (2007) Fluoride interactions: from molecules to disease. *Current Signal Transduction Therapy* 2: 190–213.
12. Valdez-Jiménez L, Fregozo CS, Beltrán MLM, Coronado OG, Vega MIP (2011) Effects of the fluoride on the central nervous system. *Neurología* 26(5): 297–300.
13. Dowd FJ (1999) Saliva and dental caries. *Dent Clin North Am* 43(4): 579–597.
14. American Academy of Pediatrics (2015) Fluorosis Facts: A Guide for Health Professionals. Available at https://ilikemyteeth.org/wp-content/uploads/2014/10/FluorosisFactsforHealthProfessionals.pdf, accessed 23 April 2019.
15. Neurath C, Limeback H, Osmunson B, Connett M, et al. (2019) Dental fluorosis trends in US oral health surveys: 1986 to 2012. *JDR Clinical & Translational Research* 4(4): 298–308.
16. United States Food and Drug Administration (2018) CFR Title 21: Part 355: Anticaries Drug Products for Over-the-Counter Human Use, Subpart C: Labeling. Available at www.accessdata.fda.gov/scripts/cdrh/cfdocs/cfcfr/CFRSearch.cfm?CFRPart=355, accessed 31 May 2021.
17. Basch CH, Rajan S (2014) Marketing strategies and warning labels on children's toothpaste. *The Journal of Dental Hygiene* 88(5): 316–319.
18. Waldbott GL, Burgstahler AW, McKinney HL (1978) *Fluoridation: The Great Dilemma*. Lawrence, KS: Colorado Press.
19. Martino JV, Limbergen JV, Cahill LE (2017) The role of carrageenan and carboxymethylcellulose in the development of intestinal inflammation. *Frontiers in Pediatrics* 5: 96.
20. Soap Detergent Association (1990) Glycerine: An Overview. Available at www.aciscience.org/docs/glycerine_-_an_overview.pdf, accessed 19 June 2019.
21. McCooey A (undated) Glycerol. Available at www.sugar-and-sweetener-guide.com/glycerol.html, accessed 31 May 2021.
22. Ibid.
23. Tada-Oikawa S, Ichihara G, Fukatsu H, Shimanuki Y, et al. (2016) Titanium dioxide particle type and concentration influence the inflammatory response in caco-2 cells. *Int J Mol Sci* 17: 576.
24. Chen XX, Cheng B, Yang YX, Cao A, et al. (2013) Characterization and preliminary toxicity assay of nano-titanium dioxide additive in sugar-coated chewing gum. *Small* 9(9–10): 1765–1774.
25. Glaser A (2004) The ubiquitous triclosan: a common antibacterial agent exposed. *Pesticides and You* 24(3): 12–17.
26. Clayton EMR, Todd M, Dowd JB, Aiello AE (2011) The impact of bisphenol A and triclosan on immune parameters in the U.S. population, NHANES 2003–2006. *Environ Health Perspect* 119: 390–396.
27. Alliance for Natural Health (2016) The FDA Bans Triclosan. Available at https://anh-usa.org/the-fda-bans-triclosan, accessed 1 June 2019.
28. Herlofson BB, Barkvoll P (1994) Sodium lauryl sulfate and recurrent aphthous ulcers. A preliminary study. *Acta Odontol Scand* 52(5): 257–259.
29. Environmental Working Group (undated) Propylene Glycol. Available at www.ewg.org/guides/substances/4889-PROPYLENEGLYCOL, accessed 1 June 2019.
30. The EWG (www.ewg.org) is an American non-profit environmental group.
31. Environmental Working Group (undated) Diethanolamine. Available at www.ewg.org/skindeep/ingredients/718373-DIETHANOLAMINE, accessed 1 June 2019.
32. Darbre PD, Harvey PW (2008) Paraben esters: review of recent studies of endocrine toxicity, absorption, esterase and human exposure, and discussion of potential human health risks. *J Appl Toxicol* 28(5): 561–578.

33. BBC (2007, July) Toxin Found in Fake UK Toothpaste. Available at http://news.bbc.co.uk/go/pr/fr/-/1/hi/business/6896182.stm, accessed 7 August 2019.
34. Haq MW, Batool M, Ahsan SH, Qureshi NR (2009) Alcohol use in mouthwash and possible oral health concerns. *J Pak Med Assoc* 59(3): 186–190.
35. Mercola J (undated) Toxic Toothpaste Ingredients You Need to Avoid. Available at https://articles.mercola.com, accessed 1 June 2019.
36. Ibid.
37. Putt MS, Milleman KR, Ghassemi A, Vorwerk LM, et al. (2008) Enhancement of plaque removal efficacy by tooth brushing with baking soda dentifrices: results of five clinical studies. *J Clin Dent* 19(4): 111–119.
38. Dewhirst S (undated) How Does Teeth Whitening Work? Available at www.tomsofmaine.com/good-matters/natural-products/how-does-teeth-whitening-work, accessed 25 May 2019.
39. Wülknitz P (1997) Cleaning power and abrasivity of European toothpastes. *Adv Dent Res* 11(4): 576–579.
40. Tada A, Nakayama-Imaohji H, Yamasaki H, Hasibul K, et al. (2016) Cleansing effect of acidic L-arginine on human oral biofilm. *BMC Oral Health* 16: 40.
41. Nascimento MM, Browngardt C, Xiaohui X, Dlepac-Ceraj V, Paster BJ, Burne RA (2014) The effect of arginine on oral biofilm communities. *Molecular Oral Microbiology* 29: 45–54.
42. Nascimento MM, Liu Y, Kalra R, Perry S, et al. (2013) Oral arginine metabolism may decrease the risk for dental caries in children. *J Dent Res* 92(7): 604–608.
43. Bovshow S (undated) Grow Mint Indoors: Spearmint and Peppermint. Available at https://foodiegardener.com/grow-mint-indoors-spearmint-and-peppermint, accessed 25 May 2019.
44. Singh R, Sushni MAM, Belkheir A (2015) Antibacterial and antioxidant activities of Mentha piperita L. *Arabian Journal of Chemistry* 8: 322–328.
45. Dagli N, Dagli R, Mahmoud RS, Baroudi K (2015) Essential oils, their therapeutic properties, and implication in dentistry: a review. *Journal of International Society of Preventive and Community Dentistry* 5(5): 335–340.
46. Cotton S (2013) Menthol – podcast with Meera Senthilingam. Available at www.chemistryworld.com/podcasts/menthol/6109.article, accessed 25 May 2019.
47. Dr. Schar (undated) Wintergreen: Gaultheria Procumbens. Available at http://doctorschar.com/wintergreen-gaultheria-procumbens, accessed 19 June 2019.
48. Kwan KY, Corey DP (2009) Burning cold: involvement of TRPA1 in noxious cold sensation. *J Gen Physiol* 133(3): 251–256.
49. Bandell M, Story GM, Hwang SW, Viswanath V, et al. (2004) Noxious cold ion channel TRPA1 is activated by pungent compounds and bradykinin. *Neuron* 41: 849–857.
50. Ibid.
51. Cortés-Rojas DF, deSouza CRF, Oliveira WP (2014) Clove (Syzygium aromaticum): a precious spice. *Asian Pacific Journal of Tropical Biomedicine* 4(2): 90–96.
52. Uju DE, Obioma NP (2011) Anticariogenic potentials of clove, tobacco and bitter kola. *Asian Pacific Journal of Tropical Medicine* 4(10): 814–818.
53. Dagli N, Dagli R, Mahmoud RS, Baroudi K (2015) Essential oils, their therapeutic properties, and implication in dentistry: a review. *Journal of International Society of Preventive and Community Dentistry* 5(5): 335–340.
54. Bandell M, Story GM, Hwang SW, Viswanath V, et al. (2004) Noxious cold ion channel TRPA1 is activated by pungent compounds and bradykinin. *Neuron* 41: 849–857.
55. Masuda H, Inoue T, Kobayashi Y (2003) Anticaries Effect of Wasabi Components. ACS Symposium Series 859. In: C-T Ho, J-K Lin, QY Zheng (eds) *Oriental Foods and Herbs: Chemistry and Health Effects*. Washington, DC: American Chemical Society, pp.142–153.
56. Bansode VJ (2012) A review on the pharmacological activities of Cinnamomum cassia Blume. *Int J of Green Pharm Apr–Jun*: 102–108.
57. Chaudhry NMA, Tariq P (2006) Anti-microbial activity of Cinnamomum cassia against diverse microbial flora with its nutritional and medicinal impacts. *Pak J Bot* 38(1): 169–174.
58. Dagli N, Dagli R, Mahmoud RS, Baroudi K (2015) Essential oils, their therapeutic properties, and implication in dentistry: a review. *Journal of International Society of Preventive and Community Dentistry* 5(5): 335–340.
59. Ranasinghe P, Pigera S, Premakumara GAS, Galappaththy P, Constantine GR, Katulanda P (2013) Medicinal properties of 'true' cinnamon (Cinnamomum zeylanicum): a systematic review. *Complementary and Alternative Medicine* 13: 275.
60. Aneja KR, Joshi R, Sharma C (2009) Antimicrobial activity of Dalchini (Cinnamomum zeylanicum bark) extracts on some dental caries pathogens. *Journal of Pharmacy Research* 2(9): 1387–1390.
61. Choi O, Cho SK, Kim J, Park CG, Kim J (2016) In vitro antibacterial activity and major bioactive components of Cinnamomum verum essential oils against cariogenic bacteria, Streptococcus mutans and Streptococcus sobrinus. *Asian Pac J Trop Biome* 6(4): 308–314.

ENDNOTES

62 Wang Y, Zhang Y, Shi Y-q, Pan X-h, Lu Y-h, Cao P (2018) Antibacterial effects of cinnamon (Cinnamomum zeylanicum) bark essential oil on Porphyromonas gingivalis. *Microbial Pathogenesis 116*: 26–32.

63 LeBel G, Haas B, Adam A-A, Veilleux M-P, Lagha AB, Grenier D (2017) Effect of cinnamon (Cinnamomum verum) bark essential oil on the halitosis-associated bacterium Solobacterium moorei and in vitro cytotoxicity. *Archives of Oral Biology 83*: 97–104.

64 Vivas APM, Migliari DA (2015) Cinnamon-induced oral mucosal contact reaction. *The Open Dentistry Journal 9*: 257–259.

65 Allen CM, Bozis GG (1988) Oral mucosal reactions to cinnamon-flavored chewing gum. *The Journal of the American Dental Association 116*(6): 664–667.

66 Prabuseenivasan S, Jayakumar M, Ignacimuthu S (2006) In vitro antibacterial activity of some plant essential oils. *BMC Complementary and Alternative Medicine 6*: 39.

67 Burhenne M (undated) Essential Oils – The Potentially Unhealthy Ingredient in your 'Healthy' Toothpaste. Available at https://askthedentist.com/essential-oils-toothpaste, accessed 11 August 2019.

68 Wyganowska-Swiathowska M, Urbanizk P, Szkaradkiewiczz A, Jankun J, Kotwicka M (2016) Effects of chlorhexidine, essential oils and herbal medicines (Salvia, Chamomile, Calendula) on human fibroblast in vitro. *Ent Eur J Immunol 41*(2): 125–131.

69 Ibid.

70 Burhenne M (undated) Essential Oils – The Potentially Unhealthy Ingredient in your 'Healthy' Toothpaste. Available at https://askthedentist.com/essential-oils-toothpaste, accessed 11 August 2019.

71 Ibid.

72 Preen C (2017) Should Anyone Take Essential Oils Internally? Available at www.complementaryhealthprofessionals.co.uk/single-post/2017/05/10/Should-anyone-take-essential-oils-internally, accessed 11 August 2019.

73 Collins J (2017) Essential Oils: The Multiple Role of the Oils in Dental Treatment. Available at www.dentistryiq.com/dental-hygiene/patient-education/article/16366392/essential-oils-the-multiple-role-of-the-oils-in-dental-treatment, accessed 11 August 2019.

74 Dagli N, Dagli R, Mahmoud RS, Baroudi K (2015) Essential oils, their therapeutic properties, and implication in dentistry: a review. *Journal of International Society of Preventive and Community Dentistry 5*(5): 335–340.

75 Halawany HS (2012) A review on miswak (Salvadora persica) and its effect on various aspects of oral health. *The Saudi Dental Journal 24*: 63–69.

76 Singh TP, Singh OM (2011) Phytochemical and pharmacological profile of Zanthoxylum armatum DC – an overview. *Indian Journal of Natural Products and Resources 2*(3): 275–285.

77 Pourabbas R, Delazar A, Chitsaz MT (2005) The effect of German Chamomile mouthwash on dental plaque and gingival inflammation. *Iranian Journal of Pharmaceutical Research 2*: 105–109.

78 Amoian B, Moghadamnia AA, Mazandarani M, Amoian MM, Mehrmanesh S (2010) The effect of Calendula extract toothpaste on the plaque index and bleeding in gingivitis. *Research Journal of Medicinal Plant 4*(3): 132–140.

79 El Ashry ESH, Rashed N, Salama OM, Saleh A (2003) Components, therapeutic value and uses of myrrh. *Pharmazie 58*: 163–168.

80 Cummins D (2009) US Patent: Oral Compositions Containing Botanical Extracts. US Patent 2009/0087501 A1. Appl no 12/243/669.

81 Al-Mobeeriek A (2011) Effects of myrrh on intra-oral mucosal wounds compared with tetracycline- and chlorhexidine-based mouthwashes. *Clinical, Cosmetic and Investigational Dentistry 3*: 53–58.

82 Scholz E, Rimpler H (1989) Proanthocyanidins from Krameria triandra root. *Planta Med 55*(4): 379–384.

83 Felter HW (1922) Krameria. From the Eclectic Materia Medica: Pharmacology and Therapeutics. Available at www.henriettes-herb.com/eclectic/felter/krameria.html, accessed 21 June 2019.

84 Tiemann P, Toelg M, Famos FMH (2007) Administration of Ratanhia-based herbal oral care products for the prophylaxis of oral mucositis in cancer chemotherapy patients: a clinical trial. *Evid Based Complement Alternat Med 4*(3): 361–366.

85 Generlich A (2008) Stop gingivitis before it starts. *Nature Vital 2008*: 36–37.

86 Kim SE, Kim TH, Park SA, Kim WT, *et al.* (2017) Efficacy of horse chestnut leaf extract ALH-L1005 as a matrix metalloproteinase inhibitor in ligature-induced periodontitis in canine model. *J Vet Sci 18*(2): 245–251.

87 Ananthathavam K, Ramamurthy J (2014) Treating periodontitis with the use of essential oil and herbs. *IOSR Journal of Pharmacy 4*(1): 39–42.

88 Elavarasu S, Abinaya P, Elanchezhiyan S, Thangakumaran, Vennila K, Naziya KB (2012) Evaluation of anti-plaque microbial activity of Azadirachta indica (neem oil) in vitro: a pilot study. *J Pharm Bioallied Sci 4*(Suppl.2): S394–S396.

89 Botelho M, dosSantos RA, Martins JG, Carvalho CO, et al. (2008) Efficacy of a mouthrinse based on leaves of neem tree (Azadirachta indica) in the treatment of patients with chronic gingivitis: a double-blind, randomized, controlled trial. *Journal of Medicinal Plants Research* 2(11): 341–346.

90 Ananthathavam K, Ramamurthy J (2014) Treating periodontitis with the use of essential oil and herbs. *IOSR Journal of Pharmacy* 4(1): 39–42.

CHAPTER 14

1 Genco RJ, Genco FD (2014) Common risk factors in the management of periodontal and associated systemic diseases: the dental setting and interprofessional collaboration. *J Evid Base Dent Pract* 14(S1): 4–16.

2 Kilian M, Chapple ILC, Hannig M, Marsh PD, et al. (2016) The oral microbiome – an update for oral healthcare professionals. *British Dental Journal* 221: 657–666.

3 Drewnowski A, Krahn DD, Demitrack MA, Nairn K, Gosnell BA (1995) Naloxone, an opiate blocker, reduces the consumption of sweet high-fat foods in obese and lean female binge eaters. *Am J Clin Nutr* 61: 1206–1212.

4 Drewnowski A, Mennella JA, Johnson SL, Bellisle F (2012) Sweetness and food preference. *Journal of Nutrition* 142(6): 1142S–1148S.

5 Esposito K, Nappo F, Marfella R, Giulgliano G, et al. (2002) Inflammatory cytokine concentrations are acutely increased by hyperglycemia in humans: role of oxidative stress. *Circulation* 106: 2067–2072.

6 Cândido FG, Valente FX, Grześkowiak LM, Moreira APB, Rocha DMUP, Alfenas RdCG (2017) Impact of dietary fat on gut microbiota and low-grade systemic inflammation: mechanisms and clinical implications on obesity. *International Journal of Food Sciences and Nutrition* 69(2): 125–143.

7 Brambilla E, Cgetti MG, Ionecu A, Campus G, Lingström P (2013) An in vitro and in vivo comparison of the effect of Stevia rebaudiana extracts on different caries-related variables: a randomized controlled trial pilot study. *Caries Research* 48(1): 19–23.

8 Mohammadi-Sichani M, Karbasizadeh V, Aghai F, Mofid MR (2012) Effect of different extracts of Stevia rebaudiana leaves on Streptococcus mutans growth. *Journal of Medicinal Plants Research* 6(32): 4731–4734.

9 Ly KA, Milgrom P, Rothen M (2006) Xylitol, sweeteners, and dental caries. *Pediatr Dent* 28(2): 154–163.

10 Isokangas P, Tiekso J, Alanen P, Mäkinen KK (1989) Long-term effect of xylitol chewing gum on dental caries. *Community Dent Oral Epidemiol* 17: 200–203.

11 Van der Lugt T, Weseler AR, Gebbink WA, Vrolijk MF, Opperhuizen A, Bast A (2018) Dietary advanced glycation endproducts induce an inflammatory response in human macrophages in vitro. *Nutrients* 10(12): 1868.

12 Uribarri J, delCastillo MD, de la Maza MP, Filip R, et al. (2015) Dietary advanced glycation end products and their role in health and disease. *Adv Nutr* 6: 461–473.

13 Poulsen MW, Hedegaard RV, Andersen JM, deCourten B, et al. (2013) Advanced glycation endproducts in food and their effects on health. *Food and Chemical Toxicology* 60: 10–37.

14 Uribarri J, delCastillo MD, de la Maza MP, Filip R, et al. (2015) Dietary advanced glycation end products and their role in health and disease. *Adv Nutr* 6: 461–473.

15 Escobosa ARC, Ojeda AG, Wrobel K, Magana AA, Wrobel K (2014) Methylglyoxal is associated with bacteriostatic activity of high fructose agave syrups. *Food Chemistry* 165: 444–450.

16 Marceau E, Yaylayan VA (2009) Profiling of α-dicarbonyl content of commercial honeys from different botanical origins: identification of 3,4-dideoxyglucoson-3-ene (3,4-DGE) and related compounds. *J Agric Food Chem* 57(22): 10837–10844.

17 Bibby BG, Mundorff SA, Zero DT, Almekinder KJ (1986) Oral food clearance and the pH of plaque and saliva. *J Am Dent Assoc* 112(3): 333–337.

18 Meletis CD (2011) Iodine: health implications of deficiency. *Journal of Evidence-Based Complementary & Alternative Medicine* 16(3): 190–194.

19 Windham B (ed.) (undated) Incidence Levels and Chronic Health Effects Related to Cavitations. Available at www.biodentistalabama.com/research/windham-cavitations.pdf, accessed 27 January 2019.

20 Cuomo R, Sarnelli G, Savarese MF, Buyckx M (2009) Carbonated beverages and gastrointestinal system: between myth and reality. *Nutrition, Metabolism & Cardiovascular Diseases* 19: 683–689.

21 Carstens E, Carstens MI, Dessirier J-M, O'Mahony M, et al. (2002) It hurts so good: oral irritation by spices and carbonated drinks and the underlying neural mechanisms. *Food Quality and Preference* 13: 431–443.

22. Simons CT, Dessirier J-M, Carstens MI, O'Mahony M, Carstens E (1999) Neurobiological and psychophysical mechanisms underlying the oral sensation produced by carbonated water. *The Journal of Neuroscience* 19(18): 8134–8144.
23. Cuomo R, Sarnelli G, Savarese MF, Buyckx M (2009) Carbonated beverages and gastrointestinal system: between myth and reality. *Nutrition, Metabolism & Cardiovascular Diseases* 19: 683–689.
24. Sánchez GA, Fernandez DePreliasco MV (2003) Salivary pH changes during soft drinks consumption in children. *Int J Paediatr Dent* 13(4): 251–257.
25. Cuomo R, Sarnelli G, Savarese MF, Buyckx M (2009) Carbonated beverages and gastrointestinal system: between myth and reality. *Nutrition, Metabolism & Cardiovascular Diseases* 19: 683–689.
26. Brown CJ, Smith G, Shaw L, Parry J, Smith AJ (2007) The erosive potential of flavoured sparkling water drinks. *International Journal of Paediatric Dentistry* 17: 86–91.
27. Cuomo R, Sarnelli G, Savarese MF, Buyckx M (2009) Carbonated beverages and gastrointestinal system: between myth and reality. *Nutrition, Metabolism & Cardiovascular Diseases* 19: 683–689.
28. Cuomo R, Grasso R, Sarnelli G, Capuano G, et al. (2002) Effects of carbonated water on functional dyspepsia and constipation. *European Journal of Gastroenterology & Hepatology* 14: 1–9.
29. Petraccia L, Liberati G, Masciullo SG, Grassi M, Fraioli A (2006) Water, mineral waters and health. *Clinical Nutrition* 25: 377–385.
30. Eweis DS, Abed F, Stiban J (2017) Carbon dioxide in carbonated beverages induces ghrelin release and increased food consumption in male rats: implications on the onset of obesity. *Obesity Research & Clinical Practice* 11: 534–543.
31. Wright KF (2015) Is your drinking water acidic? A comparison of the varied pH of popular bottled waters. *The Journal of Dental Hygiene* 89(Suppl. 2): 6–12.
32. Petraccia L, Liberati G, Masciullo SG, Grassi M, Fraioli A (2006) Water, mineral waters and health. *Clinical Nutrition* 25: 377–385.
33. Cicchella D, Albanese S, DeVivo B, Dinelli E, et al. (2010) Trace elements and ions in Italian bottled mineral waters: identification of anomalous values and human health related effects. *Journal of Geochemical Exploration* 107: 336–349.
34. Petraccia L, Liberati G, Masciullo SG, Grassi M, Fraioli A (2006) Water, mineral waters and health. *Clinical Nutrition* 25: 377–385.
35. Koufman JA, Johnston N (2012) Potential benefits of pH 8.8 alkaline drinking water as an adjunct in the treatment of reflux disease. *Annals of Otology, Rhinology & Laryngology* 12(7): 431–434.
36. Marengo K (2019) Alkaline Water: Benefits and Risks. Available at www.healthline.com/health/food-nutrition/alkaline-water-benefits-risks, accessed 29 September 2019.
37. Levine M, Rumsey SC, Daruwala R, Park JB, Wang Y (1999) Criteria and recommendations for vitamin C intake. *JAMA* 281(15): 1415–1423.
38. Padayatty SJ, Levine M (2001) New insights into the physiology and pharmacology of vitamin C. *CMAJ* 164(3): 353–355.
39. Bradfield RB, Roca A (1964) Camu-camu – a fruit high in ascorbic acid. *J Am Diet Assoc* 44: 28–30.
40. Wong JW, Gallant-Behm C, Wiebe C, Mak K, et al. (2009) Wound healing in oral mucosa results in reduced scar formation as compared with skin: evidence from the red Duroc pig model and humans. *Wound Repair and Regeneration* 17(5): 717–729.
41. Dawes C, Pedersen AML, Villa A, Ekström J, et al. (2015) The functions of human saliva: a review sponsored by the World Workshop on Oral Medicine VI. *Archives of Oral Biology* 60: 863–874.
42. Keswani SG, Balaji W, Le LD, Leung A, et al. (2013) Role of salivary vascular endothelial growth factor (VEGF) in palatal mucosal wound healing. *Wound Repair Regen* 21(4): 554–562.
43. Guo D, Murdoch CE, Xu H, Shi H, et al. (2017) Vascular endothelial growth factor signalling requires glycine to promote angiogenesis. *Scientific Reports* 7: 14749.
44. Maggio D, Polidori MC, Barabani M, Tufi A, et al. (2006) Low levels of carotenoids and retinol in involutional osteoporosis. *Bone* 38: 244–248.
45. Ahmadieh H, Arabi A (2011) Vitamins and bone health: beyond calcium and vitamin D. *Nutr Rev* 69(10): 584–598.
46. Kosanam S, Boyina R (2015) Drug-induced liver injury: a review. *International Journal of Pharmacological Research* 5(2): 24–30.
47. Huang L-G, Chen G, Chen D-Y, Chen H-H (2017) Factors associated with the risk of gingival disease in patients with rheumatoid arthritis. *PLoS ONE* 12(10): e0186346.
48. Bibby BG, Huang CT, Zero D, Mundorff SA, Little MF (1980) Protective effect of milk against in vitro caries. *J Dent Res* 59(10): 1565–1570.
49. Weiss ME, Bibby BG (1966) Some protein effects on enamel solubility. *Arch Oral Biol* 11: 59.
50. Kashket S, DePaola DP (2002) Cheese consumption and the development and progression of dental caries. *Nutrition Reviews* 60(4): 97–103.
51. Herod EL (1991) The effect of cheese on dental caries: a review of the literature. *Australian Dental Journal* 36(2): 120–125.
52. Adegboye ARA, Christensen LB, Holm-Pedersen P, Avlund K, Boucher BJ, Heitmann BL (2012) Intake of dairy products in relation to periodontitis in older Danish adults. *Nutrients* 4: 1219–1229.

53 Telgi RL, Yadav V, Telgi CR, Boppana N (2013) In vivo dental plaque pH after consumption of dairy products. *General Dentistry 61*(3): 56–59.
54 Tsang G (2010) Say Cheese: Comparing the Nutrition of Different Cheeses. Available at www.healthcastle.com/say-cheese-comparing-the-nutrition-of-different-cheeses, accessed 18 September 2019.
55 Jekl V, Krejcirova L, Buchtova M, Knotek Z (2011) Effect of high phosphorus diet on tooth microstructure of rodent incisors. *Bone 49*: 479–484.
56 Davies M (2014) The WHITE TEETH diet: dentist reveals how to EAT your way to whiter gnashers – and the good news is it even includes cheese! Available at www.dailymail.co.uk/health/article-2812971/The-WHITE-TEETH-diet-Dentist-reveals-EAT-way-whiter-gnashers-good-news-includes-cheese.html, accessed 12 June 2019.
57 Sánchez MC, Ribeiro-Vidal H, Esteban-Fernández A, Bartolomé B, *et al.* (2019) Antimicrobial activity of red wine and oenological extracts against periodontal pathogens in a validated oral biofilm model. *BMC Complementary and Alternative Medicine 19*: 145.
58 Grass J, Pabst M, Kolarich D, Pöltl G, *et al.* (2011) Discovery and structural characterization of fucosylated oligomannosidic N-glycans in mushrooms. *Journal of Biological Chemistry 286*(8): 5977–5984.
59 Sierpina VS, Murray RK (2006) Glyconutrients: the state of the science and the impact of glycomics. *EXPLORE 2*(6): 488–494.
60 Liao S-F, Liang C-H, Ho M-Y, Hsu T-L, *et al.* (2013) Immunization of fucose-containing polysaccharides from Reishi mushroom induces antibodies to tumor-associated Gobo H-series epitopes. *PNAS 110*(34): 13809–13814.
61 Sierpina VS, Murray RK (2006) Glyconutrients: the state of the science and the impact of glycomics. *EXPLORE 2*(6): 488–494.
62 Chaturvedi TP (2009) Uses of turmeric in dentistry: an update. *Indian J Dent Res 20*(1): 107–109.
63 Bakri IM, Douglas CWI (2005) Inhibitory effect of garlic extract on oral bacteria. *Archives of Oral Biology 50*: 645–651.
64 Meredith MJ (2001) Herbal nutriceuticals: a primer for dentists and dental hygienists. *J Contemp Dent Pract 2*(2): 1–24. As cited in Buggapati L (2016) Herbs in dentistry. *IJPSI 5*(6): 7–12.
65 Kakiuchi N, Hattori M, Nishizawa M, Yamagishi T, Okuda T, Namba T (1986) Studies on dental caries prevention by traditional medicines. VIII. Inhibitory effect of various tannins on glucan synthesis by glucosyltranferase from Streptococcus mutans. *Chem Pharmaceutical Bull 34*(2): 720–725.
66 Sakanaka S, Aizawa M, Kim M, Yamamoto T (1996) Inhibitory effects of green tea polyphenols on growth and cellular adherence of an oral bacterium, Porphyromonas gingivalis. *Biosci Biotech Biochem 60*(5): 745–749.
67 Fournier-Larente J, Morin M-P, Grenier D (2016) Green tea catechins potentiate the effect of antibiotics and modulate adherence and gene expression in Porphyromonas gingivalis. *Archives of Oral Biology 65*: 35–43.
68 Morin M-P, Grenier D (2017) Regulation of matrix metalloproteinase secretion by green tea catechins in a three-dimensional co-culture model of macrophages and gingival fibroblasts. *Archives of Oral Biology 75*: 89–99.
69 Kong L, Qi X, Huang S, Chen S, Wu Y, Zhao L (2015) Theaflavins inhibit pathogenic properties of P. gingivalis and MMPs production in P. gingivalis-stimulated human gingival fibroblasts. *Archives of Oral Biology 60*: 12–22.
70 Castellsagué X, Muñoz N, DeStefani E, Victora CG, Castelletto R, Rolón PA (2000) Influence of mate drinking, hot beverages and diet on esophageal cancer risk in South America. *Int J Cancer 88*: 658–664.
71 Paganini-Hill A, White SC, Atchison KA (2012) Dentition, dental health habits, and dementia: the Leisure World Cohort Study. *J Am Geriatr Soc 60*: 1556–1563.
72 Nicopoulou-Karayianni K, Tzoutzoukos P, Mitsea P, Karayiannis A, *et al.* (2009) Tooth loss and osteoporosis: the osteodent study. *J Clin Periodontol 36*: 190–197.
73 Arguin H, Tremblay A, Blundell JE, Després J-P, *et al.* (2017) Impact of a non-restrictive satiating diet on anthropometrics, satiety responsiveness and eating behaviour traits in obese men displaying a high or a low satiety phenotype. *British Journal of Nutrition 118*: 750–760.
74 Isokangas P, Tiekso J, Alanen P, Mäkinen KK (1989) Long-term effect of xylitol chewing gum on dental caries. *Community Dent Oral Epidemiol 17*: 200–203.
75 Holmes R (undated) Chewing Gum: A Sticky Question. And Is Chewing Gum Healthy? Articles are reproduced by kind permission of Vitfinder.com who originally published the articles. Available at https://www.vitfinder.com/health-articles/post/chewing-gum:-a-sticky-question and https://www.vitfinder.com/health-articles/post/is-chewing-gum-healthy, accessed 28 August 2021.
76 Mercola J (2014) 6 Disturbing Side Effects of Chewing Gum. Available at https://organic.org/6-disturbing-side-effects-of-chewing-gum, accessed 27 August 2021.
77 Bioesti (undated) Mastic (Pistacia Lentiscus). Available at http://bioesti.com/mastic, accessed 11 June 2019.

78. Paraschos S, Mitakou S, Skaltsounis A-L (2012) Chios gum mastic: a review of its biological activities. *Current Medicinal Chemistry 19*: 2292–2302.
79. Dodds MW (2012) The oral health benefits of chewing gum. *J Ir Dent Assoc 58*: 253–261.
80. Riley P, Moore D, Ahmed F, Sharif MO, Worthington HV (2015) Xylitol-containing products for preventing dental caries in children and adults. *Cochrane Database Syst Rev 3*: CD010743.
81. Nadimi H, Wesamaa H, Janket SJ, Bollu P, Meurman JH (2011) Are sugar-free confections really beneficial for dental health? *Br Dent J 211*(7): E15.
82. Brown R, Sam CH, Green T, Wood S (2015) Effect of GutsyGum™, a novel gum, on subjective ratings of gastro esophageal reflux following a refluxogenic meal. *J Diet Suppl 12*: 138–145.
83. Zoladz PR, Raudenbush B (2005) Cognitive enhancement through stimulation of the chemical senses. *North American Journal of Psychology 7*: 125–140.
84. Koparal E, Ertugrul F, Sabah E (2000) Effect of chewing gum on plaque acidogenicity. *J Clin Pediatr Dent 24*(2): 129–132.
85. Manning RH, Edgar WM, Agalamanyi EA (1992) Effect of chewing gums sweetened with sorbitol/xylitol mixture on the remineralization of human enamel lesions in situ. *Caries Res 26*: 104–109.
86. Sällsten G, Thorén J, Barregård L, Schütz A, Skarping G (1996) Long-term use of nicotine chewing gum and mercury exposure from dental amalgam fillings. *J Dent Res 75*(1): 594–598.
87. Isacsson G, Barregård L, Selden A, Bodin L (1997) Impact of nocturnal bruxism on mercury uptake from dental amalgams. *Eur J Oral Sc 105*: 251–257.
88. Moazzez R, Bartlett D, Anggiansah A (2005) The effect of chewing sugar-free gum on gastro-esophageal refluz. *J Dent Res 84*: 1062–1065.
89. Swoboda C, Temple JL (2013) Acute and chronic effects of gum chewing on food reinforcement and energy intake. *Eating Behaviours 14*(2): 149–156.
90. Mercola J (2012) Artificial Sweeteners Cause Greater Weight Gain than Sugar, Yet Another Study Reveals. Available at https://articles.mercola.com/sites/articles/archive/2012/12/04/saccharin-aspartame-dangers.aspx, accessed 11 June 2019.
91. Mercola J (undated) 6 Disturbing Side Effects of Chewing Gum. Available at https://organic.org/6-disturbing-side-effects-of-chewing-gum, accessed 27 August 2021.
92. Birkhed D (1994) Cariologic aspects of xylitol and its use in chewing gum: a review. *Acta Odontol Scand 52*(2): 116–127.
93. Nascimento MM, Liu Y, Kalra R, Perry S, *et al.* (2013) Oral arginine metabolism may decrease the risk for dental caries in children. *J Dent Res 92*(7): 604–608.
94. Ierardo G, Bossù M, Tarantino D, Trinchieri V, Sfasciotti GL, Polimeni A (2010) The arginine-deiminase enzymatic system on gingivitis: preliminary pediatric study. *Annali di Stomatologia 1*(1): 8–13.
95. Mohammadi A, Azar R (2012) Effects of dietary L-arginine on orthodontic tooth movement in rats. *African Journal of Biotechnology 11*(1): 191–197.
96. Martin LE, Nikonova LV, Kay K, Paedae AB, Contreras RJ, Torregrossa A-M (2018) Salivary proteins alter taste-guided behaviors and taste nerve signalling in rat. *Physiology & Behavior 184*: 150–161.

CHAPTER 15

1. Van der Velden U, Kuzmanova D, Chapple ILC (2010) Micronutritional approaches to periodontal therapy. *J Clin Periodontol 38*(suppl. 11): 142–158.
2. Antonietta R, Nazario B, Luigi G, Marco A, Caterina RC, Rossella P (2012) Effect of resveratrol and modulation of cytokine production on human periodontal ligament cells. *Cytokine 60*: 197–204.
3. Bhattarai G, Poudel SB, Kook S-H, Lee J-C (2016) Resveratrol prevents alveolar bone loss in an experimental rat model of periodontitis. *Acta Biomaterialia 29*: 398–408.
4. Anushri M, Yashoda R, Puranik MP (2015) Herbs: a good alternative to current treatments for oral health problems. *International Journal of Advanced Health Sciences 1*(12): 26–32.
5. Bonaterra GA, Kelber O, Weiser D, Metz J, Kinscherf R (2010) Anti-inflammatory effects of the willow bark extract STW 33-1 (Proaktiv®) in LPS-activated human monocytes and differentiated macrophages. *Phytomedicine 17*(14): 1106–1113.
6. Hannig C, Spitzmüller B, Al-Ahmad A, Hannig M (2008) Effects of Cistus-tea on bacterial colonization and enzyme activities of the in situ pellicle. *Journal of Dentistry 36*: 540–545.
7. Li X-C, Cai L, Wu CD (1997) Antimicrobial compounds from Ceanothus americanus against oral pathogens. *Phytochemistry 46*(1): 97–102.
8. Herrera DR, Yay LY, Rezende EC, Kozlowski VA Jr, Santos EB (2010) In vitro antimicrobial activity of phytotherapic Uncaria tomentosa against endodontic pathogens. *J Oral Sci 52*(3): 473–476.

9. Herrera DR, Durand-Ramirez JE, Silva DJLN, Santos EB, Gomes BPFdA (2016) Antimicrobial activity and substantivity of Uncaria tomentosa in infected root canal dentin. *Braz Oral Res* 30(1): e61.
10. Tay LY, Santos FA, Jorge JH (2015) Uncaria tomentosa gel against denture stomatitis: clinical report. *Journal of Prosthodontics* 24(7): 594–597.
11. Jiang Q, Liu P, Wu X, Liu W, et al. (2011) Berberine attenuates lipopolysaccharide-induced extracellular matrix accumulation and inflammation in rat mesangial cells: involvement of NF-κB signalling pathway. *Molecular and Cellular Endocrinology* 331: 34–40.
12. Jia X, Jia L, Mo L, Yuan S, et al. (2019) Berberine ameliorates periodontal bone loss by regulating gut microbiota. *J Dent Res* 98(1): 107–116.
13. Burdette C (2017) Dunwoody Labs Webinar: LPS, A Player in Chronic Disease. Available at https://vimeo.com/248167370, accessed 31 May 2021.
14. Femiano F, Fullo R, diSpirito F, Lanza A, Festa VM, Cirillo N (2011) A comparison of salivary substitutes versus a natural sialogogue (citric acid) in patients complaining of dry mouth as an adverse drug reaction: a clinical, randomized controlled study. *Oral Surg Oral Med Oral Pathol Oral Radiol Endod* 112(1): e15–20.
15. Robertson WGA (1903) Sialogogues: their therapeutic employment. *Trans Med Chir Soc Edinb* 22: 275–285.
16. Mardani H, Ghannadi A, Rashnavadi B, Kamali R (2017) The effect of ginger herbal spray on reducing xerostomia in patients with type II diabetes. *AJP* 7(4): 308–316.
17. Dawes C, Pedersen AML, Villa A, Ekström J, et al. (2015) The functions of human saliva: a review sponsored by the World Workshop on Oral Medicine VI. *Archives of Oral Biology* 60: 863–874.
18. Cutando A, Aneiros-Fernánez J, López-Valverde A, Arias-Santiago S, Aneiros-Cachaza J, Reiter RJ (2011) A new perspective in oral health: potential importance and actions of melatonin receptors MT1, MT2, MT3 and RZR/ROR in the oral cavity. *Archives of Oral Biology* 56: 944–950.
19. Venturi S, Venturi M (2009) Iodine in evolution of salivary glands and in oral health. *Nutrition and Health* 20: 119–134.
20. Tramontano D, Veneziani BM, Lombardi A, Villone G, Ingbar SH (1989) Iodine inhibits the proliferation of rat thyroid cells in culture. *Endocrinology* 125(2): 984–992.
21. Abraham GE (2004) The concept of orthoiodo-supplementation and its clinical implications. *Orig Internist* 11: 29–38.
22. Beyondthyca [Beyond Thyroid Cancer] (2018) Iodine, Fluoride, Chlorine, Bromine: The Health Effects of Halogens. Beyond Thyroid Cancer. Available at https://beyondthyroidcancer.com, accessed 8 December 2018.
23. Nireeksha, Hedge MN, Kumari S, Sharmila, Roopa (2020) Salivary selenium levels in dental caries. *Indian Journal of Public Health R&D 11*(6): 1141–1145.
24. Machoy-Mokrzynska A (1995) Fluoride–magnesium interaction. *Fluoride* 28(4): 175–177.
25. Sun J (2010) Vitamin D and mucosal immune function. *Curr Opin Gastroenterol* 26(6): 591–595.
26. Lechner J, Aschoff J, Rudi T (2018) The vitamin D receptor and the etiology of RANTES/CCL-expressive fatty-degenerative osteolysis of the jawbone: an interface between osteoimmunology and bone metabolism. *International Journal of General Medicine* 11: 155–166.
27. Iwamoto J, Takeda T, Sato Y (2004) Effects of vitamin K2 on osteoporosis. *Curr Pharm Des* 10(21): 2557–2576.
28. Gordeladze JO, Landin MA, Johnsen GF, Haugen HJ, Osmundsen H (2017) Vitamin K2 and Its Impact on Tooth Epigenetics. In: J Gordeladze (ed.) *Vitamin K2: Vital for Health and Wellbeing*. IntechOpen, Chapter 7. Available at www.intechopen.com/books/vitamin-k2-vital-for-health-and-wellbeing/vitamin-k2-and-its-impact-on-tooth-epigenetics, accessed 30 June 2019.
29. Bostanci N, Belibasakis GN (2012) Porphyromonas gingivalis: an invasive and evasive opportunistic oral pathogen. *FEMS Microbiol Lett* 333: 1–9.
30. Koshihara Y, Hoshi K (1997) Vitamin K2 enhances osteocalcin accumulation in the extracellular matrix of human osteoblasts in vitro. *J Bone Miner Res* 12(3): 431–438.
31. Myneni VD, Mezey E (2017) Regulation of bone remodelling by vitamin K2. *Oral Diseases* 23: 1021–1028.
32. Thaweboon S, Thaweboon B, Choonharuangdej S, Chunhabundit P, Suppakpatana P (2005) Induction of type I collagen and osteocalcin in human dental pulp cells by retinoic acid. *Southeast Asian J Trop Med Public Health* 36(4): 1066–1069.
33. Oliva A, Della Ragione F, Fratta M, Marrone G, Palumbo R, Zappia V (1993) Effect of retinoic acid on osteocalcin gene expression in human osteoblasts. *Biochem Biophys ResCommun* 191(3): 908–914.
34. Varela-López A, Navarro-Hortal MD, Giampieri F, Bullón P, Battino M, Quiles JL (2018) Nutraceuticals in periodontal health: a systematic review on the role of vitamins in periodontal health maintenance. *Molecules* 23: 1226.
35. Nielsen FH (2014) Update on the possible nutritional importance of silicon. *Journal of Trace Elements in Medicine and Biology* 28: 379–382.
36. Martin KR (2007) The chemistry of silica and its potential health benefits. *J Nutr Health Aging* 11(2): 94–97.

ENDNOTES

37. Lovett WE (2003) Patent: Vitamin formulation for enhancing bone strength. US Patent Applic US10/409,208. US6881419B2.
38. Alsenan J, Chou L (2017) Effect of silicon and calcium on human dental pulp cell cultures. *International Journal of Materials Science and Applications* 6(6): 290–296.
39. Dundar S, Eltas A, Hakki SS, Malkoc S, et al. (2016) Dietary arginine silicate inositol complex inhibits periodontal tissue loss in rats with ligature-induced periodontitis. *Drug Design, Development and Therapy* 10: 3771–3778.
40. Sastravaha G, Gassmann G, Sangtherapitikul P, Grim W-D (2005) Adjunctive periodontal treatment with Centella asiatica and Punica granatum extracts in supportive periodontal therapy. *J Int Acad Periodontol* 7(3): 70–79.
41. Meletis C, Rousett D (2010) *The Hyaluronic Acid Miracle: Instant Facelift, Anti-Aging, Rejuvenation*. Beverly Hills, CA: Freedom Press.
42. Semwal DK, Semwal RB, Combrinck S, Viljoen A (2016) Myricetin: a dietary molecule with diverse biological activities. *Nutrients* 8(2): 90.
43. Ko S-Y (2012) Myricetin suppresses LPS-induced MMP expression in human gingival fibroblasts and inhibits osteoclastogenesis by downregulating NFATc1 in RANKL-induced RAW 264.7 cells. *Archives of Oral Biology* 57: 1623–1632.
44. Editors of Encyclopaedia Britannica (undated) Lips. Available at www.britannica.com/science/lips, accessed 25 April 2019.
45. LeBell AM, Soderling E, Rantanen I, Vang B, Kallio H (2000) Effects of seabuckthorn oil on the oral mucosa of Sjogren's syndrome patients: a pilot study. Poster at the Eightieth General Session & Exhibition of International Association for Dental Research (IADR), 6–9 March, San Diego, USA. As cited in: Yang B, Kallio H (2005) Physiological Effects of Seabuckthorn (Hippophae rhamnoides) Fruit Pulp and Seed Oils. *Seabuckthorn (Hippophae L.): A Multipurpose Wonder Plant*, Vol.2 (Singh V, Editor-in-Chief). New Delhi, India, pp.363–389.
46. Smida I, Pentelescu C, Pentelescu O, Sweidan A, et al. (2019) Benefits of sea buckthorn (Hippophae rhamnoides) pulp oil-based mouthwash on oral health. *Journal of Applied Microbiology* 126(5): 1594–1605.
47. Pinto E, Vale-Silva L, Cavaleiro C, Salgueiro L (2009) Antifungal activity of the clove essential oil from Syzygium aromaticum on Candida, Aspergillus and dermatophyte species. *Journal of Medical Microbiology* 58: 1454–1462.
48. Dwivedi V, Shrivastava R, Hussain S, Ganguly C, Bharadwaj M (2011) Comparative anticancer potential of clove (Syzygium aromaticum) – an Indian spice – against cancer cell lines of various anatomical origin. *Asian Pacific J Cancer Prev* 12: 1989–1993.
49. Uju DE, Obioma NP (2011) Anticariogenic potentials of clove, tobacco and bitter kola. *Asian Pac J Trop Med* 4(10): 814–818.
50. Hosseini M, Asl MK, Rakhshandeh H (2011) Analgesic effect of clove essential oil in mice. *Avicenna Journal of Phytomedicine* 1(1): 1–6.
51. Buggapati L (2016) Herbs in dentistry. *IJPSI* 5(6): 7–12.
52. Cummins D (2009) US Patent: Oral Compositions Containing Botanical Extracts. US Patent 2009/0087501 A1. Appl no 12/243/669.
53. Al-Mobeeriek A (2011) Effects of myrrh on intra-oral mucosal wounds compared with tetracycline- and chlorhexidine-based mouthwashes. *Clinical, Cosmetic and Investigational Dentistry* 3: 53–58.
54. El Ashry ESH, Rashed N, Salama OM, Saleh A (2003) Components, therapeutic value and uses of myrrh. Pharmazie 58: 163–168.
55. Martin MD, Sherman J, VanDerVen P, Burgess J (2008) A controlled trial of dissolving oral patch containing lycyrrhiza (licorice) herbal extract from the treatment of aphthous ulcers. *General Dentistry 2008*: 206–210.
56. Anushri M, Yashoda R, Puranik MP (2015) Herbs: a good alternative to current treatments for oral health problems. *International Journal of Advanced Health Sciences* 1(12): 26–32.
57. Ibid.
58. Ibid.
59. Furiga A, Roques C, Badet C (2014) Preventive effects of an original combination of grape seed polyphenols with amine fluoride on dental biofilm formation and oxidative damage by oral bacteria. *Journal of Applied Microbiology* 116(4): 761–771.
60. Buggapati L (2016) Herbs in dentistry. *IJPSI* 5(6): 7–12.
61. Ibid.
62. Ibid.
63. Godhia ML, Patel N (2013) Colostrum – its composition, benefits as a nutraceutical: a review. *Current Research in Nutrition and Food Science* 1(1): 37–47.
64. Pedersen AM, Andersen TL, Reibel J, Holmstrup P, Nauntofte B (2002) Oral findings in patients with primary Sjögren's syndrome and oral lichen planus – a preliminary study on the effects of bovine colostrum-containing oral hygiene products. *Clin Oral Investig* 6(1): 11–20.
65. Loimaranta V, Laine M, Söderling E, Vasara E, et al. (1999) Effects of bovine immune and non-immune whey preparations on the composition and pH response of human dental plaque. *Eur J Oral Sci* 107: 244–250.
66. Uruakpa FO, Ismond MAH, Akobundu ENT (2002) Colostrum and its benefits: a review. *Nutrition Research* 22: 755–767.

67. Chinoy NJ, Sharma A (1998) Amelioration of fluoride toxicity by vitamins E and D in reproductive functions of male mice. *Fluoride 31*: 203-216.
68. Ranjan S, Yasmin S (2015) Amelioration of fluoride toxicity using amla (Emblica officinalis). *Current Science 108*(11): 2094-2098.
69. Raj GA, Sahadeb D, Chandra PR, Devendra S, Mohii S (2015) *Indian Journal of Animal Nutrition 32*(3): 329-334.
70. Blaylock RL (2004) Excitotoxicity: a possible central mechanism in fluoride neurotoxicity. *Fluoride 37*(4): 264-277.
71. Juzyszyn Z, Czery B, Myśliwiec Z, Put A (2002) Enhancement of kidney and liver respiratory activity by quercetin sulfonates in rats chronically exposed to ammonium fluoride. *Fluoride 35*(3): 161-167.
72. Sharma C, Suhalka P, Sukhwal P, Jaiswal N, Bhatnagar M (2014) Curcumin attenuates neurotoxicity induced by fluoride: an in vivo evidence. *Pharmacogn Mag 10*(37): 61-65.
73. Buggapati L (2016) Herbs in dentistry. *IJPSI 5*(6): 7-12.
74. Scherma M, Fattore L, Castelli MP, Fratta W, Fadda P (2014) The role of the endocannabinoid system in eating disorders: neurochemical and behavioural preclinical evidence. *Curr Pharm Des 20*(13): 2089-2099.
75. Scopinho AA, Guimarães FS, Corrêa FMA, Resstel LBM (2011) Cannabidiol inhibits the hyperphagia induced by cannabinoid-1 or serotonin-1A receptor agonists. *Pharmacology, Biochemistry and Behavior 98*: 268-272.
76. Fine PG, Rosenfeld MJ (2014) Cannabinoids for neuropathic pain. *Curr Pain Headache Rep 18*: 451.
77. Thirunavukkarasu V, Nandhini ATA, Anurdha CV (2005) Lipoic acid improves glucose utilisation and prevents protein glycation and AGE formation. *Pharmazie 60*: 772-775.
78. Liao S-F, Liang C-H, Ho M-Y, Hsu T-L, et al. (2013) Immunization of fucose-containing polysaccharides from Reishi mushroom induces antibodies to tumor-associated Gobo H-series epitopes. *PNAS 110*(34): 13809-13814.
79. Sierpina VS, Murray RK (2006) Glyconutrients: the state of the science and the impact of glycomics. *EXPLORE 2*(6): 488-494.
80. Heckmann SM, Hujoel P, Habiger S, Friess W, et al. (2005) Zinc gluconate in the treatment of dysgeusia – a randomized clinical trial. *J Dent Res 84*(1): 35-38.
81. Kilian M, Chapple ILC, Hannig M, Marsh PD, et al. (2016) The oral microbiome – an update for oral healthcare professionals. *British Dental Journal 221*: 657-666.
82. Haukioja A (2010) Probiotics and oral health. *Eur J Dent 4*: 348-355.
83. Wescombe PA, Heng NCK, Burton JP, Tagg JR (2010) Something old and something new: an update on the amazing repertoire of bacteriocins produced by Streptococcus salivarius. *Probiotics & Antimicro Prot 2*(1): 37-45.
84. Wescombe PA, Hale JDF, Heng NCK, Tagg JR (2012) Developing oral probiotics from Streptococcus salivarius. *Future Microbiol 7*(12): 1355-1371.
85. Ibid.
86. Burton JP, Drummond BK, Chilcott CN, Tagg JR, et al. (2013) Influence of the probiotic Streptococcus salivarius strain M18 on indices of dental health in children: a randomized double-blind, placebo-controlled trial. *Journal of Medical Microbiology 62*: 875-884.
87. Burton JP, Wescombe PA, Macklaim JM, Chai MHC, et al. (2013) Persistence of the oral probiotic Streptococcus salivarius M18 is dose dependent and megaplasmid transfer can augment their bacteriocin production and adhesion characteristics. *PLOS ONE 8*(6): e65991.
88. Scariya L, Nagarathna DV, Varghese M (2015) Probiotics in periodontal therapy. *Int J Pharm Bio Sci 6*(1): 242-250.
89. DiPierro F, Colombo M, Zanvit A, Risso P, Rottoli AS (2014) Use of Streptococcus salivarius K12 in the prevention of streptococcal and viral pharyngotonsillitis in children. *Drug Healthc Patient Saf 13*(6): 15-20.
90. Burton JP, Chilcott CN, Moore CJ, Speiser G, Tagg JR (2006) A preliminary study of the effect of probiotic Streptococcus salivarius K12 on oral malodour parameters. *Journal of Applied Microbiology 100*: 754-764.
91. Wescombe PA, Hale JDF, Heng NCK, Tagg JR (2012) Developing oral probiotics from Streptococcus salivarius. *Future Microbiol 7*(12): 1355-1371.
92. Nishihara T, Suzuki N, Yoneda M, Hirofuji T (2014) Effects of Lactobacillus salivarius-containing tablets on caries risk factors: a randomized open-label clinical trial. *BMC Oral Health 14*: 110.
93. Näse L, Hatakka K, Savilahi E, Saxelin M, et al. (2001) Effect of long-term consumption of a probiotic bacterium, Lactobacillus rhamnosus GG, in milk on dental caries and caries risk in children. *Caries Res 35*(6): 412-420.
94. Iwasaki K, Maeda K, Hidaka K, Nemoto K, Hirose Y, Deguchi S (2016) Daily intake of heat-killed Lactobacillus plantarum L-137 decreases the probing depth in patients undergoing supportive periodontal therapy. *Oral Health Prev Dent 14*: 207-214.
95. Liang S, Krauss JL, Domon H, McIntosh ML, et al. (2011) The C5a receptor impairs IL-12-dependent clearance of Porphyromonas gingivalis and is required for induction of periodontal bone loss. *The Journal of Immunology 186*: 869-877.

96 Hajishengallis G, Shakhatreh M-AK, Wang M, Liang S (2007) Complement receptor 3 blockade promotes IL-12-mediated clearance of Porphyromonas gingivalis and negates its virulence in vivo. *The Journal of Immunology* 179: 2359–2367.

97 Banerjee C, Ulloor J, Dillon EL, Dahodwala Q, et al. (2011) Identification of serum biomarkers for aging and anabolic response. *Immunity & Ageing* 8: 5.

98 Schlagenhauf U, Jakob L, Eigenthaler M, Segerer S, Jockel-Schneier Y, Rehn M (2018) Regular consumption of Lactobacillus reuteri-containing lozenges reduces pregnancy gingivitis: an RCT. *J Clin Periodontol* 43: 948–954.

99 Kraft-Bodi E, Jørgensen MR, Keller MK, Kragelund C, Twetman S (2015) Effect of probiotic bacteria on oral Candida in frail elderly. *J Dent Res* 94(9 suppl.): 181S–186S.

100 Hatakka K, Ahola AJ, Yli-Knuuttila H, Richardson M, et al. (2007) Probiotics reduce the prevalence of oral Candida in the elderly – a randomized controlled trial. *J Dent Res* 86(2): 125–130.

101 Mendonça FHBP, dosSantos SSF, deFaria IdS, Gonçalves eSilva CR, Jorge AOC, Leão MVP (2012) Effects of probiotic bacteria on Candida presence and IgA anti-Candida in the oral cavity of elderly. *Braz Dent J* 23(5): 534–538.

102 Ishikawa KH, Mayer MPA, Miyazima TY, Matsubara VH, et al. (2014) A multispecies probiotic reduces oral Candida colonization in denture wearers. *Journal of Prosthodontics* 24(3): 194–199.

103 Gleeson M, Bishop NC, Oliveira M, Tauler P (2011) Daily probiotic's (Lactobacillus casei Shirota) reduction of infection incidence in athletes. *International Journal of Sport Nutrition & Exercise Metabolism* 21(1): 55–64.

104 Ritthagol W, Saetang C, Teanpaisan R (2014) Effect of probiotics containing Lactobacillus paracasei SD1 on salivary mutans Streptococci and Lactobacilli in orthodontic cleft patients: a double-blinded, randomized, placebo-controlled study. *Cleft Palate-Craniofacial Journal* 51(3): 257–263.

105 Pérez-Cano FJ, Dong H, Yaqoob P (2010) In vitro immunomodulatory activity of Lactobacillus fermentum CECT5716 and Lactobacillus salivarius CECT5713: two probiotic strains isolated from human breast milk. *Immunobiology* 215(12): 996–1004.

106 Martin-Cabezas R, Davideau JL, Tenenbaum H, Huck O (2016) Clinical efficacy of probiotics as an adjunctive therapy to non-surgical periodontal treatment of chronic periodontitis: systematic review and meta-analysis. *J Clin Periodontol* 43(6): 520–530.

107 Mayanagi G, Kimura M, Nakaya S, Hirata H, et al. (2009) Probiotic effects of orally administered Lactobacillus salivarius WB21-containing tablets on periodontopathic bacteria: a double-blinded, placebo-controlled, randomized clinical trial. *J Clin Periodontol* 36(6): 506–513.

108 Hojo K, Nagaoka S, Murata S, Taketomo N, Ohshima T, Maeda N (2007) Reduction of vitamin K concentration by salivary Bifidobacterium strains and their possible nutritional competition with Porphyromonas gingivalis. *Journal of Applied Microbiology* 103: 1969–1974.

109 Winclove Probiotics (undated) Improvement of Oral Health and Prevention of Gingivitis. Available at www.wincloveprobiotics.com/sites/default/files/headerpics/winclove_smile.pdf, accessed 21 September 2019.

110 Kang MS, Chung J, Kim SM, Yang KH, Oh JS (2006) Effect of Weissella cibaria isolates on the formation of Streptococcus mutans biofilm. *Caries Res* 40(5): 418–425.

111 Ashwin D, Ke V, Taranath M, Ramagoni NK, Nara A, Sarpangala M (2015) Effect of probiotic containing ice-cream on salivary mutans Streptococci (SMS) levels in children of 6–12 years of age: a randomized controlled double blind study with six-months follow up. *J Clin Diagn Res* 9(2): ZC06–ZC09.

112 Terai T, Okumura T, Imai S, Nakao M, et al. (2015) Screening of probiotic candidates in human oral bacteria for the prevention of dental disease. *PLOS ONE* 10(6): e0128657.

113 Wescombe PA, Hale JDF, Heng NCK, Tagg JR (2012) Developing oral probiotics from Streptococcus salivarius. *Future Microbiol* 7(12): 1355–1371.

114 Jindal G, Pandey RK, Agarwal J, Singh M (2011) A comparative evaluation of probiotics on salivary mutans streptococci counts in Indian children. *European Archives of Paediatric Dentistry* 12(4): 211–215.

115 Chen C-H, Sheu M-T, Chen T-F, Wang Y-C, et al. (2006) Suppression of endotoxin-induced proinflammatory responses by citrus pectin through blocking LPS signalling pathways. *Biochemical Pharmacology* 72: 1001–1009.

116 Salman H, Bergman M, Djaldeti M, Orlin J, Bessler H (2008) Citrus pectin affects cytokine production by human peripheral blood mononuclear cells. *Biomedicine & Pharmacotherapy* 62: 579–582.

117 Jones DP, Coates RJ, Flagg EW, Eley JW, et al. (1992) Glutathione in foods listed in the National Cancer Institute's Health Habits and History Food Frequency Questionnaire. *Nutr Cancer* 17: 57–75.

118 Johnston CS, Meyer CG, Srilakshmi JC (1993) Vitamin C elevates red blood cell glutathione in healthy adults. *Am J Clin Nutr* 58(1): 103–105.

119 Lenton KJ, Sané AT, Therriault H, Cantin AM, Payette H, Wagner JR (2003) Vitamin C augments lymphocyte glutathione in subjects with ascorbate deficiency. *Am J Clin Nutr* 77(1): 189–195.

120 Sharma A, Kharb S, Chugh SN, Kakkar R, Singh GP (2000) Effect of glycemic control and vitamin E supplementation on total gutathione content in non-insulin-dependent diabetes mellitus. *Ann Nutr Metab* 44: 11–13.

121 Thomson CD, Steven SM, vanRij AM, Wade CR, Robinson MF (1988) Selenium and vitamin E supplementation: activities of glutathione peroxidase in human tissues. *Am J Clin Nutr* 48(2): 316–323.

122 Jiang X, Dong J, Wang B, Yin X, Qin L (2012) [Effects of organic selenium supplement on glutathione peroxidase activities: a meta-analysis of randomized controlled trials] [Article in Chinese]. *Wei Sheng Yan Jiu* 41(1): 120–123.

123 El-Hafidi M, Franco M, Ramírez AR, Sosa JS, *et al.* (2018) Glycine increases insulin sensitivity and glutathione biosynthesis and protects against oxidative stress in a model of sucrose-induced insulin resistance. *Oxidative Medicine and Cellular Longevity 2018*: 2101562.

124 Sekhar RV, McKay S, Patel SG, Guthikonda AP, *et al.* (2011) Glutathione synthesis is diminished in patients with uncontrolled diabetes and restored by dietary supplementation with cysteine and glycine. *Diabetes Care* 34(1): 162–167.

125 Zavorsky GS, Kubow S, Grey V, Riverin V, Lands LC (2007) An open-label dose-response study of lymphocyte glutathione levels in healthy men and women receiving pressurized whey protein isolate supplements. *Int J Food Sci Nutr* 58(6): 429–436.

126 Paschalis V, Theodorou AA, Margaritelis NV, Kyparos A, Nikolaidis MG (2018) N-acetyl-cysteine supplementation increases exercise performance and reduces oxidative stress only in individuals with low levels of glutathione. *Free Radical Biology and Medicine* 115: 288–297.

127 Kaneshiro Y, Nakano H, Kumada K, Boudjema K, *et al.* (1998) Augmentation of mitochondrial reduced glutathione by S-adenosyl-L-methionine administration in ischemia-reperfusion injury of the rat steatotic liver induced by choline-methionine-deficient diet. *Eur Surg Res* 30: 34–42.

128 Biswas SK, McClure D, Jimenez LA, Megson IL, Rahman I (2005) Curcumin induces glutathione biosynthesis and inhibits NF-kappaB activation and interleukin-8 release in alveolar epithelial cells: mechanism of free radical scavenging activity. *Antioxid Redox Signal* 7(1–2): 32–41.

129 Kiruthiga PV, Pandian SK, Devi KP (2010) Silymarin protects PBMC against B(a)P induced toxicity by replenishing redox status and modulating glutathione metabolizing enzymes – an in vitro study. *Toxicology and Applied Pharmacology* 247: 116–128.

130 Soto C, Pérez J, García V, Uría E, Vadillo M, Raya L (2010) Effect of silymarin on kidneys of rats suffering from alloxan-induced diabetes mellitus. *Phytomedicine* 17: 1090–1094.

131 Gould RL, Pazdro R (2019) Impact of supplementary amino acids, micronutrients, and overall diet on glutathione homeostasis. *Nutrients* 11: 1056.

132 Patrick L (2002) Mercury toxicity and antioxidants: Part I: role of glutathione and alpha-lipoic acid in the treatment of mercury toxicity. *Altern Med Rev* 7(6): 456–471.

133 Al-Madi EM, Almohaimede AA, Al-Obaida M, Awaad AS (2019) Comparison of the antibacterial efficacy of Commiphora molmol and Sodium Hypochlorite as root canal irrigants against Enterococcus faecalis and Fusobacterium nucleatum. *Evidence-Based Complementary and Alternative Medicine 2019*: 6916795.

134 Hickl J, Argyropoulou A, Sakavitsi ME, Halabalaki M, *et al.* (2018) Mediterranean herb extracts inhibit microbial growth of representative oral microorganisms and biofilm formation of Streptococcus mutans. *PLOS ONE* 13(12): e0207574.

135 Kumbar VM, Peram MR, Kugaji MS, Shah T, *et al.* (2020) Effect of curcumin on growth, biofilm formation and virulence factor gene expression of Porphyromonas gingivalis. *Odontology*, doi: 10.1007/s10266-020-00514-y

136 Moon JH, Jang EY, Shim KS, Lee JY (2015) In vitro effects of N-acetyl cysteine alone and in combination with antibiotics on Prevotella intermedia. *J Microbiol* 53(5): 321–329.

137 Tada A, Nakayama-Imaohji H, Yamasaki H, Hasibul K, *et al.* (2016) Cleansing effect of acidic L-arginine on human oral biofilm. *BMC Oral Health* 16: 40.

138 Furiga A, Roques C, Badet C (2014) Preventive effects of an original combination of grape seed polyphenols with amine fluoride on dental biofilm formation and oxidative damage by oral bacteria. *Journal of Applied Microbiology* 116(4): 761–771.

139 Hickl J, Argyropoulou A, Sakavitsi ME, Halabalaki M, *et al.* (2018) Mediterranean herb extracts inhibit microbial growth of representative oral microorganisms and biofilm formation of Streptococcus mutans. *PLOS ONE* 13(12): e0207574.

CHAPTER 16

1. Lee K, Lee JS, Kim J, Lee H, *et al*. (2020) Oral health and gastrointestinal cancer: a nationwide cohort study. *J Clin Periodontol 47*(7): 796–808.
2. Tan CXW, Brand HS, Iqbal S, DeBoer NKH, Forouzanfar T, deVisscher JGAM (2020) A self-reported survey on oral health problems in patients with inflammatory bowel disease with a stoma. *Oral Surg Oral Med Oral Pathol Oral Radiol 130*(3): e80–e86.
3. Wadia R, Booth V, Yap HF, Moyes DL (2016) A pilot study of the gingival response when smokers switch from smoking to vaping. *British Dental Journal 221*(11): 722–726.
4. Saxer U, Hassell T (2005) Periodontitis as a contagious infection: contemporary use of antimicrobial agents. Part II. *Perio 2*(1): 7–12.
5. Ciszewski A, Baraniak M, Urbanek-Brychczyńska M (2007) Corrosion by galvanic coupling between amalgam and different chromium-based alloys. *Dental Material 23*: 1256–1261.
6. Horasawa N, Takahashi S, Marek M (1999) Galvanic interaction between titanium and gallium alloy or dental amalgam. *Dental Material 15*: 318–322.
7. Sutow EL, Maillet WA, Taylor JC, Hall GC (2004) In vivo galvanic currents of intermittently contacting dental amalgam and other metallic restorations. *Dental Material 20*: 823–831.
8. Fusayama T, Katayori T, Nomoto S (1963) Corrosion of gold and amalgam placed in contact with each other. *J Dent Res 42*: 1183.
9. Sellars WA, Sellars R, Liang L, Hefley JD (1996) Methyl mercury in dental amalgams in the human mouth. *Journal of Nutritional & Environmental Medicine 6*: 33–36.
10. Koral S (undated) A Practical Guide to Compatibility Testing for Dental Materials. Available at https://iaomt.org/practical-guide-compatibility-testing-dental-materials/?cn-reloaded=1, accessed 24 March 2019.
11. Ibid.
12. Rehme MG (2013) Is There a Battery in Your Mouth? Available at https://toothbody.com/is-there-a-battery-in-your-mouth, accessed 25 July 2018.
13. Rehme MG (2009) Tinnitus Finally Gone. Available at https://toothbody.com/tinnitus-finally-gone, accessed 25 July 2018.
14. Kazantzis G (2002) Mercury exposure and early effects: an overview. *Med Lav 93*(3): 139–147.
15. U.S. Food & Drug Administration (2021) Dental Amalgam Fillings. Available at www.fda.gov/medical-devices/dental-devices/dental-amalgam-fillings, accessed 5 June 2021.
16. Haley BE (2007) The relationship of the toxic effects of mercury to exacerbation of the medical condition classified as Alzheimer's disease. *Medical Veritas 4*: 1484–1498.
17. Houston MC (2011) Role of mercury toxicity in hypertension, cardiovascular disease and stroke. *The Journal of Clinical Hypertension 13*(8): 621–627.
18. U.S. Food & Drug Administration (2021) Dental Amalgam Fillings. Available at www.fda.gov/medical-devices/dental-devices/dental-amalgam-fillings, accessed 5 June 2021.
19. Williams L (2012) Dental Cavitation Surgery. Available at www.westonaprice.org/health-topics/dentistry/dental-cavitation-surgery, accessed 2 February 2019.
20. Colson DG (2012) A safe protocol for amalgam removal. *Journal of Environmental and Public Health 2012*: 517391.
21. Roberts J (2017) Dental mercury amalgams – will their use ever end? The current state of play! *Only Natural: the Newsletter of The Natural Dispensary 26*: 10–11.
22. Cashman L (undated) Preparation for a safe and successful amalgam removal. Excerpt available at https://iowamercuryfreedentistry.com/?page_id=142, accessed 29 September 2019.
23. Cashman L (undated) Practical detoxification. Excerpt available at https://iowamercuryfreedentistry.com/?page_id=142, accessed 29 September 2019.
24. Williams L (2012) Dental Cavitation Surgery. Available at www.westonaprice.org/health-topics/dentistry/dental-cavitation-surgery, accessed 2 February 2019.
25. Radiology.org (undated) Dental Cone Beam CT. Available at www.radiologyinfo.org/en/info/dentalconect, accessed 2 February 2019.
26. Taichman LS (2014) Oral health-related complications of breast cancer treatment: assessing dental hygienists' knowledge and professional practice. *Journal of Dental Hygiene 88*(2): 102–115.
27. Taichman LS (2015) Winner: Best Paper Award: Oral health-related complications of breast cancer treatment: assessing dental hygienists' knowledge and professional practice. *Journal of Dental Hygiene 89*(suppl. 2): 22–37. Manuscript first appeared (2014) *Journal of Dental Hygiene 88*(2): 102–115.
28. Williams L (2012) Dental Cavitation Surgery. Available at www.westonaprice.org/health-topics/dentistry/dental-cavitation-surgery, accessed 2 February 2019.
29. Ibid.

30. Cashman L (undated) Coping Better with Mercury Now and Preparing for Safe Dental Amalgam Mercury Filling Removal (kindly provided by the author, L Cashman, Executive Director of DAMS).
31. Ibid.
32. Gazoni FM, Malezan WR, Santos FC (2016) B complex vitamins for analgesic therapy. *Rev Dor São Paulo* 17(1): 52–56.
33. Brockette E (2018) Infertility and inflammation: the potential connection to periodontal disease. Available at www.dentistryiq.com/dental-hygiene/student-hygiene/article/16367898/infertility-and-inflammation-the-potential-connection-to-periodontal-disease, accessed 10 October 2019.
34. Lippert F (2013) An introduction to toothpaste – its purpose, history and ingredients. *Monographs in Oral Science* 23: 1–14.
35. Karibassappa GN, Nagesh L, Sujatha BK (2011) Assessment of microbial contamination of toothbrush head: an in vitro study. *Indian Journal of Dental Research* 22(1): 2–5.
36. Deery C, Heanue M, Deacon S, Robinson PG, et al. (2004) The effectiveness of manual versus powered toothbrushes for dental health: a systematic review. *Journal of Dentistry* 32: 197–211.
37. Gujjari SK, Gujjari AK, Patel PV, Shubhashini PV (2011) Comparative evaluation of ultraviolet and microwave sanitization techniques for toothbrush decontamination. *J Int Soc Prev Community Dent* 1(1): 20–26.
38. Gondhaleker R, Richar KMJ, Jayachandra MG, Aslam S, Reddy VN, Barabde AS (2013) Effect of tongue cleaning methods and oral mutans streptococci level. *J Contemp Dent Pract* 14(1): 119–122.
39. Pedrazzi V, Sato S, deMattos MGC, Lara EHG, Panzeri H (2004) Tongue-cleaning methods: a comparative clinical trial employing a toothbrush and a tongue scraper. *J Periodontol* 75: 1009–1012.
40. Ibid.
41. Yaegaki K, Coil JM (2000) Examination, classification, and treatment of halitosis: clinical perspectives. *J Can Dent Assoc* 66: 257–261.
42. Burch JG, Lanese R, Ngan P (1994) A two-month study of the effects of oral irrigation and automatic toothbrush use in an adult orthodontic population with fixed appliances. *Am J Orthod Dentofacial Orthop* 106(2): 121–126.
43. Cutler CW, Stanford TW, Abraham C, Cederberg RA, Boardman TJ, Ross C (2000) Clinical benefits of oral irrigation for periodontitis are related to reduction of pro-inflammatory cytokine levels and plaque. *J Clin Periodontol* 27(2): 134–143.
44. Al-Mubarek S, Ciancio S, Aljada A, Awa H, et al. (2002) Comparative evaluation of adjunctive oral irrigation in diabetes. *J Clin Peridontol* 29: 295–300.
45. Khan MK, Khan AA, Hosein T, Mudassir A, Mirza KM, Anwar A (2009) Comparison of the plaque-removing efficacy of toothpaste and toothpowder. *J Int Acad Periodontol* 11(1): 147–150.
46. Dawes C (1972) Circadian rhythms in human salivary flow rate and composition. *J Physiol* 220: 529–545.
47. Humphrey SP, Williamson RT (2001) A review of saliva: normal composition, flow and function. *The Journal of Prosthetic Dentistry* 85(2): 162–169.
48. Dawes C (1972) Circadian rhythms in human salivary flow rate and composition. *J Physiol* 220: 529–545.
49. Ibid.
50. Dawes C, Pedersen AML, Villa A, Ekström J, et al. (2015) The functions of human saliva: a review sponsored by the World Workshop on Oral Medicine VI. *Archives of Oral Biology* 60: 863–874.
51. Dawes C (1972) Circadian rhythms in human salivary flow rate and composition. *J Physiol* 220: 529–545.
52. Maldarelli C (2017) Does brushing your teeth affect your appetite? *Popular Science*. Available at www.popsci.com/does-brushing-your-teeth-affect-your-appetite, accessed 10 August 2019.
53. Szarka L, Levitt M (undated) Belching, Bloating and Flatulence. The Portland Clinic, Gastroenterology Department. Available at www.theportlandclinic.com/wp-content/uploads/2017/01/10562-Belching-Bloating-and-Flatulence.pdf, accessed 20 October 2019.
54. Baulkman J (2018) Are you SURE you want a straw? They may prevent some tooth staining – but dentists warn there are more risks than benefits for your mouth, metabolism and skin. Available at www.dailymail.co.uk/health/article-5528625/Straws-provide-risks-benefits-mouth-skin.html, accessed 20 October 2019.
55. Ali MJ, Ende K, Maas CS (2007) Perioral rejuvenation and lip augmentation. *Facial Plastic Surgery Clinics of North America* 15: 491–500.
56. Godara N, Godara R, Khullar M (2011) Impact of inhalation therapy on oral health. *Lung India* 28(4): 272–275.
57. Chellaih P, Sivadas G, Chintu S, Vaishnavi Vedam VK, Arunachalam R, Sarsu M (2016) Effect of anti-asthmatic drugs on dental health: a comparative study. *J Pharm Bioallied Sci* 8(suppl. 1): S77–S80.
58. Shashikiran ND, Reddy VV, Raju PK (2007) Effect of antiasthmatic medication on dental disease: dental caries and periodontal disease. *J Indian Soc Pedod Prev Dent* 25(2): 65–68.
59. Godara N, Godara R, Khullar M (2011) Impact of inhalation therapy on oral health. *Lung India* 28(4): 272–275.

ENDNOTES

60 Ryberg M, Möller C, Ericson T (1991) Saliva composition and caries development in asthmatic patients treated with beta 2-adrenoceptor agonists: a 4-year follow-up study. *Scand J Dent Res 99*(3): 212–218.

61 Kargul B, Tanboga I, Ergeneli S, Karakoc F, Dagli E (1998) Inhaler medicament effects on saliva and plaque pH in asthmatic children. *J Clin Pediatr Dent 22*(2): 137–140.

62 Tootla R, Toumba KJ, Duggal MS (2004) An evaluation of the acidogenic potential of asthma inhalers. *Archives of Oral Biology 49*: 275–283.

63 Godara N, Godara R, Khullar M (2011) Impact of inhalation therapy on oral health. *Lung India 28*(4): 272–275.

64 Ibid.

65 American Dental Association (2019) Floss/Interdental Cleaners. Available at www.ada.org/en/member-center/oral-health-topics/floss, accessed 2 June 2019.

66 Marcotte H, Lavoie MC (1998) Oral microbial ecology and the role of salivary immunoglobulin A. *Microbiology and Molecular Biology Reviews 62*(1): 71–109.

67 Parnell C, O'Mullane D (2013) After-brush rinsing protocols, frequency of toothpaste use: fluoride and other active ingredients. *Monogr Oral Sci 23*: 140–153.

68 Auchtung TA, Fofanova TY, Stewart CJ, Nash AK, *et al*. (2018) Investigating colonization of the healthy adult gastrointestinal tract by fungi. *Sphere 3*(2): e00092-18.

69 Grand View Research (2021) *Market Research Report: Oral Care Market Size, Share & Trends Analysis Report by Product (Toothbrush, Toothpaste), by Product Type (Countertop, Cordless), by Application (Home, Dentistry), by Region, and Segment Forecasts, 2021–2028*. Summary available at www.grandviewresearch.com/industry-analysis/oral-care-market, accessed 14 June 2021.

70 Karadas M, Hatipoglu O (2015) Efficacy of mouthwashes containing hydrogen peroxide on tooth whitening. *The Scientific World Journal 2015*: 961403.

71 Lanigan RS (2001) Final report on the safety assessment of sodium metaphosphate, sodium trimetaphosphate and sodium hexametaphosphate. *Int J Toxicol 20* (suppl. 3): 75–89.

72 Walters PA, Biesbrock AR, Bartizek RD (2004) Benefits of sodium hexametaphosphate-containing chewing gum for extrinsic stain inhibition. *J Dent Hyg 78*(4): 8.

73 DrBicuspid Staff (2010) Mouthwash Staining Lawsuit Dismissed. Available at www.drbicuspid.com/index.aspx?sec=ser&sub=def&pag=dis&ItemID=305224, accessed 5 June 2019.

74 Fasig LB (2007) P&G hopes rinse effect won't wash away sales. *Cincinnati Business Courier*. Available at www.bizjournals.com/cincinnati/stories/2007/04/09/story3.html, accessed 5 June 2019.

75 Kumar T, Arora N, Puri G, Aravinda K, Dixit A, Jatti D (2016) Efficacy of ozonized olive oil in the management of oral lesions and conditions: a clinical trial. *Contemp Clin Dent 7*(1): 51–54.

76 Montevecchi M, Dorigo A, Cricca M, Checchi L (2013) Comparison of the antibacterial activity of an ozonated oil with chlorhexidine digluconate and povidone-iodine. A disk diffusion test. *New Microbiologica 36*: 289–302.

77 Indurkar MS, Verma R (2016) Effect of ozonated oil and chlorhexidine gel on plaque induced gingivitis: a randomized control clinical trial. *J Indian Soc Periodontol 20*(1): 32–35.

78 Goldberg M, Grootveld M, Lynch E (2010) Undesirable and adverse effects of tooth-whitening products: a review. *Clin Oral Invest 14*: 1–10.

79 DeMoor RJG, Verheyen J, Diachuk A, Verheyen P, *et al*. (2015) Insight in the chemistry of laser-activated dental bleaching. *The Scientific World Journal 2015*: 650492.

80 Ibid.

81 Tam L (1999) The safety of home bleaching techniques. *J Can Dent Assoc 65*: 453–455. Available at www.cda-adc.ca/jcda/vol-65/issue-8/453.html, accessed 7 March 2020.

82 Wu TT, Li LF, Du R, Jiang L, Zhu YQ (2013) Hydrogen peroxide induces apoptosis in human dental pulp cells via caspase-9 dependent pathway. *J Endod 39*(9): 1151–1155.

83 American Dental Association (2009/2010) Tooth Whitening/Bleaching: Treatment Considerations for Dentists and Their Patients, revised November 2010. Available at https://www.ada.org/~/media/ADA/About%20the%20ADA/Files/whitening_bleaching_treatment_considrations_for_patients_and_dentists.ashx, accessed 27 August 2021.

84 Greenwall L (2008) The dangers of chlorine dioxide tooth bleaching. *Aesthetic 2*(4): 20–22.

85 Ibid.

86 Basting RT, Rodrigues AL, Serra MC (2005) The effect of 10% carbamide peroxide, carbopol and/or glycerin on enamel and dentin microhardness. *Operative Dentistry 30*(5): 608–616.

87 World Health Organization (2019) WHO Model List of Essential Medicines, 21st List. Available at www.who.int/groups/expert-committee-on-selection-and-use-of-essential-medicines/essential-medicines-lists, accessed 1 June 2021.

88 Soto P (undated) Chlorhexidine Adverse Effects. Available at www.poison.org/articles/chlorhexidine-adverse-effects-172, accessed 10 June 2019.

89 Reichman DE, Greenberg JA (2009) Reducing surgical site infections: a review. *Reviews in Obstetrics & Gynecology* 2(4): 212–221.
90 James P, Worthington HV, Parnell C, Harding M, *et al.* (2017) Chlorhexidine mouthrinse as an adjunctive treatment for gingival health. *Cochrane Database Syst Rev* 31(3): CD008676.
91 Ibid.
92 Netdoctor (2017) Corsodyl Mouthwash (Chlorhexidine). Available at www.netdoctor.co.uk/medicines/mouth-teeth/a8092/corsodyl-mouthwash-chlorhexidine, accessed 10 June 2019.
93 Ibid.
94 Kolahi J, Soolari A (2006) Rinsing with chlorhexidine gluconate solution after brushing and flossing teeth: a systematic review of effectiveness. *Quintessence Int* 37(8): 605–612.
95 James P, Worthington HV, Parnell C, Harding M, *et al.* (2017) Chlorhexidine mouthrinse as an adjunctive treatment for gingival health. *Cochrane Database Syst Rev* 31(3): CD008676.
96 Netdoctor (2017) Corsodyl Mouthwash (Chlorhexidine). Available at www.netdoctor.co.uk/medicines/mouth-teeth/a8092/corsodyl-mouthwash-chlorhexidine, accessed 10 June 2019.
97 Seth S (2011) Glass ionomer cement and resin-based fissure sealants are equally effective in caries prevention. *JADA* 142(5): 551–552.
98 DeNoon DJ (2010) BPA from Dental Sealants, Fillings: Is It Safe? Available at www.webmd.com/oral-health/news/20100907/bpa-from-dental-sealants-fillings-is-it-safe, accessed 12 June 2019.
99 Olea N, Pulgar R, Pérez P, Olea-Serrano F, *et al.* (1996) Estrogenicity of resin-based composites and sealants used in dentistry. *Environ Health Perspect* 104: 298–305.
100 Joskow R, Barr DB, Barr JR, Calafat AM, Needham LL, Rubin C (2006) Exposure to bisphenol A from bis-glycidyl dimethacrylate-based dental sealants. *The Journal of the American Dental Association* 137(3): 353–362.
101 Rathee M, Malik P, Singh J (2012) Bisphenol A in dental sealants and its estrogen like effect. *Indian J Endocrinol Metab* 16(3): 339–342.
102 Fleisch AF, Sheffield PE, Chinn C, Edelstein BL, Landrigan PJ (2010) Bisphenol A and related compounds in dental materials. *Pediatrics* 126(4): 760–768.
103 DeNoon DJ (2010) BPA from Dental Sealants, Fillings: Is It Safe? Available at www.webmd.com/oral-health/news/20100907/bpa-from-dental-sealants-fillings-is-it-safe, accessed 12 June 2019.
104 Clayton EMR, Todd M, Dowd JB, Aiello AE (2011) The impact of bisphenol A and triclosan on immune parameters in the U.S. population, NHANES 2003–2006. *Environ Health Perspect* 119: 390–396.
105 Hiiri A, Ahovuo-Saloranta A, Nordblad A, Mäkelä M (2010) Pit and fissure sealants versus fluoride varnishes for preventing dental decay in children and adolescents. *Cochrane Database of Systematic Reviews* 3: CD003067.
106 Marinho VCC, Worthington HV, Walsh T, Clarkson JE (2013) Fluoride varnishes for preventing dental caries in children and adolescents. *Cochrane Database of Systematic Reviews* 7: CD002279.

CHAPTER 17

1 Mummolo S, Nota A, Caruso S, Quinzi V, Marchetti E, Marzo G (2018) Salivary markers and microbial flora in mouth breathing late adolescents. *BioMed Res Internat 2018*: 8687608.
2 Weiler RME, Fisberg M, Barroso AS, Nicolau J, Simi R, Siqueira WL (2006) A study of the influence of mouth-breathing in some parameters of unstimulated and stimulated whole saliva of adolescents. *International Journal of Pediatric Otorhinolaryngology* 70: 799–805.
3 Triana CBEG, Ali AH, León CyIBG (2016) Mouth breathing and its relationship to some oral and medical conditions: physiopathological mechanisms involved. *Revista Habanera de Ciencias Médicas* 15(2): 200–212.
4 Chiego DJ (2018) *Essentials of Oral Histology and Embryology E-Book: A Clinical Approach*. St Louis, MO: Elsevier Health Sciences, p.170.
5 Foutsizoglou S (2017) Anatomy of the ageing lip. *PFMA Journal* 4(2).
6 Jemmott JB 3rd, Borysenko JZ, Borysenko M, McClelland DC, *et al.* (1983) Academic stress, power motivation, and decrease in secretion rate of salivary secretory immunoglobulin A. *Lancet* 1(8339): 1400–1402.
7 Herbert TB, Cohen S (1993) Stress and immunity in humans: a meta-analytic review. *Psychosomatic Medicine* 55: 364–379.
8 Gleeson M (2000) Mucosal immunity and respiratory illness in elite athletes. *Int J Sports Med* 21(suppl. 1): S33–43.
9 DeBusk RM, Radler DR (2005) CAM and Oral Health. In: R Touger-Decker, DA Sirois, CC Mobley (eds) *Nutrition and Oral Medicine*. Totowa, NJ: Humana Press.
10 Ibid.

11. Imbeau J (2007) Osteoporosis and osteonecrosis of the jaws: an underestimated problem with multiple ramifications. *The New Zealand Charter Journal 2007* (summer): 14–35. Available at http://dr-jacques-imbeau.com/PDF/NZHCJ%20Part%202.pdf, accessed 25 October 2019.
12. Cheng A, Daly CG, Logan RM, Stein B, Goss AN (2009) Alveolar bone and the bisphosphonates. *Australian Dental Journal 54*(1 suppl.): S51–S61.
13. Ross R (2018) Facts about Fluorine. Available at www.livescience.com/28779-fluorine.html, accessed 19 January 2019.
14. 3M (2018) Scotchgard™ Fabric Protector (Cat. No. 4101, 4106) Safety Data Sheet. Available at https://multimedia.3m.com/mws/mediawebserver?mwsId=SSSSSuUn_zu8l00xMx_14x2GOv70k17zHvu9lxtD7SSSSSS--, accessed 23 January 2019.
15. O Ecotextiles (2010) What about Soil Resistant Finishes Like Scotchgard, GoreTex, NanoTex and GreenShield – Are They Safe? Available at https://oecotextiles.wordpress.com/2010/02/10/what-about-soil-resistant-finishes-like-scotchgard-goretex-nanotex-and-greenshield-are-they-safe, accessed 23 January 2019.
16. Fluoride Action Network (undated) Pharmaceuticals. Available at https://fluoridealert.org/issues/sources/pharmaceuticals, accessed 23 January 2019.
17. Pradhan KM, Arora NK, Jena A, Susheela AK, Bhan MK (1995) Safety of ciprofloxacin therapy in children: magnetic resonance images, body fluid levels of fluoride and linear growth. *Acta Paediatr 84*(5): 555–560.
18. Hoemberg M, Vierzig A, Roth B, Eifinger F (2012) Plasma fluoride concentrations during prolonged administration of isoflurane to a pediatric patient requiring renal replacement therapy. *Pediatric Anesthesia 22*(4): 412–413. As cited in: Fluoride Action Network (undated) Pharmaceuticals. Available at https://fluoridealert.org/issues/sources/pharmaceuticals, accessed 23 January 2019.
19. Oc B, Akinci SB, Kanbak M, Satana E, Celebioglu B, Aypar U (2012) The effects of sevoflurane anesthesia and cardiopulmonary bypass on renal function in cyanotic and acyanotic children undergoing cardiac surgery. *Renal Failure 24*(2): 135–141.
20. Baliga D, Muglikar S, Kale R (2013) Salivary pH: a diagnostic biomarker. *J Indian Soc Periodontol 17*(4): 461–465.
21. Sciencedaily (2009) Exposure to Alkaline Substances Can Result in Damaged Teeth. Available at www.sciencedaily.com/releases/2009/10/091027132424.htm, accessed 10 February 2020.
22. Taube F, Ylmén R, Shchukarev A, Nietzsche S, Norén JG (2010) Morphological and chemical characterization of tooth enamel exposed to alkaline agents. *Journal of Dentistry 38*(1): 72–81.
23. Shekarchizadeh H, Khami MR, Mohebbi SZ, Ekhtiari H, Virtanen JI (2013) Oral health of drug abusers: a review of health effects and care. *Iranian J Publ Health 42*(9): 929–940.
24. Turkyilmaz I (2010) Oral manifestations of 'meth mouth': a case report. *The Journal of Contemporary Dental Practice 11*(1): E073–E080.
25. Jackson D, Murray JJ, Fairpro CG (1973) Lifelong benefits of fluoride in drinking water. *British Dental Journal 134*(10): 419–422. As cited in: JJ Murray (ed.) (1986) *Appropriate Use of Fluorides for Human Health*. World Health Organization. Available at https://apps.who.int/iris/handle/10665/39103, accessed 3 January 2019.
26. Fluoride Action Network (2012) Medical Ethics. Available at https://fluoridealert.org/issues/water/medical-ethics, accessed 28 August 2020.
27. Fukayama H, Nasu M, Murakami S, Sugawara M (1992) Examination of antithyroid effects of smoking products in cultured thyroid follicles: only thiocyanate is a potent antithyroid agent. *Acta Endocrinol (Copenh) 127*(6): 520–525.
28. Winkler S, Garg AK, Mekayarajjananonth T, Bakaeen LG, Khan E (1999) Depressed taste and smell in geriatric patients. *J Am Dent Assoc 130*(12): 1759–1765.
29. Lie MA, Loos BG, Henskens YMC, Timmerman MF, et al. (2001) Salivary cystatin activity and cystatin C in natural and experimental gingivitis in smokers and non-smokers. *Journal of Clinical Periodontology 28*(10): 979–984.
30. Mussap M, Plebani M (2004) Biochemistry and clinical role of human cystatin C. *Critical Reviews in Clinical Laboratory Sciences 41*(5–6): 467–550.
31. Okada HC, Alleyne B, Barghai K, Kinder K, Guyuron B (2013) Facial changes caused by smoking: a comparison between smoking and non-smoking identical twins. *Plast Reconstr Surg 132*(5): 1085–1092.
32. Ali MJ, Ende K, Maas CS (2007) Perioral rejuvenation and lip augmentation. *Facial Plastic Surgery Clinics of North America 15*: 491–500.
33. Yagi T, Ueda H, Amitani H, Asakawa A, Myawaki S, Inui A (2012) The role of ghrelin, salivary secretions, and dental care in eating disorders. *Nutrients 4*: 967–989.
34. Ohta K, Laborde NJ, Kajiya M, Shin J, et al. (2011) Expression and possible immune-regulatory function of ghrelin in oral epithelium. *J Dent Res 90*(11): 1286–1292.
35. Moravec LJ, Boyd LD (2011) Bariatric surgery and implications for oral health: a case report. *The Journal of Dental Hygiene 85*: 166–176.

CHAPTER 18

1. Tiwari M (2011) Science behind human saliva. *J Nat Sci Biol Med* 2(1): 53–58.
2. Greabu M, Battino M, Mohora M, Totan A, *et al.* (2009) Saliva – a diagnostic window to the body, both in health and in disease. *Journal of Medicine and Life* 2(2): 124–132.
3. Gordon BL (1945) *The Romance of Medicine. The Story of the Evolution of Medicine from Occult Practices and Primitive Times*. Philadelphia: Davis Co. As cited in: Brandtzaet P (2013) Secretory immunity with special reference to the oral cavity. *Journal of Oral Microbiology* 5: 20401.
4. Lima DP, Diniz DG, Moimaz SAS, Sumida DH, Okamoto AC (2010) Saliva: reflection of the body. *International Journal of Infectious Diseases* 14: e184–e188.
5. Aps JKM, Martens LC (2005) Review: the physiology of saliva and transfer of drugs into saliva. *Forensic Science International* 150: 119–131.
6. Bandhakavi S, Stone D, Onsongo G, VanRiper SK, Griffin TJ (2009) A dynamic range compression and three-dimensional peptide fractionation analysis platform expands proteome coverage and the diagnostic potential of whole saliva. *J Proteome Res* 8(12): 5590–5600.
7. Lima DP, Diniz DG, Moimaz SAS, Sumida DH, Okamoto AC (2010) Saliva: reflection of the body. *International Journal of Infectious Diseases* 14: e184–e188.
8. Huang Y, Xu C, He M, Huang W, Wu K (2020) Saliva cortisol, melatonin levels and circadian rhythm alterations in Chinese primary school children with dyslexia. *Medicine (Baltimore)* 99(6): e19098.
9. Greabu M, Battino M, Mohora M, Totan A, *et al.* (2009) Saliva – a diagnostic window to the body, both in health and in disease. *Journal of Medicine and Life* 2(2): 124–132.
10. Ibid.
11. Ibid.
12. Ibid.
13. American Dental Association (2019) Oral Health Topics: Genetics and Oral Health. Available at www.ada.org/en/member-center/oral-health-topics/genetics-and-oral-health?source=VanityURL, accessed 11 August 2019.
14. Ibid.
15. Nibali L, Dilorio A, Tu Y-K, Vieira AR (2017) Host genetics role in the pathogenesis of periodontal disease and caries. *J Clin Periodontol* 44(suppl. 18): S52–S78.
16. DeVries TJ, Andreotta S, Loos BG, Nicu EA (2017) Genes critical for developing periodontitis: lessons from mouse models. *Front Immunol* 8: 1395.
17. American Dental Association (2019) Oral Health Topics: Genetics and Oral Health. Available at www.ada.org/en/member-center/oral-health-topics/genetics-and-oral-health?source=VanityURL, accessed 11 August 2019.
18. Nibali L, Dilorio A, Tu Y-K, Vieira AR (2017) Host genetics role in the pathogenesis of periodontal disease and caries. *J Clin Periodontol* 44(suppl. 18): S52–S78.
19. Adler CJ, Dobney K, Weyrich LS, Kaidonis J, *et al.* (2013) Sequencing ancient calcified dental plaque shows changes in oral microbiota with dietary shifts of the Neolithic and Industrial revolutions. *Nat Genet* 45(4): 450–455.
20. Costalonga M, Herzberg MC (2014) The oral microbiome and the immunobiology of periodontal disease and caries. *Immunology Letters* 162: 22–38.
21. Aufderheide AC, Rodriguez-Martin C, Langsjoen O (1998) *The Cambridge Encyclopedia of Human Paleopathology*. Cambridge: Cambridge University Press. As cited in: Adler CJ, Dobney K, Weyrich LS, Kaidonis J, *et al.* (2013) Sequencing ancient calcified dental plaque shows changes in oral microbiota with dietary shifts of the Neolithic and Industrial revolutions. *Nat Genet* 45(4): 450–455.
22. Adler CJ, Dobney K, Weyrich LS, Kaidonis J, *et al.* (2013) Sequencing ancient calcified dental plaque shows changes in oral microbiota with dietary shifts of the Neolithic and Industrial revolutions. *Nat Genet* 45(4): 450–455.
23. Costalonga M, Herzberg MC (2014) The oral microbiome and the immunobiology of periodontal disease and caries. *Immunology Letters* 162: 22–38.
24. Cadotte MW, Dinnage R, Tilman D (2012) Phylogenetic diversity promotes ecosystem stability. *Ecology* 93: S223–S233.
25. Petchey O, Gaston K (2009) Effects on ecosystem resilience of biodiversity, extinctions, and the structure of regional species pools. *Theoretical Ecology* 2: 177–187.
26. Loreau M, Downing A, Emmerson M, Gonzalez A, *et al.* (2002) A New Look at the Relationship between Diversity and Stability. In M Loreau, S Naeem, P Inchausti (eds) *Biodiversity and Ecosystem Functioning: Synthesis and Perspectives*. Oxford: Oxford University Press, pp.79–91. As cited in: Adler CJ, Dobney K, Weyrich LS, Kaidonis J, *et al.* (2013) Sequencing ancient calcified dental plaque shows changes in oral microbiota with dietary shifts of the Neolithic and Industrial revolutions. *Nat Genet* 45(4): 450–455.
27. Cadotte MW, Dinnage R, Tilman D (2012) Phylogentic diversity promotes ecosystem stability. *Ecology* 93(suppl. 8): S223–S233.

28. Brogden KA, Guthmiller JM (2002) Polymicrobial Diseases: Current and Future Research. In: KA Brogden, JM Guthmiller (eds) *Polymicrobial Diseases*. Washington, DC: ASM Press, Chapter 21. Available at www.ncbi.nlm.nih.gov/books/NBK2490, accessed 5 April 2019.
29. Kleinberg I (2002) A mixed-bacteria ecological approach to understanding the role of the oral bacteria in dental caries causation: an alternative to Streptococcus mutans and the specific-plaque hypothesis. *Crit Rev Oral Biol Med* 13(2): 108–125.
30. Hajishengallis G, Lamont RJ (2012) Beyond the red complex and into more complexity: the polymicrobial synergy and dysbiosis (PSD) model of periodontal disease etiology. *Mol Oral Microbiol* 27(6): 409–419.
31. Costalonga M, Herzberg MC (2014) The oral microbiome and the immunobiology of periodontal disease and caries. *Immunology Letters* 162: 22–38.
32. Baker JL, Edlund A (2019) Exploiting the oral microbiome to prevent tooth decay: has evolution already provided the best tools? *Front Microbiol* 9: 3323.
33. Ibid.
34. Kilian M, Chapple ILC, Hannig M, Marsh PD, *et al.* (2016) The oral microbiome – an update for oral healthcare professionals. *British Dental Journal* 221(10): 657–666.
35. Jorth P, Turner KH, Gumus P, Nizam N, Buduneli N, Whiteley M (2014) Metatranscriptomics of the human oral microbiome during health and disease. *mBio* 5(2): e01012–01014.
36. Zaura E, Keijser BJF, Huse SM, Crielaard W (2009) Defining the healthy 'core microbiome' of oral microbial communities. *BMC Microbiology* 9: 259.
37. Dethlefsen L, McFall-Ngai M, Relman DA (2007) An ecological and evolutionary perspective on human–microbe mutualism and disease. *Nature* 449: 811–818.
38. Turnbaugh PJ, Ley RE, Hamady M, Fraser-Liggett CM, Knight R, Gordon JI (2007) The human microbiome project: a strategy to understand the microbial components of the human genetic and metabolic landscape and how they contribute to normal physiology and predisposition to disease. *Nature* 449: 804–810.
39. Zarco MF, Vess TH, Ginsburg GS (2012) The oral microbiome in health and disease and the potential impact on personalized dental medicine. *Oral Diseases* 18: 109–120.
40. Sonnenburg JL, Fischbach MA (2011) Community health care: therapeutic opportunities in the human microbiome. *Sci Transl Med* 3(78): 1–5.
41. Dewhirst FE, Chen T, Izard J, Paster BJ, *et al.* (2010) The human oral microbiome. *J Bacteriol* 192: 5002–5017.
42. Palmer RJ Jn (2014) Composition and development of oral bacterial communities. *Periodontol 2000* 64(1): 20–39.
43. Wade WG (2013) The oral microbiome in health and disease. *Pharmacological Research* 69: 137–143.
44. Takahashi N, Nyvad B (2011) The role of bacteria in the caries process: ecological perspectives. *J Dent Res* 90(3): 294–303.
45. Guinesi AS, Andolfatto C, Bonetti Fiho I, Cardoso AA, Passaretti Filho J, Farac RV (2011) Ozonized oils: a qualitative and quantitative analysis. *Braz Dent J* 22(1): 37–40.
46. Captain J (2018) Ozonated water, ozonated oil and its products. Proceedings of the 5th WFOT Meeting, 18–20 November 2016, Mumbai, India. *J of Ozone Therapy* 2(2): 1/3.
47. Gandhi KK, Cappetta EG, Pavaskar R (2019) Effectiveness of the adjunctive use of ozone and chlorhexidine in patients with chronic periodontitis. *DBJ Open* 5: 17.
48. Pietrocola G, Ceci M, Preda F, Poggio C, Colombo M (2018) Evaluation of the antibacterial activity of a new ozonized olive oil against oral and periodontal pathogens. *J Clin Exp Dent* 10(11): e1103–e1108.
49. Gupta S, Deepa D (2016) Applications of ozone therapy in dentistry. *J Oral Res Rev* 8: 86–91.
50. Sakamoto M, Umeda M, Benno Y (2005) Molecular analysis of human oral microbiota. *J Periodont Res* 40: 277–285.
51. Cross BW, Ruhl S (2018) Glycan recognition at the saliva–oral microbiome interface. *Cellular Immunology* 333: 19–33.
52. Gilca M, Dragos D (2017) Extraoral taste receptor discovery: new light on Ayurvedic pharmacology. *Evidence-Based Complementary and Alternative Medicine 2017*: 5435831.
53. Neyraud E, Palicki O, Schwartz C, Nicklaus S, Feron G (2012) Variability of human saliva composition: possible relationships with fat perception and liking. *Archives of Oral Biology* 57: 556–566.
54. Stewart JE, Feinle-Bisset C, Golding M, Delahunty C, Clifton PM, Keast RSJ (2010) Oral sensitivity to fatty acids, food consumption and BMI in human subjects. *British Journal of Nutrition* 104: 145–152.
55. Voigt N, Stein J, Galindo MM, Dunkel A, *et al.* (2014) The role of lipolysis in human orosensory fat perception. *Journal of Lipid Research* 55: 870–882.
56. Bachmanov AA, Beauchamp GK (2007) Taste receptor genes. *Annu Rev Nutr* 27: 389–414.

57. Tepper BJ, Nurse RJ (1997) Fat perception is related to PROP taster status. *Physiology & Behavior* 61(6): 949–954.
58. Keast RSJ, Costanzo A (2015) Is fat the sixth taste primary? Evidence and implications. *Flavour* 4: 5.
59. Gilbertson TA, Baquero AF, Spray-Watson KJ (2006) Water taste: the importance of osmotic sensing in the oral cavity. *Journal of Water and Health* 4(suppl. 1): 35–40.
60. Hamzelou J (2016) There is now a sixth taste – and it explains why we love carbs. *New Scientist*, 2 Sept 2016. Available at www.newscientist.com/article/2104244-there-is-now-a-sixth-taste-and-it-explains-why-we-love-carbs, accessed 29 July 2018.
61. Lapis TJ, Penner MH, Lim J (2016) Humans can taste glucose oligomers independent of the hT1R2/hT1R3 sweet taste receptor. *Chemical Senses* 41(9): 755–762.
62. Wenner M (2008) Like the taste of chalk? You're in luck – humans may be able to taste calcium. *Scientific American*, 20 August 2008. Available at www.scientificamerican.com/article/osteoporosis-calcium-taste-chalk, accessed 29 July 2018.
63. Ohsu T, Takeshita S, Eto Y, Amino Y, et al. (2012) Kokumi-imparting agent. US Patent no US 8,173,605,B2. 8 May 2012.
64. American Chemical Society (2008) That tastes...sweet? Sour? No, it's definitiely calcium!' *ScienceDaily*, 21 August 2008. Available at www.sciencedaily.com/releases/2008/08/080820163008.htm, accessed 29 July 2018.
65. Tordoff MG, Shao H, Alarcón LK, Margolskee RF, et al. (2008) Involvement of T1R3 in calcium-magnesium taste. *Physiol Genomics* 34: 338–348.
66. Tordoff MG, Alarcón LK, Valmeki S, Jiang P (2012) T1R3: a human calcium taste receptor. *Scientific Reports* 2: 496.
67. Ward BK, Magno AL, Walsh JP, Ratajczak T (2012) The role of calcium-sensing receptor in human disease. *Clinical Biochemistry* 45(12): 943–953.
68. Brennan SC, Davies TS, Schepelmann M, Riccardi D (2014) Emerging roles of the extra-cellular calcium-sensing receptor in nutrient sensing: control of taste modulation and intestinal hormone secretion. *Br J Nutr* 111 (Suppl.1): S16–S22.
69. Ward BK, Magno AL, Walsh JP, Ratajczak T (2012) The role of calcium-sensing receptor in human disease. *Clinical Biochemistry* 45(12): 943–953.
70. Brennan SC, Davies TS, Schepelmann M, Riccardi D (2014) Emerging roles of the extra-cellular calcium-sensing receptor in nutrient sensing: control of taste modulation and intestinal hormone secretion. *Br J Nutr* 111(suppl. 1): S16–S22.
71. Ohsu T, Takeshita S, Eto Y, Amino Y, et al. (2012) Kokumi-imparting agent. US Patent no US 8,173,605,B2. 8 May 2012.
72. Hettiarachchy NS, Sato K, Marshall MR, Kannan A (eds) (2012) *Food Proteins and Peptides: Chemistry, Functionality, Interactions and Commercialization*. Boca Raton, FL: CRC Press.
73. Ohsu T, Takeshita S, Eto Y, Amino Y, et al. (2012) Kokumi-imparting agent. US Patent no US 8,173,605,B2. 8 May 2012.
74. Hettiarachchy NS, Sato K, Marshall MR, Kannan A (eds) (2012) *Food Proteins and Peptides: Chemistry, Functionality, Interactions and Commercialization*. Boca Raton, FL: CRC Press.
75. San Gabriel AM (2015) Taste receptors in the gastrointestinal system. *Flavour* 4: 14.
76. Ibid.
77. Shepherd GM (2012) *Neurogastronomy: How the Brain Creates Flavor and Why It Matters*. New York: Columbia University Press, p.110.
78. Ibid. p.30.

CHAPTER 19

1. Nazir MA (2017) Prevalence of periodontal disease, its association with systemic diseases and prevention. *International Journal of Health Science* 1(2): 72–80.
2. Sanz M, D'Aiuto F, Deanfield J, Fernandez-Avilés F (2010) European workshop in periodontal health and cardiovascular disease–scientific evidence on the association between periodontal and cardiovascular diseases: a review of the literature. *Eur Heart J Suppl* 12(suppl. B): B3–B12.
3. Dsouza SR, Ramesh A, Thomas B (2013) Risk factors of periodontal disease. *Journal of the Society of Periodontitists and Implantologists of Keral* 7(1): 8–10.
4. Ellis JS, Seymour RA, Steele JG, Robertson P, Butler TJ, Thomaso JM (1999) Prevalence of gingival overgrowth induced by calcium channel blockers: a community-based study. *J Periodontol* 70(1): 63–67.
5. Dsouza SR, Ramesh A, Thomas B (2013) Risk factors of periodontal disease. *Journal of the Society of Periodontitists and Implantologists of Keral* 7(1): 8–10.
6. Bartold PM, VanDyke TE (2013) Periodontitis: a host-mediated disruption of microbial homeostasis. Unlearning learned concepts. *Periodontol 2000* 62(1): 203–217.

APPENDIX 1

1. UK National Health Service (undated) Dental Care and Water Fluoridation. Available www.england.nhs.uk/ltphimenu/better-care-for-health-conditions-for-dental-healthcare/dental-care-and-water-fluoridation, accessed 2 June 2021.
2. Fluoride Action Network (undated) Top 10 Ways to Reduce Fluoride Exposure. Available at https://fluoridealert.org/content/top_ten, accessed 2 June 2021.
3. Götzfried F (2006) Legal aspects of fluoride in salt, particularly within the EU. *Schweiz Monatsschr Zahnmed 16*: 371–375.
4. H2O Labs (undated) Does Distilled Water Remove Fluoride? Available at www.h2olabs.com/t-does-distilled-water-remove-flouride.aspx#:~:text=Distilled%20water%20never%20contains%20fluoride,just%20about%20anything%20from%20water, accessed 4 May 2019.
5. Cade N (2021) When two tides go to war: Purified vs. distilled water. Available at https://greatist.com/health/purified-vs-distilled-water, accessed 2 June 2021.
6. Mercola J, Osmunson B (2011) A Special Interview with Dr Bill Osmunson (transcript) as part of Fluoride: The Toxic Import from China Hidden in This Everyday Beverage. Available at https://articles.mercola.com/sites/articles/archive/2011/10/11/dr-bill-osmunson-on-fluoride.aspx, accessed 20 January 2019.
7. Ibid.
8. Ibid.
9. Kohn WG, Maas WR, Malvitz DM, Presson SM, Shaddik KK (2001) Centers for Disease Control and Prevention: Recommendations for Using Fluoride to Prevent and Control Dental Caries in the United States. Morbidity and Mortality Weekly Report: Recommendations and Reports 50(RR-14). Available at www.cdc.gov/mmwr/preview/mmwrhtml/rr5014a1.htm, accessed 1 June 2019.
10. Jørgensen J, Shariati M, Shields CP, Durr DP, Proskin HM (1989) Fluoride uptake into demineralized primary enamel from fluoride-impregnated dental floss in vitro. *Pediatr Dent 11*(1): 17–20.
11. IAOMT (2017) Sources of Fluoride Exposure. Available at https://files.iaomt.org/wp-content/uploads/IAOMT-Sources-of-Fluoride-Exposure-Chart.pdf, accessed 1 June 2019.

APPENDIX 2

1. US Centers for Disease Control and Prevention (2013) Periodontal Disease. Available at www.cdc.gov/oralhealth/conditions/periodontal-disease.html, accessed 7 February 2018.
2. Ibid.

APPENDIX 3

1. Lippert F (2013) An Introduction to Toothpaste – Its Purpose, History and Ingredients. In: van-Loveren C (ed.) *Monogr Oral Sci 23*, 1–14.
2. ADA Seal of Acceptance. Available at https://www.ada.org/en/member-center/oral-health-topics/toothpastes#:~:text=All%20toothpastes%20with%20the%20ADA,enamel%20erosion%20or%20bad%20breath, accessed 29 September 2021.
3. Burt BA (2006) The use of sorbitol- and xylitol-sweetened chewing gum in caries control. *JADA 137*: 190–196.

GLOSSARY AND ABBREVIATIONS

1. Rickard AH, Gilbert P, High NJ, Kolenbrander PE, Handley PS (2003) Bacterial coaggregation: an integral process in the development of multi-species biofilms. *Trends Microbiol 11*(2): 94–100.
2. San Gabriel A, Uneyama H, Maekawa T, Torii K (2009) The calcium-sensing receptor in taste tissue. *Biochemical and Biophysical Research Communications 378*: 414–418.

3. Asea A, Kabingu E, Stevenson MA, Calderwood SK (2000) HSP70 peptide-bearing and peptide-negative preparations act as chaperokines. *Cell Stress & Chaperones* 6(5): 425–431.
4. Wolff MS, Larson C (2009) The cariogenic dental biofilm: good, bad or just something to control? *Braz Oral Res* 23(Special Issue 1): 31–38.
5. Liu L, Hansen DR, Kim I, Gilbertson TA (2005) Expression and characterization of delayed rectifying K+ channels in anterior rat taste buds. *Am J Physiol Cell Physiol* 289(4): C868–880.
6. Jamshidi N, Taylor DA (2001) Anandamide administration into the ventromedial hypothalamus stimulates appetite in rats. *Br J Pharmacol* 134: 1151–1154.
7. Tortora GJ, Derrickson B (2007) *Principles of Anatomy and Physiology* (11th edn). Hoboken, NJ: John Wiley & Sons, p.906.
8. Jain K, Parida S, Mangwani N, Dash HR, Das S (2013) Isolation and characterization of biofilm-forming bacteria and associated extracellular polymeric substances from oral cavity. *Ann Microbiol* 63: 1553–1562.
9. Flemming H-C, Wingender J (2010) The biofilm matrix. *Nature Reviews Microbiology* 8: 623–633.
10. Suri L, Gagari E, Vastardis H (2004) Delayed tooth eruption: pathogenesis, diagnosis, and treatment. A literature review. *Am J Orthod Dentofacial Orthop* 12: 432–445.
11. McLaughlin SK, McKinnon PJ, Margolskee RF (1992) Gustducin is a taste-cell-specific G protein closely related to the transducins. *Nature* 357: 563–569.
12. Suri L, Gagari E, Vastardis H (2004) Delayed tooth eruption: pathogenesis, diagnosis, and treatment. A literature review. *Am J Orthod Dentofacial Orthop* 12: 432–445.
13. Wilson MM, Bernstein HD (2016) Surface-exposed lipoproteins: an emerging secretion phenomenon in gram-negative bacteria. *Trends in Microbiology* 24(3): 198–208.
14. Dawes C, Pedersen AML, Villa A, Ekström J, et al. (2015) The functions of human saliva: a review sponsored by the World Workshop on Oral Medicine VI. *Archives of Oral Biology* 60: 863–874.
15. Tabak LA, Levine MJ, Mandel ID, Ellison SA (1982) Role of salivary mucins in the protection of the oral cavity. *J Oral Pathol* 11(1): 1–17.
16. Tortora GJ, Derrickson B (2007) *Principles of Anatomy and Physiology* (11th edn). Hoboken, NJ: John Wiley & Sons, p.906.
17. Ibid.
18. O Ecotextiles (2010) What About Soil Resistant Finishes Like Scotchgard, GoreTex, NanoTex and GreenShield – Are They Safe? Available at https://oecotextiles.wordpress.com/2010/02/10/what-about-soil-resistant-finishes-like-scotchgard-goretex-nanotex-and-greenshield-are-they-safe, accessed 23 January 2019.
19. Anders JJ (2016) Photobiomodulation. Available at www.aslms.org/for-the-public/treatments-using-lasers-and-energy-based-devices/photobiomodulation, accessed 26 October 2019.
20. Fluoride Action Network (undated) The Basics of Regulatory Toxicology: Protecting the Public from Harmful Substances. Available at www.fluoridealert.org/content/bulletin_12-14-13, accessed 23 January 2019.
21. Shiel WC (undated) Medical Definition of PYY. Available at www.medicinenet.com/script/main/art.asp?articlekey=24203, accessed 27 October 2019.
22. Levy JA (2009) The unexpected pleiotropic activities of RANTES. *Journal of Immunology* 182(7): 3945–3946.
23. Mayo Clinic (2017) Sjogren's Syndrome. Available at www.mayoclinic.org, accessed 24 February 2019.
24. Merriam-Webster (undated) Definition of Tartar. Available at www.merriam-webster.com/dictionary/tartar, accessed 16 June 2019.
25. Busch M, Dünker N (2015) Trefoil factor family peptides – friends or foes? *BioMol Concepts* 6(5–6): 343–359.
26. Bouquot JE, Roberts AM, Person P, Christian J (1992) Neuralgia-inducing cavitational osteonecrosis (NICO). *Oral Surg Oral Med Oral Pathol* 73: 307–319.
27. Bautista DM, Movahed P, Hinman A, Axelsson HE, et al. (2005) Pungent products from garlic activate the sensory ion channel TRPA1. *PNAS* 102(34): 12248–12252.
28. Johansen JS, Jensen BV, Roslind A, Nielsen D, Price PA (2006) Serum YKL-40, a new prognostic biomarker in cancer patients? *Cancer Epidemiol Biomarkers Prev* 15(2): 194–202.

Subject Index

Note: page numbers given in **bold** indicate major mentions

abrasives 128, 129, 136-7, 209
abscesses **81-2**, 83, 84, 86, 140, 159, 207
ACE-inhibitors 75
acesulfame potassium (acesulfame K) 48
Achillea millefolium 165
acidogenic bacteria 15, 54, 55, 153
acid reflux 81, 152, 153
acid-tolerant bacteria 55, 193
acini 108
Actinobacillus actinomycetemcomitans 58, 150
activated charcoal 89, **127-8**, 129, 165
acupuncture 11, 121, 122, 184
addictive behaviours 43, 116, 117, 144, 160
addictive substances **117**, 118
adjunctive therapies **122**, 123
adsorption 127
advanced glycation end-products (AGEs) 43, **63-4**, 65, 94-5, 109, 145, 160
agave syrup 50, 145
age
    hyaluronic acid changes 158
    and innate immunity 93
    life stages 107-10
    lip changes 110-11
    middle age conditions 77, 78, 79, 86, 109-10
    older age 18, **108-9**, 110-11, 112, 163, 200
    and oral health 17-18
    smell perception 19, 112
    taste perception 112
    teeth and bones as indicators of 17
    telomere length 111
ageusia 90
agglutinin 24, 27
Aggregatibacter actinomycetemcomitans 58, 104
alcohol 37, 39, 81, 82, 83, 84, 86, 90, 117, **135**, 136, 151, 177, 187, 190, 199, 211
    see also sugar alcohols
aldosterone 190
alkaline diet 185, 196
alkaline water 148
alkalinity 22, 39, 194, 196
Aloe vera 51, 140, 150, 155, 159, 165, 184

alpha 1-acid glycoprotein (AGP) *see* orosomucoid
alpha-lipoic acid 160, 165
alveolar bone 56, 57, 64, 95, 97, 100, 111, 140, 155, 158, 199
Alzheimer's disease 90, 103, 112, 168, 196, 197
amalgam fillings *see* mercury amalgam fillings
amalgam tattoo 80
amelogenin 190
American Academy of Environmental Medicine (AAEM) 213
American Dental Association (ADA) 213
amino acids 34, 59, 63, 64, 118, 196
amla (*Emblica officinalis*) 159
Amla (sour taste) 194
ammonium fluoride 159
analgesic effect 122, 158
analgesics 112, **155**
Andrographis paniculata 68, 74, 165
angiogenesis 66, 97
angiotensin II receptor blockers 75
aniseed (*Pimpinella anisum*) essential oil 139, 164
anise seed 156
anorexia nervosa 117, 187
antibacterials 21, 47, 48, 65, 111, 126, 127, 134, 137, 138, 139, 140, 150, 155, 161, 162-3, **165**, 179
antibiofilm 137, 158, 159, 163, **165**
antibiotics 22, 71, 72, 91, 161, 187, 204
anticoagulant natural substances 184
antifungals 79, 126, 137, 138, 140, 158, **165**, 187, 204
anti-inflammatories 59, 84, 95, 97, 111, **113-14**, 137, 138, 140, 154, **155**, 158, 160, 173
anti-malodour agents 209
antimicrobial considerations 22, 67, 79, 80, 83, 88, 90, 139, 164, 165, 176-7, 191
antimicrobials 15, 24, 27, 36, **114**, 122, 128, 138, 139-40, 150, 158-9, 160, **166**, 177, 189, 210, 218
antioxidant-rich foods 27, 144-5
antioxidants 46, 64, 97, 130, 138, 148, 150, 155, 156, 159, 203
antiparasitics 129, 138, **165**

— 295 —

anti-retrovirals **79**
anti-tartar/anti-calculus agents 209
antiviral considerations 75
antivirals 74, **165**
anxiety
    artificial colours linked to 135
    and bruxism 87
    and burning mouth syndrome 78
    dental 122, 171
    and dry mouth 84
    lavender essential oil for 139
    as mouth ulcer trigger 76
    and taste perception 29
aphthous mouth ulcers 75, 77
apoptosis 94, 178
apple cider vinegar 114
apples 149, 150
approximal surface 22
aquaporins 195
arabinogalactan-rich foods 51, 150
arginine 63, 65, 74, 137, 154, 157, 165, 209
arginine-rich foods 74
arnica 171
aromatherapy oils 114, 171
Artemisia absinthium 165
artemisinin 165
artificial colours **135**, 149, 211
artificial flavours 211
artificial preservatives 211
artificial sweeteners 39, 44, 46–7, **48**, 115, 116–17, **135–6**, 146, 152, 211
ascorbic acid 78, 119, 156
asparagus (*Asparagus officinalis*) 164–5
aspartame 48, 116, **136**, 152, 177, 211
aspartate 34
aspartic acid 136
Aspergillus 78
asthma 100, 175, 178, 183
astringency 37
astringents 39, 140, 150, 194
atherosclerosis 59, 98, 148
Atopobium species 54
atrophic glossitis 72
avitaminosis 79–80
Ayurvedic system of medicine 16, 49, 126, 194

babies and infants 107–8, 186
Bacillus coagulans 163
bacteria
    and activated charcoal 127
    and baking soda 136
    'beneficial' 53
    and bentonite clay 128
    binding sites 51
    black-pigmented 56–7
    and chlorhexidine 179
    entering salivary ducts 84
    and halitosis 81
    and hot compresses 171
    invasive 21, 170
    lysing 173
    methods for identifying uncultivated 193
    microwave irradiation 172
    and moist environments 172
    obligately anaerobic 22
    and oil-pulling 125
    pathogenic 22, 150
    within periodontal pockets 53
    plaque 43
    see also acidogenic bacteria; cariogenic bacteria; commensal bacteria; Gram-negative bacteria; Gram-positive bacteria; oral bacteria; periodontopathogens: bacterial
bacterial adhesion 14, 24, 126, 149, 155, 159
'bacterial challenge' 94, 190
bacterial 'clumping' 24
bacterial co-aggregation 14, 54
bacterial diseases 56, 190
bacterial dysbiosis 10, 59
bacterial endocarditis 93
bacterial endotoxins 66, 84, 95, 105, 181
bacterial enzymes/toxins 53, 84
bacterial growth 15, 24, 53, 173, 210
bacterial infection 60, 72, 73, 83, 84, 85, 94, 99
bacterial pathogens 98
bacterial pneumonia 93
bacterial products 57, 95
bacterial receptors 50
bacterial retention 183
bacterial sialadenitis 83, 87
bacterial species **23**, 53, 57–9, 93, 103, 158, 177
bacterial translocation 14
bacteriocins 161
Bacteroides forsythus 58, 59, 60
Bacteroides gingivalis see Porphyromonas gingivalis
bad breath 54, 84, 109, 127, 152, 163, 174
    see also halitosis
baking soda 89, 127, 136, 196, 212
Bambusa arundinacea 140
barberry (*Berberis vulgaris*) 140, 165
bariatric surgery 187
bathing/showering 204
beer 40
benign migratory glossitis *see* erythema migrans
bentonite clay 128–9
berberine 155–6, 165
beta-carotene 118, 148
beta-glucans 150
betel nut chewing 80
Bifidobacteria bifidum 162, 163
Bifidobacteria breve 162, 163
Bifidobacteria lactis 163
Bifidobacteria species 54, 156, 163
biofilm 14–15, **23**, 24, 48, 53, 54, 55, 57, 58, 59, 60, 71, 100, 143, 145, 160, 164, 175, 177, 191
    see also antibiofilm
biological dentistry 11, 121, 123, 201
biomarkers 63, 67, 95, 100, 101, 189–90
bisphenol-A (BPA) 180
bisphenol-a-glycidyl dimethacrylate (BIS-GMA) 180
bisphosphate use 66

bisphosphonates 110, 184–5
bitterness 18, 32, 33, **35–6**, 37, 39, 40, 48, 90, 112, 136, 149, 153, 154, 194
blackberries 149
black gums 80
black hairy tongue 78, 80
black pepper (*Piper nigrum*) 38, 40, 155, 156
black-pigmented bacteria 56–7, 59
black tea 150, 203
bleeding disorders 66
bleeding gums **56–7**, 62, 125, 207
blood-borne infections 89
blood–brain border 14
blood–cerebrospinal fluid border 14
blood circulation 122, 177
blood clots 66, 170
blood derivatives 25
blood disorders 76, 82
blood flow 94–5, 150, 153, 207
blood pressure 157
blood sugar level (BSL) 44, 45–6, 47, 48, 49, 50, 91, 95, 144, 160
blood supply 67
B-lymphocytes 61
body mass index (BMI) 100, 145, 194
boiling water 204
bone
    dental 3-D cone beam CT scan 170
    and fluoride 132, 204
    and Gingival collagenase activity 100
    hot compresses for bacterial invasion of 171
    as indicator of age 17
    jawbone cavitations 66–8
    loss of periodontal 100, 156
    melatonin promoting formation of 97
    and menopause 109
    and periodontal disease 57, 158
    regenerative capability 66
    and silicon 157
    stored toxins in 169
    vitamins important for 148, 157, 171
    see also alveolar bone
bone broth 118, 148, 170
bone destructive diseases 100, 158, 216
bone healing **66**
bone marrow defect 67
bone metabolism 97, 100, 184
bone metabolism biomarkers 101
bone mineral density (BMD) 100
bone morphogenetic protein-1 (BMP1) 101
bone remodelling 66
bone resorption 57, 59, 101
border control *see* oral border control
botanicals
    anti-inflammatories 140
    antimicrobials 27, 165–6, 218
    antiviral 74, 75, 165
    detoxification support 164, 218
    products/product ranges 217, 218
    against RANTES 68–9
    sialogogues 26–7, 156

bottled water 147, 186
bottle feeding 108
brans 51, 150
brassicas 35, 37–8, 165
breast cancer 104, 135, 169, 170, 196
breastfeeding 88, 107–8
breast milk 34, 51, 162
British Dental Association (BDA) 213
broccoli **37–8**, 164
bromelain 140
bromine 156, 186
brown oral lesions 80
brown rice 51, 150
brown staining 88, 89
brushing teeth
    cautions 175
    frequency 175, 176
    interdental 175
    timing of 174
bruxism 73, **87**, 121, 122, 185–6
buffering functions
    of alkaline water products 148
    of baking soda 89
    of casein 149
    of hyaluronic acid 111
    of saliva 21, 24, 33, 157, 183
bulimia nervosa 117, 187
burning issues 170
burning mouth syndrome **78**, 83, 90, 109, 159
burning sensations 135, 138, 168, 179
burning tongue 58
Buteyko breathing method 183, 215

calcium 33, 39, 66, 84, 95, 106–7, 137, 149, 157, 171, 194, 196
calcium bentonite 128–9
calcium carbonate 128, 209
calcium casein peptone 152
calcium channel blockers 82, 199
calcium deficiency 101, 186
calcium homeostasis 143, 157
calcium ions 38, 88
calcium metabolism 184
calcium oxalate 39
calcium phosphate 152
calcium pyrophosphate 209
calcium-rich waters 148
calcium-sensing receptor (CaSR) 196
calcium sodium phosphosilicate 209
calcium supplements 101
calcium to phosphorus ratio 149
calcium waves 36
calculus 54
    see also tartar
calendula (*Calendula officinalis*) 122, 139, 140
cancer 34, 67, 71, 78, 81, 87, 104–5, 112, 113, 138, 140, 143, 152, 169, 189, 190, 194
    see also breast cancer; gastrointestinal cancer; head/neck cancer; Kaposi's sarcoma; lip cancer; oesophageal cancer; oral cancer; pharyngeal cancer

Candida albicans 23, 48, 61, 71–2, 89, 138, 162, 176
   see also oral candidiasis
canker sores 58, 75–6
cannabis oil (CBD) 116, 160
Capnocytophaga species 58, 192
caprylic acid 165
capsaicin 32, 37, 38, 114
capsaicinoids 38
caraway seed 156
carbamide peroxide 177
carbohydrates 15, 23, 36, 41, 43, 44,
   45, 46, 54–5, 59, 60, 79, 144, 146,
   151, 153, 174, 191, 193, 194
carbohydrate sensing **41**
carbonated drinks 32, 39, 109, **146–7**
carbonic acid H_2CO_3 146–7
carbopol 178
cardiovascular disease (CVD) 10, 43, 48, 75,
   93, 98, 143, 168, 189, 190, 196, 200
caries
   anti-caries products/activities 122, 126,
      132, 137, 138, 160, 161, 191
   critical pH range 22, 55
   and dietary counselling 143
   and excessive mouth-breathing 183
   genes associated with 190–1
   and life stages 107–8, 109
   nature of **54**, 56, 57
   perio-systemic associations 102, 103, 105, 117
   prevalence 10, 11
   and salivary flow rate 95–6, 110, 151
   and salivary secretions 25
   and salivary testing 190
   terminology 29
caries-causing agents 21, 23, 43, 45, 47, 51, 53,
   54–5, 83, 87, 108, 149, 174, 175, 185, 193
caries-preventing agents 45, 46, 62,
   145, 153–4, 181, 185, 186
cariogenic bacteria 23, 45, 47, 54,
   108, 138, 145, 149, 191
cariogenic potential 146, 163
carrageenan **133**, 210, 211
carrots 51, 89, 149
casein 149, 152
castor oil 114
cauliflower 149
cavitations 18, **66–7**, 68, 146, 148,
   167, 169–70, 181, 200, 216
cayenne pepper 114
Ceanothus americanus 155
Cecropia strigosa 165
celery 149
cell membranes 14, 50, 130, 179
cementum 9, 111
Centella asiatica (gotu kola) 65, 68, 111, 140, 158
central nervous system (CNS) 67, 132, 168, 181
cephalic responses 115
cerebrovascular accidents (CVA) 99–100
cerebrovascular disease 99–100
cetylpyridinium chloride (CPC) 177
chamomile 139, 140, 156

charcoal *see* activated charcoal
cheese 34, 149–50, 162, 196–7
chemesthesis 32
chemesthetic sensations 31, 32, **38–9**, 147
chemokine ligand 5 (CCL-5) 67
chemokines 65, 67–8
chewing, act of 115, 153, 168
   see also mastication
chewing benefits 149–50
chewing capability 13
chewing difficulties 88, 89, 90, 151, 207
chewing gum 45, 133–4, 137, 138,
   145, **151–3**, 154, 175, 176
chewing sticks 139
chicken, deboned 204
childhood 108
Chinese skullcap (*Scutellaria*
   baicalensis) 74, 78, 79, 165
chlorhexidine 89, 176, 177, **179**
chloride 156
chlorine 113, 156, 186, 204
chlorine dioxide **178**
chlorophyll 68
chlorophyll-rich sources 160, 164
cholecystokinin (CCK) 33
chorda tympani (CT) 90
chromium picolinate 117, 160
chromogranin A (CHGA) 96
chronic ischaemic bone disease (CIBD)
   see ischaemic osteonecrosis
chronic obstructive pulmonary
   disease (COPD) 100, 175
cilantro (*Coriandrum sativum*) leaf 164
Cinchona bark 156
Cinchona calisaya 165
cinnamaldehyde 38, 138
Cinnamomum cassia 138
Cinnamomum zeylanicum 138
cinnamon 38, 40, 114, **138**, 152, 155, 165, 210
cinnamon aldehyde 78
cinnamon bark 156
cinnamon essential oil 114, 139
Cistus incanus 155
Cistus species 165
citric acid 156
citrus pectin 150, 164
clays **128–9**, 165
clinoptilolite 129, 169
clove essential oil 38, 139, 158
clove (*Syzygium aromaticum*) 38, 40,
   138, 150, 155, 158, 159
coaggregation 126, 193
coconut oil 114, 126, 159
coconut water 159
co-enzyme Q10 (CoQ10) 68, 119, **130**, 158, 218
cold sores **74**
collagen 57, 65, 66, 71, 101–2, 110, 148, 157, 159
collagenase 22, 24, 57, 58, 60, 65, 100, 140
collagen degradation 60, 67, 101, 130
collagen fibres 53, 60, 97
collagen glycation 63

SUBJECT INDEX

collagen metabolism 94
collagen synthesis 66, 97, 157
colloidal silver 140, 160
'colonization resistance' 23
colorectal cancer 196
colostrum 159, 189
colour
   artificial **135**, 149, 211
   of body 15–16
   of gums 80
   of oral care products 131, 210
   of teeth 17, **88–9**, 109, 122, 177, 178, 179
   of tongue 72
commensal bacteria 14, 23, 53–4, 56, 58, 93, 108, 161
commensal fungus 71–2
confidence 14, 18, 111
connective tissue 17, 18, 22, 53, 56, 57, 58, 65, 71, 76, 111, 145, 158
connective tissue destructive diseases **100–2**
connective tissue support 60, 62, 102, **118**, 148, 157
contraceptives 22, 26, 80, 82, 208
copper 80, 86, 115, 118
copper sulphate 39
Coriolus versicolor 51, 150, 160
corn syrup 46, 50
corticosteroids 66, 72, 75, 77, 79, 100, 175
cortisol 190
Covid-19 **26**, **75**, 113
cracked lips 125, 184
cranberry 159
C-reactive protein (CRP) 95, 98, **99**, 100–1, 103, 105
Crohn's disease 76, 82, 167, 192
crown 81
cruciferous vegetables 35, 37, 146
cruelty-free products 211
cryolite 203
cucumber 184
Cupid's bow 110
Curcuma longa 79, 155
   see also turmeric
curcumin 51, 150, 159–60, 165
curry leaves (*Murraya koenigii*) 114
cystatin C 186
cysteine proteinases 56, 65
cystic fibrosis 82, 83, 190
cysts **81–2**
cytokines 58, 61, 64, 65, 66, 85, 93, 155–6, 171
   IL-1β 59, 60, 95, 98, 99, 101, 162, 173
   IL-6 57, 59, 60, 67, 94, 95, 96, 99, 100, 144
   TNF-α 59, 60, 94, 95, 96, 98, 99, 101, 102, 144, 162
cytomegalovirus (CMV) 26, 61, 74, 104, 190

dairy foods 149
'dead' teeth 105
decayed, missing or filled teeth (DMFT) 105
dehydroepiandrosterone (DHEA) 190
dementia 151
demineralization *see* mineralization

dental abscesses *see* abscesses
Dental Amalgam Mercury Solutions (DAMS) 213
dental anxiety *see* anxiety
dental caries *see* caries
dental floss 133, 175, 205
   see also flossing
dental implant osseointegration 111
dental implants 66, 167, 170, 184–5
'dental,' meaning 9
dental pellicle 14, 23
dental plaque *see* plaque
dental products *see* oral healthcare products
dental pulp stem cells (DPSCs) 66
dental sealants **180**, 181
dental surgery 66, 84, 91, 143, 159, 169, 170, 171
dentifrices 127–8, 129, 136–7, 139, 171, 173, 175–6
dentigerous cysts 81–2
dentilisin 60
dentine 66, 88, 109, 148, 149, 155, 157, 168, 173, 178, 207
dentine hypersensitivity 209
dentine matrix protein-1 (DMP1) 101–2
dentistry *see* biological dentistry; functional dentistry
dentures 22, 72, 75–6, 79, 81, 82, 109, 110, 122, 151, 155, 162, 207
Desmodium molliculum 164
desquamative gingivitis 77
detoxification 64, 118, 119, 127, 128, 129, 151, 156, 169, 183
detoxification considerations **164–5**
detoxification support 27, 67, 68, 115, 169, 218
devitalized teeth 169
diabetes 10, 36, 40, 43, 45–6, 54, 63–4, 71, 78, 81, 93, **94–6**, 99, 100, 113, 117, 143, 173, 192, 200, 207
   see also Type 2 diabetes mellitus (T2DM)
diabetic gingiva 64
diabetic nephropathy 94
diatomaceous earth (DE) 128, **129**
dietary AGEs 64
dietary choices 31, 37, 41, 91
dietary considerations **144–54**
dietary counselling 143
diethanolamine (DEA) 134–5, 211
diethylene glycol 135
digestion 24, 35, 36, 147, 148, 152
distilled water 204
dopamine 39, 115, 117, 118, 119
drugs
   fluorinated 204
   illicit 118, 185–6, 190
   and mouth ulcers 76
   and oral swellings 82
   and periodontal disease 199
   pharmaceutical 22, 33–4, 56, 83, 185, 190
   and taste dysfunction 112
   and taste loss 90
   transfer into saliva 216
dry mouth 11, 15, 17, 18, 111, 158, 167, 179, 208
   see also salivary hypofunction; xerostomia

'dry socket' 66, 170
dysbiosis 10, 14, 23, 27, 54, 55, 57, 59, 103–4, 146, 160, 163
dysgeusia 34, 90, **113**, 117, 160, 184, 187, 198

eating dangerously **144**
eating disorders 40–1, 113, **117**, 144, 160, 187
Echinacea 51, 118, 165
ecosystem 21, 191, 192
edentulous (lacking teeth) 18, 80, 94, 99
elastase 65, 71
elastin 110
electrolytes 157, 164
emotions 87, 110, 121, 122, **123**, 197, 200
enamel 17, 53, 66, 88, 89, 108, 109, 127, 128, 129, 136–7, 149, 152–3, 173, 176, 178, 185, 190
enamel-attacking acids 15, 45, 55, 109, 145, 153, 156, 193
endocannabinoids **116**, 144, 160
endocrine cells 96
endocrine cephalic response 115
endocrine disorders 71–2, 80, 113
endocrine-disrupting compounds 134, 180
endocrine function 190
endodontic(s) 104, 122
endotoxemia 104
endotoxins 60, 66, 84, 95, 100, 105, 155, 160, 164
 see also toxins
Entamoeba gingivalis 61
Enterococcus faecium W54 163
enzymes 50, 53, 57, 58, 63, 64, 65, 84, 118, 148, 153, 158, 161, 192, 210
 see also co-enzyme Q10
epidermal thinning 110
epidermolysis bullosa 76
epigallocatechin gallate (EGCG) 150, 158
epithelial cells 24, 25, 61, 97, 150, 189
epithelialization 66
epithelial layer 18, 60, 108
epithelial lining 14
Epstein-Barr Virus (EBV) 26, 61, 74, 79, 104, 190
epulis 82
erectile dysfunction **102**
erosion prevention agents 209
eruptive lingual papillitis 73
erythema migrans 77, 78
erythema multiforme 76
erythematous candidiasis 79
erythritol **46–7**, 50, 51, 136, 145, 210, 211
essential oils 74, 133, 138, **139**, 171
'essential saccharides' 44, 50
ethanol 38, 48, 66, 135, 145, 210
Eubacterium nodatum 58
eucalyptus essential oil 114, 139
eugenol 38, 89, 138, 158
everyday mouth and dental hygiene **171–6**
evolutionary changes research **191–2**
exercise
 for detoxification 164, 183
 as dopamine-booster 115
 effect on saliva **27**
 improving cell oxygenation 68

performance 41
 and salivary IgA and IgM concentrations 184
extracellular matrix (ECM) 64, 65, 101, 102, 111
extra-oral taste receptors **35–6**, 196

facial femininity 110
fat-burning 41
fat, dietary 113, 144, 195, 196
fat distribution and droop 110
fat loss 116, 164
fat perception 39, 40, **194–5**
fat storage 153
fat taste receptors 198
fat tissue 96, 134, 145, 164
fatty acids (FAs) 66, 68, 119, 144, 184, 194–5
fatty degenerative osteolysis of jawbone (FDOJ) 67, 157
fennel 140
fertility, factors impacting 107, 132, 135, 186
fertility treatment 171
fetal brain development 107, 132, 135
fetal inflammatory response 102
fetal organ formation 112
fibroblasts 64, 94, 95, 101, 107, 158
fibrous lumps 82
fight or flight 123
filiform papillae 77
fimbriae 60
fish bones 151
fizzy drinks 39, 146–7
flavonoids 79, 118, 139, 159
flavour 31, 41, 115–16, **197–8**
flavoured waters 146, 147
flavourings 138, 152
flavour perception
 and food temperature 39–40
 functions 19
 nature of 32, 197
flavours 32, 194, 210, 211
flossing 23, 54, 171, 174, 175
 see also dental floss
fluoridated salt 204
fluoride 88, 89, 95, 103, 107, 108, **131–3**, 135–6, 157, 159, 180, 181, 185, 186, **203–5**, 209, 213–15
Fluoride Action Network 214–15
fluorosis 88, 132, 159, 186
foaming agents 134–5, 209–10, 211
folate deficiency 72, 78
food debris 24, 25, 81, 84, 173
food molecule translocation 14
food temperature 39–40
food texture hardness 115
Forsythia suspensa 68
fructose 45, 46, 47, 50, 51, 63, 145
functional dentistry **121–3**
fungiform papillae 37, 90, 195
Fusobacterium nucleatum 55, 58, 150, 159, 192

GABA agonists 78
GABA release 39

galactose 50, 51, 63, 85
Galvanic current 168
Galvanic reactions 167-8
gangrene 67
garlic 38, 40, 68, 81, 114, 150, 166, 184, 196
gastric cells 33, 35
gastric disease 58, 76
gastric emptying 35, 46
gastric HCl 36
gastric mucosa 132
gastroesophageal reflux 86, 147
gastrointestinal cancer 167
gelatine 148, 159
genetics
   and oral health 216
   and pigmentations 80
   research directions **190-1**
   and taste 37-8
Gentiana lutea root 156
geographic tongue *see* erythema migrans
German chamomile 140
ghrelin 35, 115, 117, 147, 187, 200
ginger 38, 40, 114, 138, 152, 155, 156, 184
gingipains 56, 60, 65
gingivae 77, 111, 118
gingival bleeding 170, 173
gingival collegenase activity 100
gingival crevices 22, 23, 175
gingival crevicular fluid (GCF) 23, **25-6**, 54, 94, 100, 105, 107, 193
gingival disease 149
gingival fibroblasts 64, 101, 158
gingival fibromatosis 82, 199
gingival health 54, 158, 177
gingival inflammation 14, 45, 53, 56, 58, 107, 140, 170, 173, 186
   see also gingivitis; gum disease
gingival lumps 82, 167
gingival margin 175
gingival overgrowth 82, 199
gingival papillae 82
gingival pocket sites 61
gingival recession *see* receding gums
gingival sulcus 53
gingival tissue 57, 58, 60, 65, 130, 148, 177
gingivitis 10, 11, 22, 23, 26, 54, 56, 58, 77, 81, 82, 107, 109, 110, 111, 113, 117, 140, 143, 148, 150, 152, 154, 158, 159, 160, 161-2, 167, 172, 175, 179, 184, 185, 190, 207
   see also gingival inflammation; gum disease
Ginkgo biloba 184
glandular fever 26, 61
gleeking **29**
glossitis **72**, 77, 78
glossodynia/glossopyrosis *see* burning mouth syndrome
glucans 55, 150
glucitol *see* sorbitol
glucosamine 118, 150, 160
glucose 36, 43, 45, 46, 47, 48, 49, 50, 51, 63, 144, 145, 160, 174, 195, 210

glucose-fructose syrup 50
glucosensing 33
glucuronic acid 111, 118
glutamate 34, 159
glutamic acid 34
glutathione 27, 64, 68, 165, 169, 196
glutathione-rich foods 165
glycaemic control 64, **94-6**, 98
glycaemic index (GI) 44
glycanbiology **193**
glycan-rich foods 27, 150
glycans 44, 50-1, 193
glycated haemoglobin 64, 96
glycated matrix 64
glycation **63-5**, 160
glycerine/glycerol 47, **133**, 152, 178, 195, 210, 211
glycine 101, 118, 148, 165
glyconutrients 215
glycoproteins 14, 24, 27, 44, 50, 85, 96
glycosaminoglycans (GAGs) 110, 111, 118, 157, 158
glycosylation 63, 102
Glycyrrhiza glabra (liquorice root) 49, 89, 140, 159
Glycyrrhiza uralensis (Chinese liquorice) 68
glycyrrhizin 49
goldenseal (*Hydrastis canadensis*) 165
golden syrup 50
Gore-Tex 185
G-protein coupled receptors (GPCRs) 18, 32, **33-4**, 36, 41, 196
Gram-negative bacteria 23, 53, 56, 57-8, 59, 60-1, 159, 179, 216
Gram-positive bacteria 54, 56, 58, 138, 159, 179, 216
grapefruit juice 35
grapefruit seed extract 165
grape juice, organic 203
grape seed extract (*Vitis vinifera*) 159, 165
green tea 34, 68, 78, 115, 150, 203
guaraná 184
'gum-base' 151-2
gum disease 81, 89, 93, 104, 105, 108, 135
   see also gingival inflammation; gingivitis
gums
   botanicals for 140
   discoloured 80
   'leaky' 56
   soft 105
   susceptibility to plaque 109
   see also bleeding gums; receding gums
gustation **31-2**, 183
gustatory cortex (GC) 31-2
gustatory dysfunction 115
gustatory nerve responses 40
gustatory receptor cells 33
gustatory system 32, 195
gustducin **33**, 35
gustin 91
gut 9, 10, 14, 35-6, 46, 56, 148, 152, 153, 161, 169, 192
gut inflammation **103-4**, 133
gut microbiota 54, 109, 144, 156
Gymnema sylvestre 49, 160

hairy leucoplakia (hairy tongue) 78–9, 80
halitosis 58, **81**, 125, 138, 159, 160, 161, 172, 175, 183, 207
   see also bad breath
halogens 156
hand, foot and mouth disease (HFMD) 76
head/neck cancer 22, 72, 83, 91, 105
healthcare providers/practitioners 19, 200
healthy mouth
   features of **19**
   importance of 13
   and oral microbiome health 14
Helicobacter pylori 45, 58–9, **76**, 81, 104, 190
hepatitis 79, 90, 190
hepatoprotective herbs 160, 164
herbal extracts 210
herpes simplex virus (HSV) 72, 74, 76, 97, 104, 108, 172
herpes viruses 61, 72, 74, 75, 90, 97, 113, 156, 183, 190
herpetiform ulcers 75
Herxheimer reactions 164, 169
high-density lipoproteins (HDL) 96, 98
high-fat diets 144, 195
high fructose corn syrup (HFCS) 50
Himalayan salt 126–7, 151
histadine-rich proteins 24
histatins 65
Holistic Dental Association (HDA) 213
holistic dentistry 121
holobiont 143, 160, 192
homeopathy 122, 170, 171, 184, 216
honey 47, 114, 145
   see also Manuka honey
hormonal changes 22, 76, 107, 199, 208
hormone imbalance 184
hormone replacement therapy (HRT) 110
horse chestnut (*Aesculus hippocastanum*) 140
horseradish 38, 40, 138, 156
host defence mechanisms 22, 130, 193
hot beverages 40, 90, 150
hot compresses 171
hot foods 39, 40, 65, 150
hot pepper 116, 119, 151
'hot' sensation 38
Houttuynia cordata 165
human cytomegalovirus (hCMV) 26
human immunodeficiency virus (HIV) 71, 76, 79, 83, 104, 138, 190
human microbiome project (HMP) **192–3**
Human Oral Microbiome Database (HOMD) 192
human papillomavirus (HPV) **73–4**
humectants 131, 133, 210
humic/fulvic acid 165
hyaluronic acid (HA) 25, 53, 65–6, 68, **111**, 118, 130, 158, 159
hyaluronidase 22, 25, 60, **65**, 111
hydrated silica 128, 136–7, 209
hydration 27, 41, 68, 84, 115, 126, 151, 164, 186
hydrogen peroxide 47, 90, 176, 177, **178**
hydroxyapatite 60, 88, 209

Hypericum perforatum 165
hyperlipidaemia 98
hyperpigmentation 80
hypersalivation 85–6
hypogeusia 90, 91
hypoglycaemia 64
hyposalivation 112, 162

ice-cream 163
illegal drugs 118, 185–6, 190
immune-mediated oral conditions 75
immune response 14, 34, 36, 53–4, 56, 57, 61, 94–5, 98, 108, 122, 157, 162, 177, 187, 200
immunoglobulins 9, 53, 60, 105, 159
   see also secretory immunoglobulin A
immunological effects 68
immunological responses 10, 54
immunologic salivary component 24
immunomodulatory activity 69, 97
immunomodulatory effects 113–14, 164
impacted teeth 17, 88, 107
infants 107–8
infectious mononucleosis 26, 61
infertility **102**, 200
inflammation
   and AGE formation 64
   and ageing 108–9
   associated with poor oral health and chronic illness propensity 200
   as defining characteristic of periodontitis 93, 95
   dental considerations 167
   and dysbiosis **53–62**
   generalized 43
   immune system with limited ability to fight 10
   measures to ameliorate 144–5, 147, 161, 164
   and oxidative stress 105, 111
   'silent' **67–8**
   systemic 40, 60, 63, 67, 68, 85, 100, 103, 104, 144
   see also gingival inflammation; stomatitis
inflammatory bowel disease (IBD) 48, 103, 133, 167
inflammatory chemokine 67–8, 194
inflammatory conditions 82, 87, 105, 133, 190
inflammatory cytokines 58, 61, 64, 66, 67, 94, 98, 102, 144, 155, 171, 173
inflammatory exudate 26
inflammatory liquefaction 67
inflammatory mediators 23, 95, 96, 100, 104, 107, 194
inflammatory processes 15, 27, 58, 65, 67, 93, 145
inflammatory response 10, 23, 53–4, 57–8, 59, 64, 94, 95, 100, 102, 103, 133, 134, 150, 155, 157, 164, 175, 190
The Institute for Functional Medicine (IFM) 214
insulin 41, 46, 49, 81, 83, 95, 96, 98, 117, 153, 190
interdental brushing 175
interleukins 57, 59, 60, 67, 94, 95, 96, 98, 99, 100, 101, 110, 144, 161, 162, 173, 191
   see also cytokines
International Academy of Biological Dentistry and Medicine (IABDM) 213

SUBJECT INDEX

International Academy of Oral Medicine and Toxicology (IAOMT) 213-14
International College of Integrative Medicine (ICIM) 214
intestinal barriers 56, 156
intestinal glucose uptake 49
intestinal lumen 36
intestinal mucosa 33, 34
intestinal permeability 144
inulin 50, 150, 160
iodine 131-2, 146, 151, **156**, 186
iodine-rich foods 156
ion channels 18, 32, 33, 38, 137-8
ion-exchange resins 204
ions 32, 38, 84, 88, 108
iron 56, 68, 72, 76, 78, 80, 89
iron sulphate 89
irritable bowel syndrome (IBS) 45, 46, 152, 153
Isatis indigotica 68
ischaemic osteonecrosis 67, 68, 216
    see also cavitations
isothiocyanates 35, 38, 138

jawbone 13, **66-8**, 109, 157
jaw cysts 82
jaw movement 87
jaw problems 86, 153, 167-8, 170
Juglans nigra 165

kaolin clay 128
Kaposi's sarcoma 80
Kashaya (astringent taste) 194
Katu (pungent taste) 194
keratosis (leucoplakia) 78-9, 80
kinesiology 121, 122
'kissing diseases' 26
Klebsiella species 103
kokumi 39, 196
Krameria triandra (rhatany/ratanhia) 122, 140
kryptopyrroluria 105

labelling **132**, **210-12**
lactilol 47
Lactobacilli 45, 47, **54-5**, 108, 156, 162
Lactobacillus acidophilus 162, 163
Lactobacillus casei 162
Lactobacillus fermentum 162, 163
Lactobacillus gasseri 163
Lactobacillus paracasei 162
Lactobacillus plantarum 161, 163
Lactobacillus reuteri 161-2
Lactobacillus rhamnosus 55, 159, 161, 162, 163
Lactobacillus salivarius 161, 162-3
lactoferrin 22, 159, 210
lactoperoxidase 210
lantibiotics 161
L-arginine 137, 154, 165
Lavana (salty taste) 194
lavender essential oil 139, 171

L-cysteine 165
'leaky gums' 56
'leaky gut' 14, 56
leishmaniasis 76-7
lemon 114, 145, 149, 210
lemon balm (*Melissa officinalis*) 74, 165
lemon essential oil 139
leptin 96-7, **116**, 153
leucoplakia *see* keratosis
lichen planus 16, 75, 76, 77, **78-9**, 159, 160
lie bumps 73
lifestyle options **183-7**
lingual lipase 24, 195
lingual papillitis 73
lip cancer 183
lipids 43-4, 50, 63, 98, 194-5
lipopolysaccharides (LPS) 60, 63, 64, 155, 164
lips
    changes in **110-11**, 158
    cold sores 74
    components 158
    cracked 125, 184
    dry 148, 184
    need for protection 183-4
    salivary glands in 25
    'smokers' 186
    vermillion of 183-4
    see also stomatitis
liquorice *see Glycyrrhiza*
liver cirrhosis 83, 103
L-lysine 165
longevity 18
low-calorie sweeteners 116
low-density lipoproteins (LDL) 64, 98
low-inflammatory diet 144-5
L-theanine 78, 115
lubricating function
    of hyaluronic acid 25, 66, 111
    of saliva 13, 21, 24, 151
lucuma 48, 145, 198
lung cancer 105
lupus erythematosus 79, 85
Lyme disease 73, 87-8, 90
lymphatic drainage 184
lysozyme 15, 22, 173, 210

macrophages 66
Madhura (sweet taste) 194
magnesium 39, 123, 147-8, 157, 159, 164, 169, 171, 196
Mahonia aquifolium 165
Maillard reaction 63
malabsorption syndromes 36
male reproductive organs 102, 159
malic acid 156
malocclusion 88
maltilol 47
mannitol 46, 47
Manuka honey 47, 65, 145, 159
maple syrup 47, 48

mastication 13, 25, 65-6, 85, 87, 103, 143
　see also chewing, act of
mastic gum (*Pistacia lentiscus*) 152
matrix glycation 64
matrix metalloproteinase (MMPs) 24, 57, 61,
　65, 66, 67, 95, 100-1, 150, 158, 190
melanin 80, 183
melatonin 25, 66, 68, **97**, 156, 190
Melissa officinalis see lemon balm
'menopausal glossitis' 72
menopause 37, 91, **109-10**, 112
menstrual cycle 37, 112
menthol 32, 38, 78, 137
mercury 80, 86, 105, 121, 165, 167,
　168, 169, 181, 213-14
mercury amalgam fillings 10, 18, 63, 66, 68,
　89, 103, 153, 164, 168-9, 200, 215
metabolic syndrome 48, 96, **98-9**, 143
metallic taste **39**, 49, 167, **168**
metalloproteinases 57, 58, 64, 140
methadone 117
methamphetamine ('meth'/'speed') 186
methylcobalamin 169
methylglyoxal (MG) 47, **64-5**, 145
methyl salicylate 137
MG1 and MG2 (mucins) 50
mGluR1 taste receptors 34
mGluR4 taste receptors 34
mica 210
microbeads **135**, 177, 211
microbial adherence 24
microbial alteration 53, 55
microbial colonization 24
microbial communities 57, 160-1, 173, 191-2
microbial composition 23
microbial defence 26, 54
microbial ecology 21, **22**, 54, 107
microbial homeostasis 23, 53, 56
microbial interactions 193
microbial metabolism 45
microbial products 100
microbial species 192
microbiota see gut microbiota; oral microbiota
microorganisms 14, 18, 22, 23, 24, 32, 53,
　55, 58, 65, 66, 98, 149, 172, 192, 199
microwave irradiation 172
milk 149, 161, 175
milk teeth 17
milk thistle 164, 165
mineralization 17, 21, 102, 157, 190
　demineralization 15, 21, 22, 43, 55, 57, 132, 149
　remineralization 15, 55, 122, 128, 132, 149, 152
mineral water **147-8**
mints **137**
miracle berry (*Synsepalum dulcificum*) 49
miraculin 48-9
misalignment 88, 123, 167
mitochondrial energy 130, 159
modified sugars **50**
monk fruit (*Siraitia grosvenori*) 48, 145
monolaurin 165

monosodium glutamate (MSG) 34
monounsaturated fatty acids (MUFA) 144
montmorillonite 128, 129
mood-boosting therapies 87, 187
Moringa oleifera 159
mouth-breathing 84, 183
mouth cancer see oral cancer
mouth-feel (touch) 32
mouthguards 173
mouth ulcers 11, **75-7**, 86, 134, 140, 158-9
mouthwashes 75, 84, 89, 90, 122, 130, 132, 134,
　135, 139, 140, 158, 172, 174, 176-7, 178, 179
mucins see salivary mucins
mucopolysaccharides 45, 145, 157
mucosal dysplasia 186, 187
mucosal immunity 184
mucosal infections 84, 104, 175
mucosal layer 160
mucosal lesions 72, 117, 187
mucosal surfaces 24, 32
mucosal tissue 25, 148, 157
mucosal transudations 25
mucosal wound healing 25, 148
mucous membranes 39, 71, 72, 76, 77, **80**,
　85, 86, 111, 122, 138, 147, 158
mumps (paramyxovirus) 82, 86
mushrooms 40, 46, 51, 150, 160, 165
mustard oil 38, 138, 150
mutualism 14
myoglobin 72
myricetin 158
myrrh (*Commiphora molmol*) 140, 158, 165

N-acetylcysteine 165
N-acetylglucosamine 50, 85, 111
nano-TiO$_2$ 133-4
National Institute of Dental and Craniofacial
　Research (NIDCR) 214
National Institute of Dental Research (NIDR) 214
natural anticoagulants 184
natural calorific sweeteners **47-8**, 198
natural oral healthcare ingredients **136-41**
natural sialogogues 156
'natural' toothpaste ingredients **136-7**
natural whitening methods 89
natural zero-calorie sweeteners **48-50**, 198, 211
neem (*Azadirachta indica*) 140, 155, 166
nerve damage **90**, 115
neuralgia inducing cavitational
　osteonecrosis (NICO) 67, 216
neurogastronomy 197-8, 215
neuroinflammation **103**
neurotransmitters 33, 38-9, 184
nickel 167
nidus 84
NMDA glutamate receptors 159
non-bacterial periodontopathogens **61**
non-communicable diseases (NCDs) 10
noni (*Morinda citrifolia*) 155
non-stick pans 185

SUBJECT INDEX

nutrient appetite 196
nutrient deficiency 71, 72, 76, 101
nutrients
    foods rich in 148, 149, 197
    glyconutrients 215
    helpful for taste loss 115
    helping post-surgery bone growth 171
    immune-boosting 146
    macronutrients 194
    source for oral bacteria 193
nutrient sensing 35
nutrient–toxin detection system 32
nutritional therapy
    ageing, telomere length, satiety
        and sugar detox 118-19
    holistic dentistry 123
    oral border control 27
    oral healthcare product ingredients 141
    periodontal disease, caries and gum bleeding 62
    perio-systemic associations 105
    sugar 51
    taste 40-1
    wound repair, cavitations, RANTES 68-9
    see also Chapter 14; Chapter 15

obesity 35, 40-1, **96-8**, 99, **115-17**, 144, 146, 147, 151, 192, 194-5, 196, 200
obstructive sleep apnoea (OSA) 85
odontoblasts 166
odontogenic cysts 82
oesophageal cancer 105, 150, 158
oestradiol/oestriol 190
oestrogen 72, 100, 101, 107, 109, 110, 135, 156, 170, 184
oil-pulling 87, 114, **125-6**, 171, 172
older age *see* age
olfaction 31, 32, 183, 197
olfactory dysfunction 115
olfactory system 32, 40, 197
oligofructose 50, 150, 160
olive leaf extract 165
olive oil 126, 144
olive pits 127
omega-3 fatty acids 66, 68, 119, 144, 155, 184
opiates 117
opioids 117, 118
oral bacteria 22, 56, 93, 137, 179, 193
oral border control
    nutritional support for 27
    oral microbiome 14-15
oral cancer 73, 74, 77, **86-7**, 97, 156
oral candidiasis 61, **71-2**, 77, 78, 79, 84, 87, 109, 113, 175, 187
    see also Candida albicans
oral cavity
    anatomy resource 215
    database of taxa present in 192
    definition 29
    factors detrimental to 26, 145, 184
    inflammation 95, 187, 200
    microbial homeostasis 56

probiotics 160-3
quantity of bacterial species in 23, 57, 58
quantity of salivary glands in 25
role of **13-14**
and 'taste ability' 9, 18-19
temperature 40
warm and moist environment 65
oral cavity health
    association with systemic health 15, 143, 200-1
    factors important for 17, 21-2, 29, 97, 156, 179
    resources 215-17
oral cysts *see* cysts
oral dysaesthesia *see* burning mouth syndrome
oral health
    and age-related changes 17-18
    conclusions 200-1
    conditions affecting **71-91**
    diet for optimal 143-54
    and genetics 190, 216
    infant 107-8
    and melatonin **97**
    perio-systemic links 98, 104, 105
    protecting **21-7**
    recognition of 10
    research directions 193
    resources 213-18
    and whole-body health 121-2
oral healthcare products
    choice 176-7
    ingredients 131-41, 209-10
    labels 210-12
Oral Health Foundation 214
oral hygiene
    alternatives 125-30
    considerations 167-88
    everyday 171-6
oral irrigators 173
oral microbial ecology 21, **22**, 54, 107
oral microbiome 9, 14-15, 19, 21-2, 23, 27, 53, 57, 85, 104, 109, 139, 163, 171, 186, 191, 192, 193, 200, 218
oral microbiota 22, 57, 58, 103, 104, 109, 161, 191, 193
oral mucositis **86**, 87, 140
oral piercings **89-90**
oral soreness, non-ulcerative causes 75, **77**, 78
oral surgery *see* dental surgery
oral swellings **82-3**
orange peel 156
oranges 89, 149
orbicularis oris muscle 174, 186
oregano essential oil 139
oregano (*Origanum vulgare*) 165, 166
organic disease 78, 87
organic drinks 203
organic foods 47, 151, 164
organic oral care products 211, 217
'organofluorines' 185
orofacial pain **87-8**
oropharynx 25
orosensory perception 195
orosensory stimulation 115

305

orosomucoid 98
orthodontic appliances 72, 162
orthodontics 205
osteocalcin 157
osteoclast activation 61, 64
osteoclast activity 97, 101
osteoclastogenesis 101, 138, 158
osteogenesis 102
osteonecrosis 67, 68, 216
osteoporosis 100, 101, 102, 110,
    148, 151, 156, 196, 199
Osteoporotic Fractures in Men (MrOS) study 101
Otoba parvifolia 166
overeating **115-17**
ovulation 26, 107
oxidative stress 63, 64, 96, 97, 105, 111
ozonated oils 177, 193
ozone therapy 122

palantine tonsils 83
palate 25, 74, 88, 162, 186
pancreatic cancer 104
papaine 159
papaya 140
papillae 37, 72, 73, 77, 82, 90, 195
parabens 135, 210, 211
parathyroid hormone (PTH) 101
Parkinson's disease (PD) 78, 86, 90, 103
parotid gland 25, 86
parsley (*Petroselinum crispum*) 164
pathobionts 57, 59
pathogenic organisms 14, 22, 23, 24, 53,
    56, 60, 61, 149, 150, 191, 193
pectin 51, 136, 150, 164
pemphigoid 75, 76, 77
pemphigus 75, 76
peppermint 38, 114, 137, 155
peppermint essential oil 74, 114, 137, 139
peptides 24, 33, 36, 96, 115, 196
Peptostreptococcus micros 58
perfluorooctane sulfonate (PFOS) 185
perfluorooctanoic acid (PFOA) 185
periapical cysts 82
periapical inflammation 64, 82
pericoronititis 82
periodontal disease
    aetiology of 53
    and bariatric surgery 187
    beneficial treatments 140, 156, 158, 161, 173, 191
    and Co-enzyme Q10 130
    as communicable 26
    and diet-associated disorders 36, 40, 94-8
    and fertility 171
    and genetics 190-1
    and hyaluronic acid 111
    illicit drug use associated with 185
    including gingivitis and periodontitis 56
    and matrix metalloproteinases 65, 67
    microbiome complexity of 57
    and non-bacterial periodontopathogens 61
    and periodontopathic ecology 57-8
    as polymicrobial 57, 191
    prevalence and potential impact **199-200**
    and 'red complex' 59-61
    salivary components influencing 25
    salivary testing for 190
    and sleep apnoea 85
    species diversity within biofilm
        associating with 14
    systemic disease association 10, 93-105, 143
    and vitamin K 157
periodontal health
    associated with systemic health 181
    dietary sugar impacting 63
    glycaemic control/diabetes link 94
    products/product ranges **217-18**
periodontal infection 59, 64, 94, 98, 102
periodontal inflammation 57, 64, 101
periodontal ligament 66, 95, 111, 140, 155
periodontal pockets 22, 53, 58, 59, 60,
    61, 103, 122, 161, 170, 193
periodontics 122
periodontitis **56, 58-9**
    altered salivary pH 22
    beneficial foods, drinks and
        nutrients 149, 150, 158
    beneficial treatments 27, 65, 130, 140, 175
    biofilms responsible for 23
    and eating disorders 117
    elevated collegenase activity in 24
    and *Entamoeba gingivalis* 61
    and human herpes viruses 74, 113
    as infectious disease 167
    and menopause 109-10, 156
    and metabolic syndrome 143
    as part of periodontal disease 56
    prevalence and treatability 199
    preventative 152
    probiotics for 161
    and 'Red Complex' 59-60
    research into 189-90
    risk factors **207-8**
    and sleep apnoea 85
    symptoms **207**
    systemic disease associations 93-105
    telomere length and oxidative stress 111
periodontium 59, 95, 100, 102, 199
periodontopathic ecology **57-9**
periodontopathogens
    bacterial 23, 53-61
    non-bacterial **61**
perioral wrinkles 110
periosteum 66
perio-systemic associations 93-105, 200
peritonsillar abscesses 83, 86
peritonsillar cellulitis 83
pH
    adjusters 135, 210
    and biofilm formation 54
    effect of miraculin 49
    gastric HCl reducing 36

importance of 55
and lactic acid production 149
MMPs functioning at neutral 65
mouth 117, 127, 128
plaque 43, 55, 145-6, 175
salivary 22, 24, 43, 55, 83, 84, 109-10, 147, 175, 185
vomiting altering 187
phagocytosis 59, 94, 168
pharmaceuticals 22, 27, 31, 33-4, 41, 56, 82, 133, 174, 184, 185, 190, 199, 204, 216
pharyngeal cancer 87
pharynx 29
phenylalanine 136
phospholipase C (PLC) 33
phosphorous 66, 149
phylogenetic diversity 191
pigmentation 56-7, 59, **79-80**
Pimpinella anisum see aniseed
pineapple 80, 149
Piper nigrum see black pepper
placental-fetal exposure 102
Plantago tincture 140
plaque
  amyloid 103
  atherosclerotic 98
  bacteria found in 60
  and caries 54, 55, 57
  and gingivitis 56
  and halitosis 81
  and inflammatory processes 58
  and menopause 109
  remedies 125-6, 127, 128, 136, 140, 152, 159, 161, 163, 172, 173-4, 175, 179, 210
  research into 191
  and xylitol 45
plaque accumulation 53, 54, 161, 175
plaque biofilms 57, 58, 71, 175, 191
plaque formation 14, 22
plaque pH 43, 55, 145-6, 175
platelet activation 66
platelet receptor 191
Polygonum cuspiatum (Japanese knotweed) 165
polymicrobial diseases 57, 191
polyols *see* sugar alcohols
polyphenols 64, 79, 150
polytetrafluoroethylene (PTFE) 185
polyunsaturated fats (PUFA) 144
pomegranate (*Punica granatum*) 65, 68, 140, 158
porphyrin 56-7
Porphyromonas gingivalis 48, 56-7, 58, **59-61**, 64, 65, 100, 103, 104, 138, 150, 155, 157, 159, 161, 163, 177, 199
prebiotic-rich foods 50, 149
pre-eclampsia 102
pregnancy 10, 26, 37, 58, 80, 82, 86, 88, 91, **102**, 107, 139, 156, 162, 171, 196, 208
preservatives 135, 152, 179, 210, 211
preterm birth 102
Prevotella species 56, 58, 192
proanthocyanidin-rich foods 140, 150

probiotic-rich foods 149
probiotics 27, 54, 62, 74, **160-3**, 177, 187, 191, 218
processed foods 203, 204
procollagen-1 101-2
products *see* oral healthcare products; periodontal health: products/product ranges
progesterone 109, 190
proline 101, 118
proline-rich proteins (PRPs) 24
prominent gag reflex 122
propolis 140, 155, 159
propylene glycol 78, 134, 210, 211
protein absorption 36
protein deficiencies 66
protein folding 50
protein glycation 160
protein-induced satiety 35
proteins 15, 24, 25, 26, 37, 43-4, 50, 63, 64, 71, **81**, 84, 101-2, 105, 108, 116, 118, 145, 165, 170, 171, 189-90, 194
  see also C-reactive protein (CRP)
proteolytic activity 24
proteolytic bacteria 53, 57
proteolytic enzymes 57, 118
psychogenic pain 87, 187
ptyalism 85-6
pulmonary links to periodontal disease 99-100
pulp 66, 82, 157, 168, 178, 207
pulpal necrosis 82
pungency *see* spicy sensation
pycnogenol 155

Quassia amara 166
quercetin 68, 140, 158, 159

radiotherapy 22, 26-7, 34, 72, 80, 83, 84, 86-7, 90-1
RANTES 65, **67-8**, 68-9, **194**, 200, 216
ratanhia *see Krameria triandra*
reactive oxygen species (ROS) 63-4, 95, 130, 144, 173, 177
rebaudioside A 48
receding gums 17, 54, 89
receptors for AGEs (RAGEs) 64
'The red complex' **59-61**
red lips 183-4
red oral lesions **79-80**, 86
redox potential 22
redox regulator 27
redox status 27
red pepper 116, 151
red tongue conditions 73, 77
red wine 39, 150, 177
referred pain 87, 187
refined sugars 44
refiners syrup 50
regulated on activation, normal T-cell expressed and secreted *see* RANTES
reishi mushrooms 51, 150, 160
relative dentine abrasivity (RDA) 173, 215
remineralization *see* mineralization

research directions **189-98**
resveratrol 155
retinoic acid 157
retronasal smell **197-8**
reverse osmosis 204
rheumatoid arthritis (RA) 59, 85, 100, 102, 105, 149
Rhodiola rosea 115, 119
root canals 18, 66, 68, 82, 89, 104, 105, 122, 169, 170, 214
Rosmarinus officinalis 165

saccharides 44, 45, 46, 50-1, 55, 59, 60, 64, 145, 157, 160, 164, 215
saccharin 48, 116, 210
Safe Mercury Amalgam Removal Technique (SMART) 121, 169, 213-14
sage 140, 159
salicylic acid 137
saliva
   and age 108, 109
   assessment/testing 189-90
   as buffer 21, 24, 33, 157, 183
   communicable diseases associated with 26
   conditions affecting **83**
   effect of exercise 27
   flow of 26-7, 173-4
   functions and nature of 21, 24-5, 150, 173, 189-90
   healthy 15, 173-4
   red 80
salivary amylase 24, 27, 40, 43
salivary bifidobacteria 163
salivary components 22, 24, 65-6
salivary defence **24**, 27, 108
salivary duct obstruction **83-4**
salivary flow rate 22, 26, 27, 55, 83, 95-6, 109, 183
salivary gland disorders 82-3, **85-6**, 156
salivary glands 13, **25**, 26, 82, 83, 84, 86, 179
salivary gland secretion 25
salivary gland swelling 82, 83
salivary health 21-2, 71
salivary histatins 65
salivary hypofunction 72
   see also dry mouth; xerostomia
salivary IgA 24, 25, 184
   see also secretory immunoglobulin A (sIgA)
salivary IgM 184
salivary microbiota 103
salivary minerals 66
salivary mucus 25, 148
salivary mucins 22, 27, 50, 85, 108, 134, 193
salivary pH *see* pH: salivary
salivary proteins 24, 37
salivary secretion 115, 168
salivary secretion rate 22, 27, 184
salivary VEGF (vascular endothelial growth factor) 25, 97, 148
salt
   fluoridated 204
   iodized 156
   potassium 209

   sodium chloride 212
   strontium 209
   zinc 209
   see also Himalayan salt; sea salt
saltiness (taste) 18, 32-3, 115, 168, 194
salt intake 151
salt paste 150
salt rinses 73, 90, **126-7**, 159, 171, 174
salts 39, 84, 122, 147, 151, 174, 216
salty foods 90, 113, 115, 184
Salvadora persica (toothbrush tree) 139
salvia essential oil 139
Salvia miltiorrhiza 79
Salvia sclarea 165
Sambucus nigra 165
SAMe (S-adenosyl-*L*-methionine) 165
SARS-COV-2 **26**, **75**, 113
satiety 9-10, 35, 40, **115-16**, 119, 144, 146, 147, 184, 195, 196, 198, 200
saturated fatty acid (SAFA) 144
savouriness *see* umami taste
scalloped tongue 73
Scutellaria baicalensis (Chinese skullcap) 74, 78, 79, 165
sea buckthorn (*Hippophae rhamnoides*) 158
sealants *see* dental sealants
sea salt 90, 126-7, 136, 151
seasoning 154
seaweed 34, 133, 156
secretory immunoglobulin A (sIgA) 15, 17, 22, 24, 25, 27, 51, 57, 83, 107, 108, 162
selenium 119, 156-7, 165
seleno-methionine 169
self-esteem 14, 111, 200
seromucous coating 21
serotonin 117, 160
serotonin syndrome 86
serrapeptase 165
sesame seed oil 114, 126
sex hormones 26
shiitake mushrooms 40, 51, 150, 160
sialadenitis 82-3, 84, 87
sialochemistry **189-90**
sialogogues **26-7**, 84, 85, 110, 156, 186
sialolithiasis 83-4
sialoliths 84
sialorrhoea 85-6
sialosis 82
signalling cascades 41
'silent' inflammation **67-8**
silicon 129, **157**
single nucleotide polymorphisms (SNPs) 191
sixth taste 39, 194, **195-7**
Sjögren's syndrome (SS) 82-3, 85, 86, 113, 190
sleep apnoea 73, **85**, 121, 183
sleep issues 183
smell
   of food 84, 197
   loss of 26, 91, 112, 113, 197
   orthonasal 197
   retronasal 197-8
   sense of 19, 31, 32, 113-14

unusual 82
smell disorders 91, 112
smell perception **112**
smile 9, 14, 17, 19, 110, 111, 200
smoking 21, 22, 26, 64, 66, 72, 78, 79, 80, 81, 89, 90, 99, 100, 101, 104, **113**, 152, 167, 174, 177, **186**, 187, 199, 200, 207
snacking 146
sodium chloride 212
sodium hexametaphosphate 176
sodium hydroxide 210
sodium laureth sulphate (SLES) 134, 210
sodium lauryl sulphate (SLS) 77, 134, 173, 177, 209, 210
soft palate 74
Solobacterium moorei 138
sorbitol **46**, 135, 210, 211
sorghum syrup 48
'sound enamel' 55
sour foods 49, 86, 114
sour taste 18, 32–3, 115, 147, 194, 196
spacer devices 175
spermatogenesis 102
spices 81, 136, **138**, 147
spicy foods 39, 72, 77, 90, 184
spicy sensation **38–9**, 194
spore-formers 163
sports drinks 41
spring water 203, 204
staining causes 88–9, 109, 177, 179
staining foods 80, 89, 149, 150
stain removal 127–8, 136–7, 149, 150, 174, 176, 177, 209
Staphylococcus aureus 128, 177
'starchiness' 39, 194, 195
starchy foods 145–6, 195
statherins 24
stevia (*Stevia rebaudiana*) 36, **48**, 51, 136, 145, 165, 211, 218
stomatitis 34, 74, 75, 79, 138, 155, 184
'strawberry tongue' 73
straws, use of **174**
Streptococcus mitis 163
Streptococcus mutans 45, 47, 48, 54, 55, 71, 105, 107, 108, 138, 145, 150, 155, 158, 161, 162, 163, 172
Streptococcus pyogenes 150, 161
Streptococcus salivarius 161, 163
Streptococcus sobrinus 138, 159
Streptococcus thermophilus 163
stress 22, 29, 51, 54, 73, 76, 86, 87, 109, 112, 115, 118, **123**, 139, 146, 170, 184, 199–200, 208
Strobilanthes cusia 68
subgingival biofilm 100
subgingival crevices 59
subgingival environment 25, 53
subgingival plaque 60
sublingual gland 25, 84
submandibular gland 25, 83
subnucleus caudalis (Vc) 39
sucralose 48, 116–17, 210
sucrose 22, 44, 46, 47, 48, 55, 63, 116–17, 133, 174
sugar-addictive behaviours 116, 117, 118

sugar alcohols 44, **45–7**, 152, 153
sugar-based inhalers 175
sugar craving **117–18**
sugar fibres 44, **50**
sugar-free chewing gum 152
sugars
 advantages and disadvantages 43–4
 avoidance of 17, 21, 119, 144–5
 beneficial **50–1**
 and childhood caries 108
 conversion to lactic acid 54
 destroyer of **49**, 160
 excess consumption 98
 high-sugar diet 21, 116
 industrially processed 191
 modified **50**
 natural alternatives to 215
 nutritional therapy relating to **51**
 reducing 63, 64
 resources 215, 216
 and salivary flow 83
 and starchy foods 145–6, 195
 and *Streptococcus mutans* 55
 and sweeteners **44**, 47–50, 116, 146, 215
 and sweet taste 36, 40, 116–17
 and telomere length 111
sugar-sensing mechanisms 40
sulphur-rich foods 165
'supertasters' **37–8**, 195
supplement considerations **155–63**
supragingival environment 25
surface adhesion capacity 127
surfactants 134, 209–10
sweat glands 183–4
sweat therapies 164, 183
sweeteners 36, 43, **44**, 45, 47–50, 51, 108, 145, 152, 153, **198**, 210, 211, 215
 see also artificial sweeteners; low-calorie sweeteners; natural calorific sweeteners; natural zero-calorie sweeteners
sweetness
 as addictive 117, 144
 cephalic responses 115
 cravings 49, 117–18, 119, 160
 as distinct from starchiness 195
 taste 18, 32, 33, **36**, 37, 115, 194
sweetness perception 40, 196
sweetness sensing 36, **116–17**
sweetness suppressant 49
sweet taste receptors 33, 35–6, 49, 116, 196
syphilis 73, 78
systemic health
 association with oral cavity health 15, 143, 200–1
 dietary considerations in promoting 144–54
 nerve damage impacting 90
 periodontal health associated with 181
 protecting 21–7
 teeth and dental health as highly relevant to 29

3-D cone beam CT (computed tomography) scanner 169–70
Tabebuia impetiginosa (pau d'arco) 155, 165, 166

table salt 151
Tannerella forsythia 60, 162
    see also *Bacteroides forsythus*
tannin-rich teas 150
tannins 39, 140, 177
tap water 147, 186, 203
tartar 54, 179, 209
tastants 33
taste
    ability to 9, **18-19**
    addressing loss of **113-15**
    five primary **32-6**, 194
    importance of research **198**
    issues with **90-1**
    nutritional therapy in relation to **40-1**
    research into number of **194**
    'sixth' 39, 194, **195-7**
    see also metallic taste
taste bud receptors 18, 31-2, 33
taste buds 13, **31-2**, 33, 34, 37, 40, 49, 91, 108, 114, 172
taste gene 37
taste integration **197-8**
taste perception 9, 19, 31-2, 38, 41, **112**, 115, 154, 196, 200
taste receptors 31, 33-7, 102, 196, 198
'taste tripping' 49
tea plants 203
tea tree (*Melaleuca alternifolia*) essential oil 74, 130, 139
teeth
    colour of 17, **88-9**, 109, 122, 177, 178, 179
    as indication of age 17-18
    issues with **88**
    revealing health **16-18**
    'toxic' 181
teeth cleaning see brushing teeth
teeth whitening see whitening
Teflon 185, 203
telomere length **111**, 119
temporal headache 167, 168
temporomandibular joint pain dysfunction syndrome (TMJD) 87
temporomandibular joint (TMJ) 87-8, 122, 123, 153, 167, 170
testosterone 109, 132, 184, 190
tetracycline 88
thiocyanate 186
thrush see *Candida albicans*
Thymus longicaulis 165
Tikta (bitter taste) 194
tinnitus 167, 168
tissue inflammation 53
tissue inhibitors of metalloproteinases (TIMPs) 24, 65
tissue salts 122, 216
titanium dioxide (TiO$_2$) **133-4**, 135, 152, 211
tongue
    and ageing 108
    burning sensation in 58, 78, 168
    characteristics of healthy 15-16
    chlorhexidine mouthwashes 179
    colour of 72, 80
    diagnosis and TCM **15-16**
    and halitosis 81
    issues with 72-3, 77-8, 79, 80, 119
    roles 13
    salivary glands in 25
    sweet receptors on 49
    see also hairy leucoplakia
tongue biofilm 24
tongue biting **73**
tongue cancer 73
tongue cleaning 172, 174, 217
tongue papillae 72, 77, 90
tongue piercings 89-90
tonsils 81, **83**, 170, 172, 183
tooth bleaching 89, **177-8**, 215
toothbrushes
    and charcoal application 128
    and cold sores 74
    decontamination 122
    protocols **171-2**
    resources 217
tooth decay 45, 48, 82, 108, 132, 152, 174, 180, 200, 207
tooth discolouration **88-9**, 177, 179
tooth eruption 17, 22, 88, 145
tooth extraction 25, 66, 68, 148, 170, 171
tooth healing 66
tooth integrity 24, 55
tooth issues **88**
tooth loss 98, 100, 103, 105, 110, 151, 157, 186
tooth misalignment 88
'tooth or consequences' **181**
toothpaste
    alternatives 122, 127, 128, 129, 130
    aspartame in 48, 136
    clove seed extract use 158
    fluoride in 108, 132, 157, 203, 204
    'free-from' ingredients 210-11
    'natural' ingredients **136-7**
    possible cause of glossitis 72
    products/product ranges 217-18
    recommended amount 176
    sodium lauryl sulphate in 77
    xylitol in 45, 145
toothpaste abrasiveness 173, 215
toothpaste dispensers 131
toothpaste ingredients 132-9, 176, 179, 210-12
toothpastes 205
tooth powders see dentifrices
tooth reflexology **16-17**
tooth regeneration 66
tooth-supporting tissues 23
tooth wear 109, 110, 185
tooth whitening see whitening
toxic dental materials 167
toxic ingredients **134-5**
toxins 13, 14, 18, 19, 32, 53, 66, 82, 84, 86, 119, 123, 125, 126, 127, 128, 141, 144, 145, 151, 164, 165, 169
    see also endotoxins
trabecular bone 100

SUBJECT INDEX

Trachyspermum ammi seeds 114
Traditional Chinese Medicine (TCM)
   body meridians 170
   five defined flavours 194
   oral lichen planus efficacy 79
   saliva 189
   tongue diagnosis **15–16**
   xerostomia efficacy 85
transduction cascade 102
transient lingual papillitis (TLP) 73
transient receptor potential (TRP) cation channels 33, **38–9**, 40, 137–8
Treponema denticola 60–1
triclosan **134**, 177, 211
triethylene glycol 180
trigeminality 32
trigeminal nerve 31, 38, 195, 197
trigeminal pain 39, 40
trigeminal receptor activation 38
Triplaris peruviana 166
turmeric 150, 159
   see also Curcuma longa
Type 2 diabetes mellitus (T2DM) 35, 48, 49, 63, 64, 81, 82, 83, 90, 94, 95, 96, 105, 156, 173, 196, 199
   see also diabetes

Ulmo honey 47
umami receptors 33, 34, 35, 196
umami resource 217
umami-rich foods 40, 119
umami taste 32, 33, **34**, 37, 40, 196
Uncaria tomentosa 155, 165
Unique Manuka Factor (UMF) 47
upper-lip wrinkles 186
Usnea barbata 165
uvula 89

vagus nerve 90
Valeriana officinalis 78
vanilloid receptors 38, 40, 135
vaping 167
varnishes 181
vascular endothelial growth factor (VEGF) 148
vasoconstriction 66, 168
vegan products 211
vegetables 116, 136, 145, 146, 148, 149–50, 153, 158, 164, 165, 170
   see also brassicas
VEGF *see* salivary VEGF (vascular endothelial growth factor)
vermillion 183–4
vermillion border 110
virulence factors 56, 59–61, 65, 71, 72, 98
viscosity and rheology modifiers 210
vitamin A 66, 68, 78, 115, 118, 148, 157
vitamin B1 76
vitamin B2 76
vitamin B3 115
vitamin B6 76, 105, 115

vitamin B12 36, 72, 76, 78, 115
vitamin B complex 169, 171
vitamin C 56, 74, 79, 114, 118, 123, 146, **148**, 149, 159, 165, 169, 171, 186
vitamin D 64, 68, 101, 119, 146, 149, 157, 159, 169, 186
vitamin D3 157, 159, 171
vitamin D receptor (VDR) 157, 192
Vitamin E 74, 159, 165, 184
vitamin K2 **157**
vomiting 81, 86, 117, 187

wasabi 38, 40, 138
water 210, 212
water distillation 204
water filters 186, 204
water flossers 173
water fluoridation 108, 157, 186, 203
water homeostasis 195
water taste detection 195
Weissella cibaria 163
white adipose tissue (WAT) 96
'white' fillings 180
whitening 172, 209
   see also tooth bleaching
whitening products 89, 128, 129, 137, 171, 176, 177, 178, 211
white oral lesions 72, **78–9**, 86
white willow bark (*Salix alba*) 155
wintergreen (*Gaultheria procumbens*) 137
wisdom teeth 21, 68, 88, 107
wound healing **25**, **65–6**, 94, 95, 97, 109, 122, 138, 148, 159

xenoestrogens 180
xerogenic pharmaceuticals 22
xerostomia 16, 26, 34, 45, 71, 78, 79, 81, **84–5**, 86, 87, 91, 109, 112, 117, 135, 143, 156, 159, 170, 175, 184, 185–6, 187
   see also dry mouth; salivary hypofunction
xylitol 45–7, 131, 136, 145, 152–3, 210

yacón syrup (*Polymnia sonchifolia*) 47–8, 50, 145
Yale Food Addiction Scale 118
yerba maté 184
YKL-40 105
yoghurt 149, 156

Zanthoxylum armatum ('toothache tree') 139–40
zeolite **129**, 165, 169
zinc 74, 77, 91, 105, 115, 118, 123, 146, 159, 165, 171
zinc gluconate 160
zinc picolinate 169
zinc salts 209
zinc sulphate 39
Zingiber officinale (ginger root) 156

Author Index

A~ P 128
Aas JA 23
Abbruscato T 36
Abdullahi SL 128
Abed F 147
Abraham GE 156
Acharya AB 95
Adams JU 33
ADA.org 209
Addy M 88, 89
Adegboye ARA 149
Adler CJ 191
Adler I 58–9, 76
Agalamanyi EA 152
Agere SA 67
Aguirre-Zero O 45
Ahmadieh H 148
Ahmadi-Motamayel F 47
Ahmad R 89
Ahmed N 63
Aickin DR 107
Ajithkumar KC 57–8, 95, 100
Akobundu ENT 159
Albander JM 58
Ali AH 183
Ali E 58
Ali MJ 174, 186
Alken RG 74
Allen AL 37
Allen CM 138
Allen IE 110
Alliance for Natural Health 134
Allin KH 105
Al-Madi EM 165
Al-Majid A 67
Almén MS 34
Al-Mobeeriek A 140, 158
Al-Mubarek S 173
Alqahtani MQ 88, 89
Alramadhn E 78
Al-Romaiyan A 49
Alsenan J 157
AlShoubaki RE 80

Alwan AH 57
Alzahrani AA 74, 104
AlZahrani AS 80
American Academy of Pediatrics 132
American Chemical Society 196
American Dental Association 175, 178, 190
Amir E 80
Amoian B 140
Anand R 80
Ananthathavam K 140
Anders JJ 232
Aneja KR 138
Anggiansah A 153
Anguah KO-B 115–16
Antonietta R 155
Anurdha CV 160
Anushri M 155, 159
Appay V 67
Aps JKM 83, 108, 189
Arabi A 148
Arguin H 116, 151
Arifa SS 83–4
Arizona State University 43, 44, 50
Arreola R 114
Asai D 61
Aschoff J 157
Asea A 222
Ashwin D 163
Asl MK 158
Asokan S 125, 126
Association for Psychological Science 31, 90
Assos-Soares JS 101
Atarashi K 103
Atchison KA 151
Auchtung TA 176
Audu AA 128
Aufderheide AC 191
Avcu N 76
Avila WM 108

Axe J 46
Azarpazhooh A 75, 93
Azar R 153

Bachmanov AA 195
Badet C 159, 165
Baik I 119
Bailey AJ 63
Bains A 98
Bains R 27
Bains VK 27
Baker JL 191–2
Bakri IM 150
Baliga D 22, 185
Baltz ML 99
Banbula A 65
Bandell M 38, 137, 138
Bandhakavi S 190
Bandyopahyay SK 115
Banerjee C 161
Bansode VJ 138
Baquero AF 195
Barahoyee A 114
Baraniak M 168
Barkvoll P 77, 134
Barnum CJ 103
Barrett S 17
Barros SP 102
Bartizek RD 176
Bartlett D 153
Bartold PM 53, 54, 200
Bartoshuk LM 29, 37, 78, 90
Basch CH 132
Bashirelahi N 127
Basset C 85
Basting RT 178
Baulkman J 174
Bautista DM 38, 40, 238
BBC 135
Beauchamp GK 34, 116, 195
Becker Y 74
Beck J 107

AUTHOR INDEX

Behrens M 35
Bekeleski GM 125-6
Beklen A 101
Belibasakis GN 59, 157
Belkheir A 137
Ben-Baruch A 67
Bengmark S 64
Bennett PH 94
Benno Y 193
Bergeron C 85
Bernstein HD 229
Bernstein KN 96
Bertoldo BB 107
Beyondthyca (Beyond Thyroid Cancer) 156
Bezençon C 33
Bhattacharjee MK 58
Bhattarai G 155
Bibby BG 145-6, 149
Biesbrock AR 176
Bioesti 152
Birkhed D 153
Bishop NC 27
Biswas SK 165
Blaylock RL 159
Bluestone R 85
Blumberg JB 114
Bobetsis VA 102
Böhm M 63, 64
Bolscher JGM 25
Bonaterra GA 155
Bond A 85
Bonner M 61
Borgnakke WS 94
Bostanci N 59, 157
Botelho M 140
Bouquot JE 67, 82, 238
Bovshow S 137
Boyce JM 113
Boyd LD 187
Boyina R 148
Bozis GG 138
Bozkurt FY 98
Bozoglan A 98
Bradbury J 37
Bradfield RB 148
Bradford A 87, 125
Brala PM 49
Brambilla E 48, 145
Brand JG 33
Brennan SC 196
Bridge MW 41
British National Formulary 88
Brockette E 171
Brogden KA 191
Bronte-Stewart B 113
Brooks JK 127
Brown CJ 147
Brownfield E 86
Brownley KA 117
Brown R 152

Buduneli N 26, 93
Buggapati L 158, 159, 160
Bui DT 25
Bullon P 96
Burch JG 173
Burch TA 94
Burdette C 156
Burgstahler AW 132
Burhenne M 127, 139
Burt BA 46, 211
Burtner AP 34
Burton JP 161
Busch M 237
Byun R 54

Cade N 204
Cadotte MW 191
Caglar E 55
Cahill LE 133
Cai L 155
Cairns BE 87
Calkins CC 56, 60
Calmes R 26
Caló C 91
Campbell E 50
Campbell LA 98
Campisi J 109
Campolattaro MM 49
Cândido FG 144
Cappetta EG 193
Captain J 193
Carinci F 93
Carpenter GH 24
Carpentieri AR 97
Carratù B 34
Carreras-Presas C 26
Carson CF 74
Carstens E 39, 147
Casale M 111
Casey R 99
Cashman L 169, 170
Castellani RJ 103
Castellsague X 150
Castro MR 45, 46
Caufield PW 55, 107-8
CDC 61
Centers for Disease Control and Prevention 74, 207-8
Cerami C 64
Chaffee BW 96
Challacombe SJ 17, 22, 108-9
Chambers ES 41
Chamundeswari R 125
Chang PC 64
Chan KG 56
Chapple ILC 155
Chatterjee A 115
Chatterjee S 115
Chaturvedi TP 150
Chaudhari N 34

Chaudhary SR 109
Chaudhry NMA 138
Chauhan A 96
Chellaih P 175
Chempakam B 114
Chen C-H 164
Chen XX 134
Cheng A 184-5
Chiego DJ 183
Childs CB 58
Chinoy NJ 159
Chiou WF 68
Chitra S 122
Chitsaz MT 140
Choi DH 24
Choi O 138
Chou L 157
Christensen CM 33
Christian J 67
Cicchella D 147
Cicciù M 84
Çiçek Y 80
Cirino E 73
Ciszewski A 168
The Clay Cure 129
Clayton EMR 134, 180
Cle MF 105
Cohen NA 33, 36
Cohen S 22, 184
Coil JM 172
Cole MF 108
College of Dental Hygienists of Ontario 87
Collins J 139
Collyer CA 65
Colson DG 169
Conforti FD 50
Connett P 107
Córdova A 123
Corey DP 137
Cortés-Rojas DF 138
Costalonga M 23, 24, 57, 191
Costanzo A 32, 195
Cotton S 137
Coventry J 77
Craig RG 100-1
Crawford JM 25
Cross BW 193
Crough T 61
Crowther G 105
Cui M 116
Culty M 111
Cummins D 140, 158
Cuomo R 146, 147
Cury JA 47
Cutando A 97, 156
Cutler CW 173

Dagli N 137, 138, 139
Dahiya P 111

D'Aiuto F 98
Damak S 33, 116
Dandona P 95
Darbre PD 135
Darby I 56
Darling-Fisher CS 94
Darveau RP 59
Dashper SG 60
DaSilva Dantas A 71
Davies M 150
Dawes C 24, 25, 45, 83, 97, 148, 156, 173–4, 230
Dawson-Hughes B 100
deAraujo IE 32
DeBusk RM 184
De Cock P 46
Dede FO 98
Deepa D 122, 193
Deery C 172
deGraaf C 115
Delazar A 140
DellaCorte KW 63
DeMoor RJG 89, 177
denHartog GJ 46
DeNoon DJ 180
DePaola DP 149
Depoortere I 35
Derin S 115
Derrickson B 224, 231, 232
DeSilva S 36
DeSimone JA 33
deSmit M 100
deSouza CRF 138
Dethlefsen L 192
Devi KP 165
DeVries TJ 190
Dewhirst FE 192
Dewhirst S 137
Diabetes Canada 45
Diabetes UK 46
DiNicolantonio JD 117, 118
Dinis-Oliveira RJ 87
Dinnage R 191
DiPierro F 161
Discepoli N 66
Divya VC 83, 84
Dřízhal I 111
Dodds MW 152
Dodman T 93
Dong H 162
Douglas CWI 93, 150
Dowd FJ 132
Drago SR 24
Dragos D 194
DrBicuspid Staff 177
Drenckhahn D 35
Drewnowski A 37, 116, 117, 144
Dr. Schar 137
Dryden M 87
Dsouza SR 199–200
Duffill M 76

Duffy VB 37
Duggal MS 175
Du L 132
Dulguerov P 84
Dumlu A 80
Dundarov S 74
Dundar S 157
Dünker N 237
Dunning T 94
Dutchen S 44
Dutt P 109
Dwivedi V 158
Dziedzic A 75

Ebersole JF 60
Edgar WM 22, 55, 152
Edlund A 191–2
Edmonds M 49
Egan JM 116
Eissa SAL 67
Elahi S 104
El Ashry ESH 140, 158
Elavarasu S 140
Elenkova M 64
El-Hafidi M 165
Ellis JS 199
Ellis ME 76
Emmadi P 125
Encyclopaedia Britannica 158
Ende K 174, 186
Engelen L 24, 40
English Oxford Living Dictionaries 29
Eni Juliana A 66
Environmental Working Group (EWG) 134–5
Ercalik-Yalcinkaya S 80
Eren K 57
Ericson T 175
Erkner A 115
Ertugrul F 152
Escobosa ARC 145
Esposito K 144
Evans JJ 107
Evans P 17
Evert J 18
Eweis DS 147
Eylgor H 84

Fábián TK 24
Fairpro CG 186
Falsetta M 71
Famos FMH 140
Farquar DR 104
Fasig LB 177
Feeney EL 37
Feingold KR 96
Felter HW 140
Femiano F 156
Fentoglu O 98

Ferguson MM 117
Fernandez DePreliasco MV 147
Ferrell RE Jr 128
Fine PG 160
Finger TE 35
Fischbach MA 192
Fitzpatrick AL 111
Fleisch AF 180
Fleming TH 64
Flemming H-C 54, 224
Flötra L 89
Fluoride Action Network 185, 186, 203–4, 233
Folkers K 130
Food and Drug Administration 48, 132, 168
Fournier-Larente J 150
Foutsizoglou S 110, 184
Fowler SPG 48
Franceschi C 109
Franco C 65
Frank GKW 117
Fraunberger EA 27
Freed SH 49
Freni SC 132
Freudenheim JL 104
Friedman PK 18
Froom P 85
Fukayama H 186
Furiga A 159, 165
Furuta M 98
Fusayama T 168

Gagari E 224, 228
Galland L 123
Gandhi KK 193
Gan SH 114
Gao S 104
Garcia RI 100
Gardana C 48
Garrigue-Antar L 101
Gaston K 191
Gazoni FM 171
Gedikli O 90
Genco CA 59
Genco FD 143
Genco RJ 94, 143
Generlich A 140
Gerhold KA 40
Getchell TV 90
Gevorgyan A 114
Gibbons RJ 24
Gibson FC III 59
Gilbertson TA 195
Gilca M 194
Gilchrist A 33
Ginsburg GS 192
Gkogkolou P 63, 64
Glaser A 134
Gleeson M 27, 162, 184

AUTHOR INDEX

Glenville M 44, 48, 118, 119
Go Ask Alice! Columbia University Health Q&A 89, 90
Godara N 175
Godara R 175
Godhia ML 159
Gokmenoglu C 98
Goldberg M 177
Golub LM 58, 100
Gomes-Filho IS 99, 103
Gondhaleker R 172
González JA 33
Goodson A 49
Gordeladze JO 157
Gordon BL 189
Gorovic N 37
Götzfried F 204
Gould RL 165
Graham BG 90, 112
Grand View Research 176
Grant DA 21
Grass J 150
Graves DT 101
Greabu M 24, 25, 189, 190
Greenberg JA 179
Greenwall L 127, 178
Grembecka M 46, 47
Grenier D 150
Griffen AL 59
Griffith RS 74
Grootveld M 177
Grossi SG 64
Grube BD 104
Grynpas M 17
Guan X-b 16, 79
Guillemin GJ 27
Guinesi AS 193
Gujjari SK 172
Gunthorpe MJ 38
Guo D 148
Guo Y 65
Gupta S 122, 193
Gurav AN 63, 95
Gurgan S 109–10
Gurgan T 109–10
Gussy MG 108
Guthmiller JM 191

H2O Labs 204
Haffajee AD 53, 58
Hagen RL 49
Hajishengallis G 57, 59, 93, 161, 191
Hakashima H 61
Halawany HS 139
Haley BE 103, 168
Hallemeier CL 83
Halpern BP 49
Hamid Q 85

Hammett JT 83, 84
Hamzelou J 195
Hanaoka A 103
Handelman SL 112
Hanifl PH 111
Hanioka T 130
Hannig C 155
Hansen LL 96
Han YW 58, 93
Haq MW 135
Hardikar S 115
Harding A 103
Haririan H 96
Harrison JD 84
Hartigan N 101
Harvey PW 135
Hassell T 167
Hatakka K 162
Hatipoglu O 176
Haukioja A 161
Haydel SE 128
Hayes JE 37
Hazuda HP 48
Heath TP 29, 115
Hebling E 17, 108
Heckmann SM 160
Helmerhost EJ 24
Henderson SA 37
Henkin RI 91
Herbert TB 22, 184
Herlofson BB 77, 134
Hernández M 58
Herness S 29
Herod EL 149
Heron SE 104
Herrera DR 155
Hert KA 63
Herzberg MC 23, 24, 57, 191
Hettiarachchy NS 196
He W 33
He X-Y 111
Hickl J 165
Hiele M 46
Hiiri A 181
Hileman B 107, 132
Hilton HB 88
Hino H 46
Hiraki A 105
Hirasawa M 47–8
Hirschfield GM 99
Hoemberg M 185
Höfer D 35
Hojo K 163
Holder BL 128
Holmes R 151
Holmstrom SB 67
Holsinger FC 25
Holt SC 53, 58, 59, 60
Holzer P 38
Honkala S 46
Horasawa N 168

Hoseinishad M 122
Hoshi K 157
Hosseini M 158
Hotamisligil GS 96
Houston MC 168
Hovan AL 34
How KY 56
Hsu P-Y 16, 85
Huang L-G 149
Huang Y 190
Huang Y-F 101
Humphrey SP 21, 22, 24, 26, 55, 173
Humphreys I 26
Hurtig S 126–7

IAOMT (International Academy of Oral Medicine and Toxicology) 67, 129, 205
Ide M 102, 103
Ierardo G 154
Ignacimuthu S 139
Ikeda T 47–8
Ilievski V 103
Imbeau J 184
Indurkar MS 177
Ingram MJ 89
Inoue T 138
Isacsson G 153
Ishihara K 60
Ishikawa KH 162
Ishimaru Y 36
Ismail A 55
Ismond MAH 159
Isokangas P 145, 151
Iwamoto J 157
Iwasaki K 161

Jabr F 63
Jackson D 186
Jackson JA 113
Jacob JA 104
Jacob RA 56
Jain K 224
James P 179
Jamshidi N 116, 224
Janket SJ 98
Janssen S 35
Japan Patent Office 34
Jawed M 95–6
Jayakumar M 139
Jekl V 149
Jemmott JB 3rd 22, 184
Jenness R 34
Jethanandani P 132
Jiang Q 155–6
Jiang X 165
Jiao S 21
Jia X 156
Jindal G 163

Jockers D 105
Joffe DJ 49
Johansen JS 105, 240
Johnson JM 50
Johnston CS 165
Johnston N 148
Jones DA 41
Jones DP 165
Jordt S-E 38
Jorge JH 155
Jørgensen J 205
Jorth P 192
Joshi A 113
Joshi R 138
Joskow R 180
Jurkić LM 129
Juzyszyn Z 159

Kadir AKMS 130
Kadler KE 101
Kakiuchi N 150
Kale R 22, 185
Kamal R 111
Kamat M 49
Kaminski LC 37
Kaneshiro Y 165
Kanetkar P 49
Kang MS 163
Karadas M 176
Karesek M 97
Kargul B 175
Karibassappa GN 172
Kärkkäinen S 127
Kashihara K 103
Kashket S 149
Katayori T 168
Katz J 64
Kaufman LB 18
Kazantzis G 168
Keast RSJ 32, 195
Keles ZP 105
Kennedy BA 128
Kesic L 58
Keswani SG 25, 97, 148
Kettner NM 97
Khandelwal V 45
Khan MK 173
Khanna R 61
Khorsand A 100
Khosravi R 96
Khullar M 175
Kilian M 143, 160-1, 192
Kim JM 114
Kim SE 140
Kimoff J 85
Kiruthiga PV 165
Kitei M 44, 50, 85
Kleinberg I 57, 191
Klinger MM 111
Knowler WC 94

Kobayashi Y 138
Kogawa EM 96
Ko HC 68
Kohn WG 205
Koizumi K 38
Kolahi J 179
Kolenbrander PE 14
Kong L 150
Koo H 55
Koparal E 152
Koral S 168
Kosanam S 148
Koshihara Y 157
Ko S-Y 158
Koufman JA 148
Koytchev R 74
Kraft-Bodi E 162
Krall EA 100
Krut LH 113
Kumar M 96
Kumar P 109
Kumar PS 56
Kumar T 177
Kumbar VM 165
Kurapati KRV 79
Kurihara K 34
Kurita T 47-8
Kuzmanova D 155
Kwan KY 137
Kwan S 18

Lalla E 64
Lamey J 78
Lamont RJ 57, 191
Lamster IB 18
Lanese R 173
Langsjoen O 191
Lanigan RS 176
Lapis TJ 195
Larjava H 66
Larson C 14, 15, 223
Lasschuijt MP 115
Lavoie MC 21, 22, 24, 56, 57, 58, 175
Law Smith MJ 110
Layton S 87
Leake JL 75
LeBel G 138
LeBell AM 158
Lechner J 67, 68, 157
leCoutre J 33
Lee J 60, 96
Lee J-H 101, 102
Lee K 167
Lehmann W 84
Leimola-Virtanen R 109
Lenton KJ 165
León CyIBG 183
Leonard RH Jr 88
Leonhardt K 74

Lerner UH 109
Leukfeld I 100
Leung CW 111
Levine M 148
Levine RS 98
Levitt J 74
Levitt M 174
Levy JA 67, 234
Levy T 104
Liang S 59, 161
Liao S-F 150, 160
Liao WC 68
Li DX 95
Li J 103
Li N 65
Li RQ 76, 104
Li T-L 27
Li X-C 155
Li Y 107-8
Lie MA 186
Lim J 195
Lima DP 189, 190
Limbergen JV 133
Lipatova O 49
Lippert F 171, 209-10
Lisi O 76-7
Listgarten MA 21
Littarru GP 130
Liu L 223
Lobbezoo F 122
Lockhead E 112
Löe H 94
Loimaranta V 159
Long H 107, 132
Long SD 96
Longas MO 111
Loprinzi CL 83
Loreau M 191
Lotz M 100
Lovegrove JM 57
Lovett WE 157
Low JYQ 36
Low MA 25, 66
Lu P 36
Luddi A 102
Luke J 132
Luther F 87
Ly KA 45, 145
Lynch E 177

Ma X 99
Maas CS 174, 186
Machoy-Mokrzynska A 157
Maciocia G 16
MacLachlan A 44
Madison Avenue Dentists 47-8
Maes FW 112
Mager DL 24
Maggio D 148
Mainland JD 36

AUTHOR INDEX

Majtan J 64
Mäkinen KK 45, 47
Mak NK 68
Malamud D 33
Malaty IAC 115
Malaty J 115
Maldarelli C 174
Malezan WR 171
Malik P 180
Mandel ID 21, 24
Manikandan GR 57–8, 95, 100
Manning RH 152
Marceau E 145
Marchal F 84
Marcotte H 21, 22, 24, 56, 57, 58, 175
Mardani H 156
Marek M 168
Marengo K 148
Margolskee RF 36, 116, 227
Marincola M 66
Marinho VCC 181
Markou E 107
Marsh PD 17, 22, 23, 53, 54, 55, 56, 57, 108–9
Martens LC 83, 108, 189
Martin KR 157
Martin LE 37, 154
Martin MD 159
Martin-Cabezas R 162
Martínez-Pérez EF 84
Martino JV 133
Mascarenhas P 109
Mashhadi NS 114
Masi S 111
Masic U 40, 119
Masuda H 138
Matsunami H 36
Mayanagi G 162–3
May Medical Laboratories 32
Mayer W 68
Mayo Clinic 32, 76, 85, 235
Mayrand D 60
McCauley LK 101
McCombs G 125–6
McCooey A 44, 133
McDermid AS 22
McDonald F 87
McFall-Ngai M 192
McKay DL 114
McKee AS 22, 59
McKenna CJ 17
McKinney HL 132
McKinnon PJ 227
McLaughlin SK 227
McNamara FN 38
McRee JT 130
Meiselman HL 49
Melamed S 85
Meletis C 111, 146, 158
Melvin WL 125–6

Mendonça FHBP 162
Mennella JA 34
Menzies A 129
Meraz-Ríos MA 103
Mercola J 136, 152, 153, 204, 205
Meredith MJ 150
Merriam-Webster 237
Messina P 109
Meyer CG 165
Meyerhof W 35
Mezey E 157
Micklem HS 107
Migliari DA 138
Mignogna MD 86
Milanovich N 128
Miletic ID 17, 108
Milgrom P 45, 145
Miller DW 131–2
Miller IJ 37
Miller M 94
Mimi Sakinah AM 45
Mitakou S 152
Miyamoto M 60
Moallem SA 114
Moazzez R 153
Moffitt JM 88
Mohamad I 83
Mohammadi A 154
Mohammadi-Sichani M 48, 145
Molan PC 47
Möller C 175
Möller P 32
Mondoa EI 44, 50, 85
Montevecchi M 177
Moon JH 165
Moore LVH 23
Moore WEC 23
Moosavi M 128
Moravec LJ 187
Morin M-P 150
Morishita M 107
Moritani T 96
Mouth Healthy/American Dental Association 126
Muglikar S 22, 185
Mummolo S 183
Murray JJ 186
Murray RK 150, 160
Mussap M 186
Mustapha IZ 99
Myneni VD 157
Mysak J 59, 60
Mysels DJ 117

Nadimi H 152
Nagarathna DV 161
Nagesh L 172
Nandan N 125, 126
Nandhini ATA 160
Narayanan A 126

Nascimento MM 137, 154
Näse L 161
National Cancer Institute 34
National Institutes of Health 91
Navas FJ 123
Nayak PA 45
Nayak UA 45
Nazir MA 10, 199
Nelson GM 90, 91
Nema NK 65
Netdoctor 179
Neurath C 132
Neuvonen PJ 127
Neyraud E 24, 194
Ngan P 173
Nguyen HA 111
Nguyen K-A 65
NHS (National Health Service) 76, 203
Nibali L 190–1
Nicopoulou-Karayianni K 151
Nielsen FH 157
Nieman DC 27
Nieuw Amerongen AV 24
Niki M 116
Nilius B 38
Nireeksha 157
Nishihara T 161
Noack B 99
Nogales CG 122
Nokhbehsaim M 96–7
Nolan A 111
Nomoto S 168
Norat T 87
Nordblad A 45
Nordestgaard BG 105
Nurse RJ 195
Nutting PG 129
Nyvad B 193

Oakley A 76
Obioma NP 138, 158
Oc B 185
O'Connor CM 33
O'Connor DT 96
O Ecotextiles 185, 232
Offebacher S 102
Ohkoshi N 112
Oho T 27
Ohsu T 196
Ohta K 187
Okada HC 186
O'Keefe JH 117, 118
Oksenberg A 85
Okuda K 60
Olea N 180
Oliva A 157
Oliveira WP 138
Olsen I 104
Olshevsky U 74

O'Mullane D 176
Ono Y 103
Orgill C 129
Osmunson B 204, 205
O'Sullivan I 93, 105
Oteri G 84
Oudhoff MJ 65
Ozbayrak S 80
Öztekin G 100

Padayatty SJ 148
Paganini-Hill A 151
Pagnacco A 111
Paknejad M 100
Palmer RJ Jn 192
Pandian SK 165
Pandit N 60
Pandor S 121
Papapanou PN 102
Paraschos S 152
Park K 114
Park S-R 58
Parnell C 176
Parthasarathy VA 114
Paschalis V 165
Patel N 159
Patel NN 33, 36
Patrick L 165
Paul RG 63
Pavaskar R 193
Pazdro R 165
Pedersen AM 159
Pedrazzi V 172
Peedikayi FC 126
Pekala PH 96
Penner MH 195
Pepelassi E 89
Pepys MB 99
Percival RS 17, 22, 108–9
Pereira LJ 26
Peres MA 10
Pérez-Cano FJ 162
Perrin MJ 113
Petchey O 191
Petersen PE 18
Petraccia L 147–8
Phalipon A 24
Pietrocola G 193
Pietropaoli D 64
Pilch PF 96
Pincus D 93
Pinto E 158
Pitigoi-Aron G 88
Pitts NB 55
Plebani M 186
Plessas A 89
Pogrel MA 25, 66
Pol A 81
Politis C 65, 66
Polyzos NP 102

Porter S 72, 78, 79, 80, 82, 86, 87
Posch G 60
Potempa J 65
Pothuraju R 49
Poulsen MW 145
Pourabbas R 140
Poyraz O 57
Prabuseenivasan S 139
Pradhan KM 185
Práger N 102
Prandi S 35
Preen C 139
Priyadarshini C 17
Procopio RM 84
Proskin HM 45
Prutkin J 37, 112
Puranik MP 17, 155, 159
Pure Circle Stevia Institute 48
Püschel B 35
Putt MS 136

Qin N 103
Qin XF 48

Rabbani N 64
Rabbi AA 130
Radiology.org 170
Radler DR 184
Rafiqul ISM 45
Rahman MM 130
Raj GA 159
Raj S 125, 126
Rajan S 132
Raju PK 175
Rakhshandeh H 158
Ramamurthy J 140
Ramesh A 199–200
Ranasinghe P 138
Randal A 38
Rangé H 98
Ranjan S 159
Rao G 113
Rao PV 114
Rashid MA 98
Rask-Andersen M 34
Rathee M 180
Raudenbush B 152
Raut CP 130
Redding SW 72, 84
Reddy VV 175
Redmer J 115
Reece AS 117
Rehme MG 168
Reichling C 35
Reichling J 74
Reichman DE 179
Reinhardt RA 110
Relman DA 192
Ren X 33
Ren YF 26

Reynolds MA 127
Riboli E 87
Rickard AH 14, 220
Riera CE 39
Riley P 45, 152
Rimpler H 59, 140
Ritthagol W 162
Roberts J 169
Robertson WGA 156
Robson J 93
Roca A 148
Rodrigues AL 178
Rodriguez-Martin C 191
Roper SD 34
Roques C 159, 165
Rosenfeld ME 98
Rosenfeld MJ 160
Ross R 185
Rothen M 45, 145
Roth G 26
Rousett D 111, 158
Rowland-Jones SL 67
Rowltt G 41
Royle L 51
Rozengurt E 35
Rüdiger SG 26
Rudi T 157
Ruhl S 193
Russell CS 111
Ryberg M 175

Sabah E 152
Saetang C 162
Sahin IO 98
Said HS 103
Saini R 122
Saito T 96
Sakamoto M 60, 96, 193
Sakanaka S 150
Sällsten G 153
Salman H 164
San Gabriel A 196, 221
Sánchez GA 147
Sánchez MC 150
Sánchez-Domínguez B 64
Sangeetha M 26
Santos FA 155
Santos FC 171
Sanz M 199
Sarari AS 76
Saremi A 94
Saruta J 96
Sastravaha G 65, 158
Sathasivasubramanian S 83, 84
Sato Y 157
Saxer U 167
Scannapieco FA 93
Scardina GA 109
Scariya L 161
Schatzman AR 91

Scheid RC 110
Scheinin A 45
Schemehorn BR 128
Scherma M 160
Schiffman SS 39, 90, 112
Schiöth HB 34
Schlagenhauf U 161–2
Schmid U 126
Schmidt AM 64
Schnitzler P 74
Scholz E 140
Schuett S 68
Schuhmacher A 74
Schulman H 33
Schulze-Späte U 101
Schwartz RA 77
Sciencedaily 185
Scopinho AA 160
Scott J 18, 108
Scully C 72, 75, 76, 77, 78, 79, 80, 82, 86, 87, 90
Sekhar RV 165
Sellars WA 168
Selvam P 125, 126
Selwitz RH 55
Semwal DK 158
Seo WH 85
Serra MC 178
Seth S 180
Sethi KS 130
Shah K 36
Shahid Z 75
Shanbhag VKL 126
Shang-Rong JI 99
Shariff JA 102
Sharma A 159, 165
Sharma C 138, 159
Sharma V 130
Shashikiran ND 175
Shekarchizadeh H 185–6
Shepherd GM 197–8
Shiel WC 233
Shih M 49
Shimazaki Y 96
Shimizu K 49
Shin C 119
Shin Y-H 114
Shoji S 112
Shone GR 113
Shotts R 75, 76, 77, 78, 87, 90
Sideras K 83
Sierpina VS 150, 160
Simon SA 32
Simons CT 147
Simón-Soro A 23
Singhal R 49
Singh BB 74
Singh J 180
Singh N 33, 35
Singh OM 139–40
Singh R 137

Singh TP 139–40
Sircus M 126
Skaltsounis A-L 152
Slots J 58, 61
Smalley JW 59, 65
Smeets PA 115
Smida I 158
Smith DJ 17, 25
Smith KR 116
Smith QT 58
Smith RG 34
Smithsonian National Museum of Natural History 17
Snyder DJ 29, 90
Soap Detergent Association 133
Soares RV 15
Socransky SS 53, 58
Söder B 104
Söderling E 45
Song KP 56
Soni S 130
Sonnenburg JL 192
Sood P 125
Soolari A 179
Soory M 27
Soria G 67
Soto C 165
Soto P 179
Sotoudeh G 56
Soukos NS 57
Spector AC 116
Spijkervet FK 108
Spray-Watson KJ 195
Sprouse-Blum AS 39
Sreenivasan P 126
Srilakshmi JC 165
Srinivasan K 122
Sroka A 56
Stanford Medicine 72, 78
Stanley M 73–4
Steele J 93, 105
Stephens JM 96
Stern IB 21
Stern R 25, 66, 111
Stewart JE 24, 194
Stiban J 147
Stice E 115
Strienz J 105
Strunecka A 132
Su Y 96
Subrahmanyam MV 26
Suez J 48
Sujatha BK 172
Sukumar S 111
Sulieman M 88, 89
Sullivan MA 117
Sun J 157
Sun Y 102
Suri L 224, 228
Suri V 110
Susanto H 100

Susheela AK 132
Sushni MAM 137
Sutow EL 168
Swithers SE 48
Swoboda C 153
Szarka L 174

3M 185
Tabak LA 230
Tada A 137, 165
Tada-Oikawa S 133–4
Taichman LS 170
Takahashi N 193
Takahashi S 168
Takeda M 63
Takeda T 157
Talavera K 40
Tam L 178
Tamer TM 111
Tan CXW 167
Tan KH 60–1
Tanaka M 65
Tang H-B 39
Tanner ACR 60
Tansey MG 103
Tariq P 138
Tatemoto K 96
Taube F 185
Taubman MA 25
Tay LY 155
Taylor DA 116, 224
Teanpaisan R 162
Teixeira FB 99, 103
Teles RP 58
Telgi RL 149
Telles-Araujo GdeT 75
Temple JL 153
Tenenbaum HC 93
Tepper BJ 195
Terai T 163
Thatcher BJ 91
Thaweboon S 157
Thirunavukkarasu V 160
This Green 128
Thomas B 199–200
Thomson CD 165
Thomsson KA 27, 50
Thornalley PJ 64
Tiemann P 140
Tilman D 191
Tirado-Lee L 38, 39
Titsas A 117
Tiwari M 24, 189
Tiwari S 122
Tobias PS 60
Toelg M 140
Toker H 57
Tootla R 175
Tordoff MG 196
Torres-Lagares D 84

Tortora GJ 224, 231, 232
Touger-Decker R 43, 57
Toumba KJ 175
Tramontano D 156
Travis J 65
Treesukosol Y 116
Triana CBEG 183
Trim RD 61
Tsang G 149
Tsoukalas D 119
Turkyilmaz I 186
Turnbaugh PJ 192

Ueno M 18
Uju DE 138, 158
Umamaheswari G 115
Uma SR 17
Umar S 114
Umeda M 193
Umeki H 96, 97
Underhill CB 111
Urbanek-Brychczyńska M 168
Uribarri J 63, 64, 65, 145
Uruakpa FO 159

Valdez-Jiménez L 132
Välimaa H 109
Van der Bijl P 88
Van der Lugt T 64, 145
Van der Velden U 155
Van Loveren C 43, 45, 47
Van Nieuw Amerongen A 25, 108
VanDyke TE 53, 54, 200
VanWinkelhoff AJ 59
Varela-López A 157
Varghese M 161
Vastardis H 224, 228
Veerman ECl 24, 25
Vennekens R 38
Venturi M 156
Venturi S 156
Verma R 177
Vess TH 192
Vieira C 114
Vissink A 108
Vivas APM 138
Vlassara H 63
Voigt N 195
von Baehr V 67, 68
Vriens J 38

Wade WG 193
Wadia R 167
Waldbott GL 132
Walker C 83, 84
Wallman IS 88
Walters PA 176
Wang C-W 101
Wang J 101
Wang P-L 60
Wang W 107-8
Wang X 93
Wang Y 138
Ward BK 196
Watts A 88, 89
WebMD 90
Wei BL 68
Wei SHY 89
Weiler RME 183
Weiss ME 149
Wenner M 196
Wescombe PA 161, 163
Weston SJ 96
White SC 151
Wilkinson AR 107
Willershausen I 104
Williams K 48
Williams L 67, 168-9, 170
Williams LB 128
Williams RC 24
Williamson RT 21, 22, 24, 26, 55, 173
Wilson M 23
Wilson MM 229
Wilson WL 117, 118
Winclove Probiotics 163
Windham B 66, 105, 146
Wingender J 54, 224
Winkler S 186
Woelfel JB 110
Wojtyczka R 75
Wölbling RH 74
Wolff MS 14, 15, 223
Wölnerhanssen BK 46
Wong JW 25, 148
Wooding S 37
Workman AD 33, 36
World Dental Federation 122
World Health Organization 127, 179
Wormer EJ 126
Wright KF 147

Wu CD 155
Wu IB 77
Wu SV 35
Wu T 99
Wu TT 178
Wu Y 99
Wülknitz P 137
Wyganowska-Swiathowska M 139

Xiang Q 132
Xu H 39
Xu J 26

Yaegaki K 172
Yaghobee S 100
Yagi T 117, 187
Yalçin F 109-10
Yale New Haven Health Hospital 46
Yamaguchi S 34
Yamamoto K 36
Yamazaki K 104
Yaqoob P 162
Yaroko AA 83
Yashoda R 155, 159
Yasmin S 159
Yaylayan VA 145
Yeomans MR 40, 119
Yilmaz M 100
Ylitalo K 45

Zachariah TJ 114
Zachariasen RD 22
Zadik Y 89
Zambon JJ 22
Zarco MF 192
Zaura E 192
Zavorsky GS 165
Zero DT 45
Zervakis J 112
Zhang Y 33
Zheng A 96
Zheng P 58
Zheng Y 48
Zhou W 58
Zhou X 98
Zoladz PR 152
Zou QH 76, 104